AF411999

# Neoplastic Transformation in Human Cell Culture

# Experimental Biology and Medicine

# Neoplastic Transformation in Human Cell Culture

## Mechanisms of Carcinogenesis


Edited by

### Johng S. Rhim

*Laboratory of Cellular
and Molecular Biology
National Cancer Institute
Bethesda, MD*

### Anatoly Dritschilo

*Department of Radiation Medicine
Georgetown University Medical Center
Washington, DC*


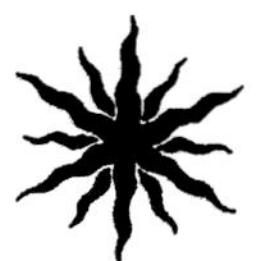

## Humana Press • Totowa, New Jersey

Library of Congress Cataloging-in-Publication Data

Neoplastic transformation in human cell culture: mechanisms
of carcinogenesis / edited by Johng S. Rhim, Anatoly Dritschilo.
     p.    cm. — (Experimental biology and medicine)
   Papers from a workshop held at Georgetown University Medical
Center, Washington, DC, on April 25–26, 1991, sponsored by the
Georgetown University Dept. of Radiation Medicine and the University
of Chicago, Dept. of Radiation and Cellular Oncology.
   Includes index.
   ISBN 0-89603-227-2
   1. Carcinogenesis—Congresses. 2. Cell transformation–
–Congresses. 3. Human cell culture—Congresses. I. Rhim, Johng S.
II. Dritschilo, Anatoly. III. Georgetown University. Dept. of
Radiation Medicine. IV. University of Chicago. Dept. of Radiation
and Cellular Oncology. V. Series: Experimental biology and medicine
(Clifton, N.J.)
   [DNLM: 1. Cell Transformation, Neoplastic—congresses. 2. Cells
Cultured—congresses.    QZ 202 N4385 1991]
RC268.5.N46    1991
616.99'4071—dc20
DNLM/DLC
for Library of Congress                                        91-35328
                                                                   CIP

# Preface

The role of carcinogenic agents in the deveolopment of human cancers is now being defined using a variety of human cells as experimental model systems. A workshop on "neoplastic transformation in human cell systems in vitro: mechanisms of carcinogenesis" was held at the Georgetown University Medical Center, Washington, DC, on April 25–26, 1991. The aims of the workshop were to present the state-of-the-art in the transformation of human cells in culture, as well as to provide insight into the molecular and cellular changes involved in the conversion of normal cells to a neoplastic state of growth.

The following topics were closely related to the theme of the workshops:

1. Derivation of in vitro model systems (epithelial, fibroblastic, and hematopoietic).
2. Factors modulating cellular transformation.
3. Usefulness of defined in vitro model systems for viral, chemical, and radiation carcinogenesis.
4. Multistep nature of human cell carcinogenesis.
5. Role of activated and suppressor oncogenes in neoplastic transformation.

The workshop was organized by J. S. Rhim and A. Dritschilo (cochairmen), G. Jay, J. Little, M. McCormick, R. Tennant, and R. R. Weischelbaum. There were 32 speakers, 30 poster presentations, and about 190 participants.

The workshop was well received and was perhaps the first one devoted solely to the subject of humaan cell transformation systems in vitro. It is our privilege to have an opportunity to edit these proceedings and also on behalf of all the contributors to thank everyone who has helped us produce this book. We particularly wish to thank Ms. Sandra Hawkins for her exceptional effort to assure the success of both, the workshop and this text. The excellent typing of Mrs. Frances Hyman is also greatly appreciated.

Johng S. Rhim  
Anatoly Dritschilo

*v*

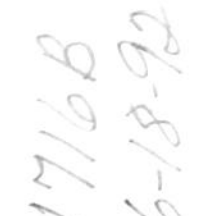

# Acknowledgments

This workshop was sponsored by:

Georgetown University
Department of Radiation Medicine
Washington, DC 20007

and

University of Chicago
Department of Radiation and Cellular Oncology
Chicago, Illinois 60637


Financial support for this publication came from:

Center for Radiation Therapy
Chicago, Illinois 60637

# Contents



## I. Preneoplastic Events



## II. Radiation Transformation and Oncogenes

## III. Viral Transformation and Oncogenes

## IV. Multistep Models

# NEOPLASTIC TRANSFORMATION IN HUMAN CELL SYSTEMS - AN OVERVIEW

J. S. Rhim[1] and A. Dritschilo[2]

[1]National Cancer Institute, Bethesda,
MD 20892 USA, [2]Department of Radiation
Medicine, Georgetown Medical Center,
Washington, D.C. 20007 USA

It is now well accepted that cancer arises in a
multistep fashion and that environmental exposures to
physical, chemical, and biological agents, are major
etiological factors (1,2).  Besides irradiation,
chemicals, and viruses, other influences such as genetic,
hormonal, nutritional and multifactor interactions are
also involved.  While the majority of studies of
carcinogens have relied on the use of rodent cells in
culture, experimental models to define the role of these
agents in the development of human cancer must be
established using human cells.  Thus, the study of human
cell transformation in culture by carcinogenic agents is
of particular importance for understanding the cellular
and molecular mechanisms underlying human carcinogenesis.

Knowledge of the mechanisms of carcinogenesis in
human cells will have obvious implications on strategies
for cancer therapy and cancer prevention  Since the
development of cancer is a multistage process that
generally takes several years, opportunities exist to
stabilize, reverse and inhibit the preneoplastic stages.
Damage to cellular DNA by carcinogens is considered an
important initial step in carcinogenesis in both human and
experimental animals.  Once "initiated" by a carcinogen,
the cell can be stimulated by promoters and/or cocarcino-
genes to progress to an invasive malignant state of
growth.  The molecular and cellular mechanisms of tumor
development involve point mutations, chromosomal
rearrangements and loss of suppressor genes.  Recent

studies have shown that several gene changes appear to be necessary to cause most common cancers. Not only do one or more growth-stimulatory oncogenes have to be activated, but the growth-inhibitory genes that would otherwise suppress tumor formation have to be inactivated.

Unlike rodent cells, normal human cells in culture do not or rarely undergo spontaneous transformation and have generally proven resistant to neoplastic transformation by carcinogens (3). Previous transformation of human cells have mostly been with fibroblastic cells, which are relatively easy to culture. While the use of DNA tumor viruses (4,5), X-ray (6) and chemical carcinogens (7,8) has led to the development of established, biologically abnormal lines of fibroblasts, neoplastic transformation has proven very difficult to achieve. Recently, neoplastic conversion of immortalized, non-tumorigenic human fibroblasts expressing the $SV_{40}$ tumor antigen (9) or induced by irradiation (10) was achieved by infection with murine sarcoma viruses. Possibly, transformation of human fibroblasts is complicated by the requirement, similar to that observed in primary rodent fibroblasts, of two separate genetic events, one for rescue from senescence and another for conversion to the tumorigenic phenotype (11,12).

For initial studies, a flat, nontumorigenic clonal line (TE85 clone F-5), originally derived from human osteosarcoma cells (13), was used. This cell system was found to be very useful for viral and chemical carcinogenesis since nonproducer Kirsten murine sarcoma virus (Ki-MSV) transformed human cells (14) and chemically transformed human cells (15) have been derived using this cell system.

Since most human cancers are of epithelial origin it is important to obtain a better understanding of this cell type. We used primary human foreskin epidermal keratinocytes to ascertain whether prototypic RNA (Ki-MSV) or DNA (Ad12-SV40 hybrid virus) tumor viruses could confer the malignant phenotype to normal primary human epithelial cells. In doing so, we were able to develop for the first time an *in vitro* multistep model suitable for the study of human epithelial cell carcinogenesis (16).

The neoplastic transformation in human cells will be reviewed. To do so, we shall attempt to put in perspective the history of human cell transformation by carcinogenic agents and to discuss the current state-of-the-art in transformation of human cells in culture. We hope this will provide further insight into the molecular and cellular mechanisms involved in the conversion of normal cells to a neoplastic state of growth.

## *History of human cell transformation*

More than 30 years ago, Shein (17) and Koprowski *et al.* (18) demonstrated for the first time that $SV_{40}$, a DNA tumor virus of the papova virus family which was isolated by Sweet and Hillman (19), could morphologically transform human fetal and adult skin fibroblasts, respectively. The transformation of mammalian cells by $SV_{40}$ is known to require expression of only the early region of the viral genome, which encodes two proteins, large T-antigen (94 kd) and small t-antigen (17 kd). Subsequently, Girardi *et al.* (4) showed "crisis" and recovery in $SV_{40}$-transformed human fibroblasts. Usually only rare variant $SV_{40}$-transformed human cells ever escape crisis to become progenitors of immortal lines.

## *Neoplastic transformation of nontumorigenic human osteosarcoma clonal (TE-85 clone F-5) line by Ki-MSV*

Based on the rapidly expanding knowledge in tumor virus research in the 1970's, the Virus Cancer Program (VCP), an intensive targeted and coordinated research program on the role of viruses in cancer, with particular emphasis on RNA tumor viruses was implemented. An intensive search for human tumor viruses has begun.

To develop an *in vitro* human cell system for the detection of possible human RNA tumor viruses, we have studied normal and malignant human cells for their susceptibility to focus formation by Ki-MSV, and whether nonproducers (NP) could be obtained from the transformed foci. About 20 normal and malignant cells were tested. Variation in susceptibility of individual human cells to transformation by Ki-MSV was noted (20). A flat, nontumorigenic human osteosarcoma (HOS) line (TE-85 clone F-5) was found to be highly sensitive to transformation (14). The fibro epithelial like TE85 clone F-5 line formed foci consisting of spindle-shaped or stellar cells and three-dimensional clumps of round cells (Fig. 1B). Subsequently, nonproducer (NP) cells were isolated from the transformed foci (14). These morphologically altered NP cells induced tumors when injected into nude mice and produced neither infectious virus nor complement-fixation antigens of the murine sarcoma-leukemia virus complex.

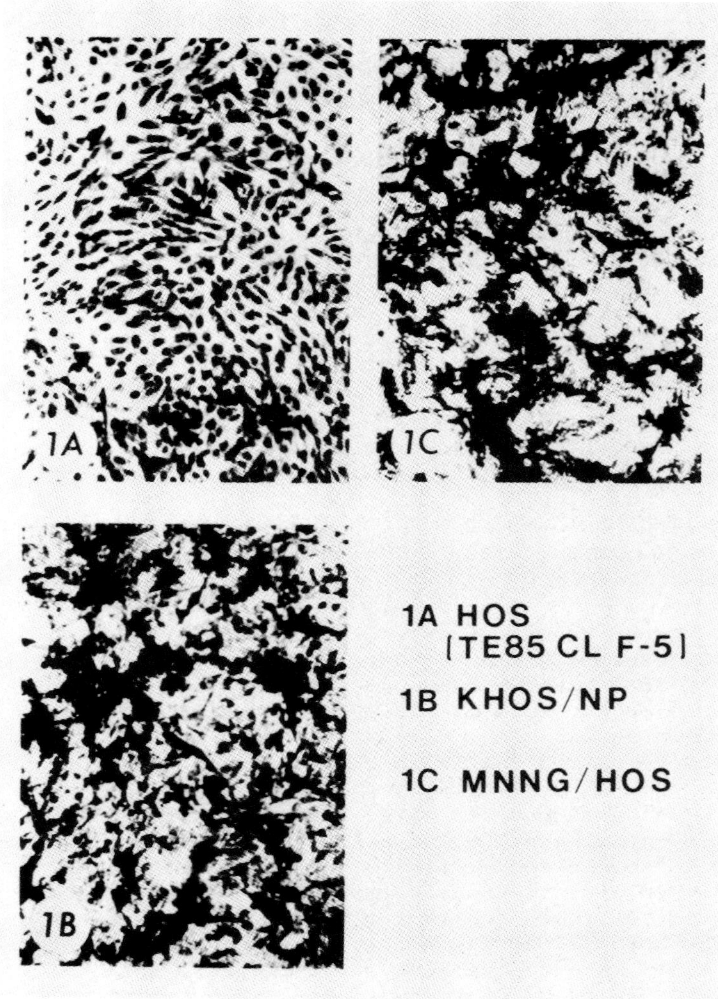


Figure 1.    Human osteosarcoma clonal line (TE85, clone F-5) (A).  Ki-MSV-transformed NP HOS line (B) and MNNG (0.01mg/ml) transformed HOS line (c).

However, the sarcoma virus genome could be rescued from these NP cells by co-cultivation with cells carrying "helper" Kirsten murine leukemia virus. The possible usefulness of these cells in efforts designed to detect, covert or repressed RNA tumor viruses in various human tissues has been examined without success. Subsequent studies have shown that this HOS cell line was sensitive to viruses and chemical carcinogens (Table 1).

## Neoplastic transformation of human osteosarcoma cells by chemical carcinogens

*In vitro* chemical transformation of various rodent cells has been well established (21,22,23). Since certain carcinogenic polycyclic hydrocarbons have been identified in our environment, it is important to test the response of human cells to such compounds. Many attempts have been made to transform various cultured normal or genetically abnormal human cells with chemical carcinogens, but without success (24). The possibility of using continuous lines of human sarcoma cells for chemical transformation was investigated since certain human sarcoma cell lines are susceptible to transformation by DNA and RNA tumor viruses (25,26). We studied the characteristics of the HOS line after treatment with N-methyl-N-nitro-N-nitrosoguanidine (MNNG) and 7.12-dimethyl-benz (a) anthracene (DMBA). The chemically-treated cells underwent morphological alterations (Fig. 1C) and the resulting transformed cells produced tumors when injected into nude mice (14,15). This provided the first evidence that human cells can be neoplastically transformed by chemical carcinogens. Subsequently, we have shown that 3-methylcholanthrene (3MC) also induced transformation of the revertant 312H-HOS nonproducer cells (27) and that these transformed cells produced tumors when injected into nude mice (28). The flat 312H cells, like the parent HOS cells, were not tumorigenic in nude mice and did not contain the Ki-MSV-specific gene sequences (29) (Table 1). These chemically-treated malignantly-transformed HOS cell lines were later found to be useful for the studies of activated oncogenes and tumor suppressor genes.

## Activation of transforming genes met and c-H-ras in chemically-transformed HOS cell lines

The detection and identification of cellular transforming genes from chemical carcinogen-induced animal tumors and chemically transformed cells *in vitro* (30,31) by DNA-mediated gene transfer studies with NIH/3T3 cells

**Table 1:  Human osteosarcoma clonal (HOS) cells and their transformants**

| Cell Designation | Cell description | Remarks |
| --- | --- | --- |
| HOS (TE85 C1-F-5) | Human osteogenic sarcoma clonal cells (3) | P53 (low) |
| KHOS/NP | Nonproducer cells from KiMSV transformed HOS cells (14) | Rescuable sarcoma genome (+) |
| MNNG/HOS | MNNG transformed HOS cells (15) | met (+), P53 (high) |
| DMBA/HOS | DMBA transformed HOS cells (61) | |
| Revertant 240S | Revertant from KHOS cells (27) | |
| $S^{+}L^{-}$ HOS | Sarcoma-positive, leukemia-negative HOS cells induced by Mo-MSV (FLV) (62) | |
| RSV/HOS | RSV-SR transformed HOS cells (63) | |
| Revertant 312H | Revertant from KHOS cells (27) | |
| 3MC/312H | 3MC transformed 312H cells (28) | cH-*ras*, 61st (+), P53 (high) |
| DMBA/312H | DMBA transformed 312H cells (28) | P53 (high) |

have made it possible to understand the molecular and genetic basis of chemical carcinogenesis. Most transforming genes so far detected by these studies are related to three highly-conserved members of the *ras* gene family, H-, Ki- and N-*ras*, all of which encode closely-related proteins that are designated p21. Members of the *ras* gene family have been detected in a variety of human tumors (30,31). Most *ras* oncogenes analyzed have been activated by point mutations in the codons for amino acids 12 or 61. The carcinogen-activated *ras* oncogenes have the same type of activating mutation as those present in human tumors (32).

A non-*ras* cellular transforming gene, *met*, was also isolated and identified by transfection of DNA from a late passage (>150) MNNG/HOS cell line using the NIH/3T3 cell transfection assay (33,34). We have also detected and identified the *met* oncogene in an earlier passage (p98) of MNNG/HOS cells (unpublished data). However, DNA from malignantly-transformed DMBA/HOS cells has so far been negative in our transfection assay (34). The *met* gene is activated by gene rearrangement, resulting in the fusion of a tpr (translocated promoter region) locus on chromosome 1 to the 5' region of sequence derived from the *met* locus on chromosome 7 (35,36) which is closely-linked to the genetic marker for cystic fibrosis (37). Additional studies have demonstrated that the region of the activated *met* gene is homologous to a family of genes that encode protein kinases. The met gene encodes a 190-kd transmembrane glycoprotein, whose transcript is expressed in many tissues and in cell lines, such as spontaneous NIH/3T3 transformants and certain human gastric carcinoma cells. Recently the *met* gene was identified as the hepatocyte growth factor receptor (38).

DNA prepared from the 3MC-transformed 312H-HOS cell line induced foci on NIH/3T3 cells, whereas DNAs prepared from DMBA-transformed and control 312H-HOS cell lines did not. The transformed gene from the 3MC-transformed 312H-HOS cells was identified as an activated form of the human H-*ras* oncogene. Analysis of the *ras* oncogene product p21 in this transformant by immunoprecipitation and gel electrophoresis showed altered mobility , suggesting that this oncogene is likely to have been activated by a point mutation. These findings demonstrate that activation of a member of the *ras* gene family can occur in a chemically-transformed human cell line (39).

## *Viral transformation of human skin fibroblasts*

Most carcinogenesis studies of human cells have used fibroblasts which are easy to culture. However, neoplastic transformation of human skin fibroblasts in culture has not been readily achieved (3).

Infection by certain DNA tumor viruses ($SV_{40}$ and adenovirus) and rarely chemical carcinogens had led to the development of karyologically-abnormal fibroblast lines which are tumorigenic in nude mice. So far, no successful neoplastic transformation of human skin fibroblasts by RNA tumor viruses has been reported, except those by the combined effects of two viruses and of radiation plus viruses (9,10).

Ki-MSV induced distinct transformed foci in human skin fibroblasts. However, the same KiMSV-induced foci gradually disappeared following subcultivation, and the cells eventually died. Thus another step is necessary for these cells to become neoplastic. Human skin fibroblasts derived from genetically predisposed individuals, such as those with ACR (adenomatosis of the colon and rectum) and Gardner's syndrome, are more highly sensitive to Ki-MSV transformation (40). There are genetic differences in viral susceptibility. Steroid hormones (hydrocortisone, dexamethasone) also enhance Ki-MSV transformation of human skin fibroblasts (41). However, all of these fibroblastic lines become senescent.

## *Chemical transformation of human skin fibroblasts*

Most human fibroblasts treated with chemical carcinogens showed morphological alteration, extended life span and growth in soft agar, but did not become permanent lines. In 1977, Kakunaga reported for the first time the neoplastic transformation of human diploid fibroblasts (KD) by chemical carcinogens (42). However, McCormick *et al.* (1988) examined the karyological markers of the normal fibroblastic cell line (KD) and the transformed HuT cell lines developed by Kakunaga and found marked differences, indicating that the KD cells and HuT cells were derived from different individuals. He further demonstrated that the HuT series of "carcinogen-transformed" human fibroblast cell lines were derived from the human fibrosarcoma cell 8387 (43). These findings tell us how important it is to examine carefully the karyological identity of cells with which we are working.

## *Human epithelial cell carcinogenesis*

Since the majority of human tumors are of epithelial origin, it is important to study the epithelial cell system.  However, because of our inability until recently to grow human epithelial cells and to transform them *in vitro,* it has been difficult to define the process of neoplastic transformation of human epithelial cells.  When we began our studies, there had been a few reports describing altered growth and differentiation of human keratinocytes following $SV_{40}$ infection and $SV_{40}$ DNA transfection but in both reports, the tumorigenicity of the altered cells was not demonstrated (44,45).

We began by asking several simple questions: 1) Do highly oncogenic RNA or DNA tumor viruses induce morphological alteration or alter the growth properties of primary human epithelial cells?  2) Can virus-transformed human epithelial cells be maintained as stably-established cell lines?  3) Do virus-transformed cell lines induce carcinomas when transplanted into nude mice?  We used primary human foreskin epidermal keratinocytes to ascertain whether prototypic RNA (Ki-MSV) or DNA (Ad12-$SV_{40}$ hybrid virus) tumor viruses could induce the malignant phenotype.  In doing so, we were able to develop for the first time an *in vitro* multistep model suitable for the study of human epithelial cell carcinogenesis (16).  We describe the derivation of our *in vitro* multistep human epidermal model, the factors involved in modulating this cellular transformation system, the usefulness of this model system for viral, chemical and radiation carcinogenesis, and the multistep nature of human epithelial cell carcinogenesis.

## *Derivation of nontumorigenic human epidermal keratinocyte line (RHEK-1) by infection with the Ad12-$SV_{40}$ virus*

In an attempt to alter the growth properties of primary human epidermal keratinocytes, we used Ki-MSV, a prototype retrovirus whose K-*ras* oncogene has been detected in many human epithelial malignancies, (30,31) and the Ad12-$SV_{40}$ hybrid virus, which induces malignant transformation of fibroblasts in culture.  Neither control nor Ki-MSV-infected human epithelial cultures could be propagated serially beyond two or three subcultures.  In contrast, infection of primary cultures of human epithelial cells with Ad12-$SV_{40}$ led to the appearance of actively growing colonies by weeks 3 to 4. By week 6, $SV_{40}$ tumor (T) antigen was detected in the nuclei of a large fraction of the infected cultures by indirect immunofluorescence staining. A number of cell lines were obtained by limiting dilution from colonies that proliferated. All lines but one released Ad12-$SV_{40}$ virus, as indicated by the induction of cytopathic effect in Vero cells. We selected the nonproducer line, designated RHEK-1 for further characterization. The RHEK-1 line had a flat epithelial morphology, showed a number of epithelial cell markers, and was not tumorigenic in nude mice, although in some cases, regressing small cystic nodules containing epidermoid cells appeared at the site of inoculation (Fig. 2).

In experiments to determine which, if any, of the transforming genes in the Ad12-$SV_{40}$ hybrid virus was actively transcribed in the altered human epithelial cells, molecular characterization of the RHEK-1 line was carried out. It had no detectable transcripts from the early region of Ad12 but had substantial amounts of messenger RNA (mRNA) from the transforming region of $SV_{40}$. Analysis by immunoprecipitation and sodium dodecyl sulfate-polyacrylamide gel electrophoresis revealed that both large T and small t antigens of $SV_{40}$ were expressed in this human epithelial cell line. Thus, the $SV_{40}T/t$ antigens could be responsible for inducing and maintaining the growth properties of the RHEK-1 cell line. This "flat" nonproducer cell line has proven useful in our laboratory for studying multistage carcinogenesis.

### *Neoplastic transformation of human epidermal keratinocytes by Ad12-$SV_{40}$ and Ki-MSV*

The flat epithelial morphology and lack of tumorigenicity of the RHEK-1 cell line led us to inquire whether its growth properties might be further altered by addition of a virus containing an activated *ras* oncogene. Infection of the RHEK-1 line at passage 10 with Ki-MSV (BaEV) resulted in a striking alteration in cell morphology. As early as 5 to 6 days after infection, the cells began to pile up in focal areas, forming small projections, and releasing round cells (Fig. 2B). The absence of any detectable alterations induced by the helper virus (BaEV) alone implied that Ki-MSV was responsible for the rapid induction of the transformed morphology.

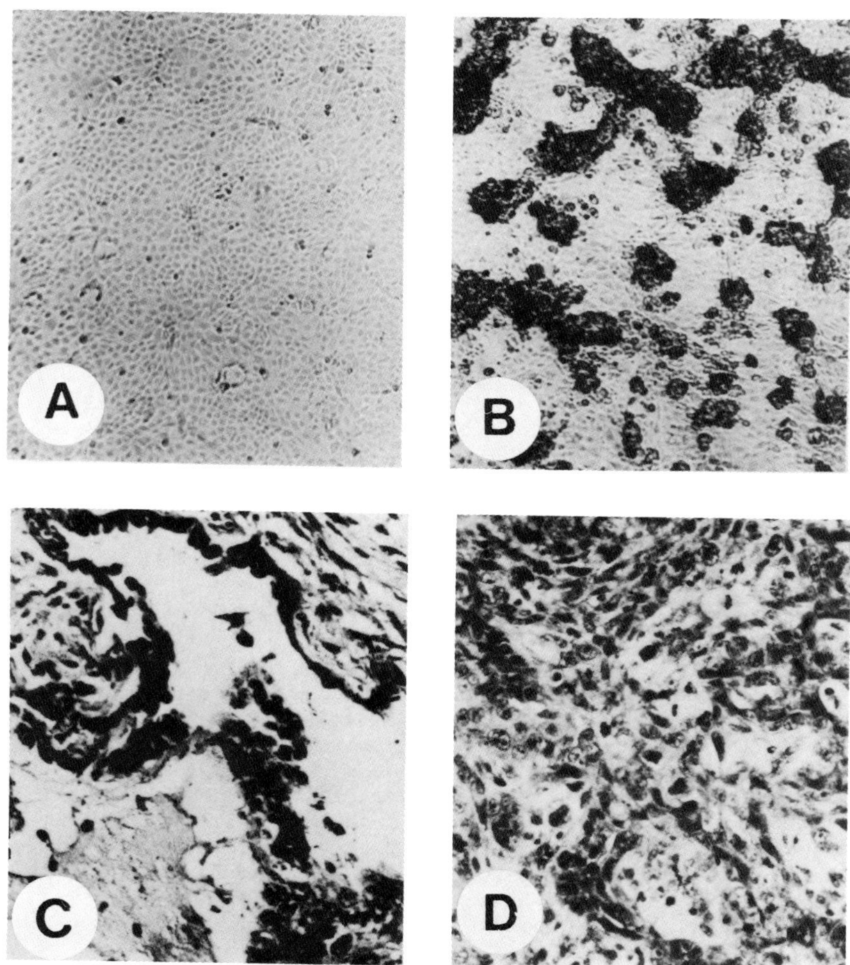

Figure 2. Human epidermal keratinocyte line (RHEK-1) (A) and Ki-MSV transformed RHEK-1 line (B). Regressing cystic nodules containing epidermal cells induced by RHEK-1 cells (C). *In vivo* tumor induced by Ki-MSV transformed RHEK-1 cells (D) Invasive squamous cell carcinoma with central necrosis.

The Ki-MSV-altered RHEK-1 cells expressed the K-*ras* p21 protein. They not only produced colonies in soft agar but were tumorigenic in nude mice. When athymic nude mice were inoculated with as few as $10^6$ Ki-MSV transformed RHEK-1 cells, the animals developed invasive, rapidly progressive tumors within 3 weeks. Such tumors were diagnosed as squamous cell carcinomas with characteristic keratin pearls (Fig. 2D). Cell lines established from the tumors were readily transplantable and were confirmed to be derived from the parental RHEK-1 cells by karyological analysis. These findings demonstrate the malignant transformation of primary human epithelial cells in culture by the combined action of $SV_{40}$ T antigen and Ki-MSV p21, and support a multistep process for neoplastic conversion (16).

Several investigators have reported that primary rodent fibroblasts can undergo neoplastic conversion in response to the combined action of two viral or cellular oncogenes (11,12). To our knowledge, our study is the first to show neoplastic conversion of human epithelial cells in culture and to define the minimum number of transforming genes that appeared to be required.

## *Hydrocortisone enhances Ki-MSV induced focus formation in RHEK-1 cells*

In an attempt to achieve maximum transformation efficiency, the effect of hydrocortisone on focus formation by Ki-MSV in human epidermal keratinocytes was examined. Hydrocortisone has previously been shown to significantly enhance Ki-MSV-induced transformation of human skin fibroblasts (41). The results showed that hydrocortisone significantly enhances focus formation in RHEK-1 cells. The maximum effect, a 20-fold increase in focus formation, was seen at a hydrocortisone concentration of 5 mg/ml. In the hydrocortisone-treated human epidermal cells, Ki-MSV produced larger and well-defined foci which could be counted seven days after infection. In contrast, in untreated human epidermal cells, foci were small and barely visible and could not be counted until 14 days after infection. Therefore, medium containing hydrocortisone concentration at 5 mg/ml was used in our transformation experiments (3).

## *Usefulness of the RHEK-1 cell model for viral, chemical and radiation carcinogenesis*

Since certain carcinogenic polycyclic hydrocarbons have been identified in our environment and some are known definitely to cause cancers in humans, it is important to study the response of human cells to such compounds. However, there was no reproducible human cell systems for carcinogen-induced neoplastic transformation in culture (3). In addition, the carcinogenic action of ionizing radiation in humans has been well recognized from epidermiological data. Despite this fact, there has been no model to study the radiation-induced neoplastic transformation of human cells, particularly those of epithelial cells. We have, therefore, examined the susceptibility of the RHEK-1 cell line to chemical carcinogens and X-ray irradiation. Subsequent treatment of chemical carcinogens (MNNG or 4NQ)) or X-ray irradiation induced morphological alterations and the acquisition of neoplastic properties (46,47). Subsequently it was found that this line could be transformed neoplastically by a variety of retrovirus-containing H-*ras*, *bas*, *fes*, *fms*, *erb*B and *src* oncogene (48) and by transfection with an activated human *ras* oncogene (49). Thus, this *in vitro* system may be useful in studying the interaction of a variety of carcinogenic agents and human epithelial cells. These findings demonstrated the malignant transformation of human primary epithelial cells in culture by the combined action of viruses, oncogenes, chemical carcinogens, or X-ray irradiation and support a multistep process for neoplastic conversion.

## *Ras oncogenes were not activated in the chemically-transformed human epidermal (RHEK-1) line*

Since RHEK-1 cells can be transformed by Ki-MSV infection and become tumorigenic (16) we analyzed the *ras* p21 product in the chemically-transformed as well as in the Ki-MSV-transformed RHEK-1 cells by using antibody to p21 and sodium dodecyl sulfate-polyacrylamide gel electrophoresis. In contrast to the findings in the Ki-MSV-transformed cells, neither altered mobility nor increased expression of p21 was observed in the chemically-transformed RHEK-1 cells. Moreover, the DNA from these chemically altered cells failed to induce detectable transformed foci upon transfection of NIH 3T3 cells. These results indicate that the *ras* oncogenes, which have been implicated in chemical carcinogen-induced animal tumors, spontaneous human tumors and 3MC-induced human transformed cell line, were not activated in the

chemically-transformed human epithelial cell lines so far
analyzed.  Thus, this system may be useful in efforts to
detect and characterize other cellular genes that can
contribute to the neoplastic phenotype of human epithelial
cells.

## Transforming genes from radiation-transformed human epidermal keratinocytes detected by a tumorigenicity assay

DNA-mediated gene transfer studies using rodent cells
as recipients have demonstrated the presence of transforming genes in radiation-induced rodent tumors and rodent
cells transformed by radiation (30,31).  As described
above, there was no detectable transformed foci upon
transfection of NIH 3T3 cells with the DNA's from the
radiation altered human epidermal cells (47).  Therefore,
we tested the DNA's from these transformants by a
tumorigenicity assay since the tumorigenicity assay has
been shown to detect weak transforming genes (50,51).  The
DNA from a highly tumorigenic radiation-altered soft agar
clone (8 Gy) induced *Alu*-positive tumors in nude mice.
Positive primary nude mouse tumor DNA's were submitted to a
second round of analysis in the tumorigenicity assay with
high frequency and short latency and were found to be *Alu*-
positive.  The DNA's from the *Alu*-positive secondary nude
mouse tumors were screened for homology with probes for the
*ras* gene family.  None of the *Alu*-positive bands were found
to be N-, K- or H-*ras*.  Subsequent analysis has also
eliminated the c-*raf* gene.  Further characterization of
these transforming genes is in progress.  The results so
far indicate that members of the *ras* oncogene family are
not activated in the radiation-transformed human epidermal
lines (52).

## Immortalization of other human epithelial cells by the Ad12-SV40 virus

Recent advances in the cultivation of human
epithelial cells has made it possible to study problems
related to carcinogenesis and differentiation in cell
culture systems.  Primary cultures of epithelial cells can
now be established from various human tissue biopsies
without difficulty even in the absence of serum
supplement.  However, the usefulness of such cell cultures
is limited by factors including cellular "senescence,"
slow growth rates, and small numbers of available cells.
Many of these limitations can now be overcome by our
ability to transform epithelial cells.

Besides the human foreskin epidermal cells described above, we were able to successfully establish lines from primary cultures by $Ad12-SV_{40}$ virus infection of: 1) human bronchial epithelial cells, (53) human salivary gland epithelial cells, (54) nasal polyp epithelial cells from cystic fibrosis (CF) patients, and (55) normal and CF bronchial epithelial cell lines (56).

*Evidence for the multistep nature of in vitro human epithelial cell carcinogenesis*

In addition to $Ad12-SV_{40}$ immortalized human epidermal (RHEK-1) model already described, we have shown another multistep models for human epithelial cell transformation.

1. Neoplastic conversion of normal human epidermal (11367) line established by $pSV_3$-neo transfection was achieved with Ki-MSV infection (57).

2. Neoplastic transformation was obtained in a $SV_{40}$ T antigen-immortalized human bronchial epithelial cell line by v-Ki-*ras* (58).

3. Malignant conversion of human foreskin keratinocytes by human papilloma virus type 16 DNA and v-K-*ras* oncogene (59). These findings demonstrate the malignant conversion of human primary epithelial cells in culture by the cooperation of a HPV DNA and a retroviral gene, and support a multistep process for neoplastic conversion.

Since our initial report (16), the list of successful reports on the neoplastic transformation of normal human cells including fibroblasts have been growing (Table 2). These were achieved in a stepwide fashion. Human primary cells immortalized by a variety of means (viruses, chemicals, irradiation, or spontaneously without any treatment) could be transformed neoplastically by a carcinogenic agent. Thus, these studies demonstrate that neoplastic transformation of normal human cells in culture is indeed a multistep process. In all these cases, the initial event seemed to be immortalization of the cells followed by neoplastic conversion. As postulated for rodent fibroblasts (60), the immortalization step is a critical initial step and rate limiting for *in vitro* neoplastic transformation of human epithelial cells.

**Table 2:   In Vitro Multistep Models for Human Cell Carcinogenesis**

| Cells | Stage of carcinogenesis | | Ref. |
|---|---|---|---|
| | Immortalization Step | Transformation Step | |
| **Epithelial Cells** | | | |
| Keratinocytes | Ad12-SV$_{40}$ | Ki-MSV | 16 |
| | Ad12-SV$_{40}$ | MNNG or 4NQO | 46 |
| | Ad12-SV$_{40}$ | x-ray | 47 |
| | Ad12-SV$_{40}$ | Retroviruses | 48 |
| | Ad12-SV$_{40}$ | c-H-*ras* | 49 |
| | pSV$_3$ neo | Ki-MSV | 57 |
| | spontaneous | c-H-*ras* | 64 |
| | HPV-16 | KI-MSV | 59 |
| Bronchial | Ad12-SV$_{40}$ | Ki-MSV | 58 |
| | Ad12-SV$_{40}$ | v-H-*ras* | 65 |
| Mammary | BP | retroviruses | 66 |
| Amnlotic | SV$_{40}$ | KI-MSV | 67 |
| Cervical | HPV-16 | v-H-*ras* | 68 |
| Urinary tract | SV$_{40}$ | 3MC | 69 |
| | SV$_{40}$ | c-H-*ras* | 70 |
| Liver | SV$_{40}$ | - | 71 |
| Kidney | Nickel | v-H-*ras* | 72 |
| Thyroid | Adeno EIA | - | 73 |
| | SV$_{40}$ Orl- | - | 74 |
| Colon | SV$_{40}$ Orl- | - | 75 |
| | MNNG & Sod. butyrate | - | 76 |
| Tracheal gland | Ad12-SV$_{40}$ | - | 77 |
| Letinal pigment | SV$_{40}$ | - | 78 |
| Esophagus | SV$_{40}$ | - | 79 |

Table 2:   In Vitro Multistep Models for Human Cell
           Carcinogenesis   (continued)

| Cells | Stage of carcinogenesis | | Ref. |
|-------|-------------------------|------------------------|------|
|       | Immortalization Step | Transformation Step |      |
| Melanocyte | $SV_{40}$ | – | 80 |
| Prostate | $SV_{40}$ | – | 81 |
| Fibroblasts | $SV_{40}$ | KI-MSV | 9 |
|  | gamma ray | H-MSV or c-H-*ras* | 82 |
|  | v-myc | H-*ras* | 83 |

## Summary

The immortalization and transformation of cultured
human cells has far-reaching implications for both cell
and cancer biology.  Human cell transformation studies
will increase our understanding of the mechanisms
underlying carcinogenesis and differentiation.  The neoplastic process can now be studied in a model human cell
culture system.  The accompanying biochemical and genetic
changes, once identified, will help define the
relationship between malignancy and differentiation.

The present studies indeed demonstrate that the
neoplastic process can now be studied in a human cell
model system.  Primary human cells treated with various
carcinogens became immortalized in culture but were not
tumorigenic.  Additional exposure to either retroviruses,
chemical carcinogens or X-ray irradiation to these cells
induced morphological alterations associated with the
acquisition of neoplastic properties.  These findings
demonstrate the malignant transformation of human primary
cells in culture by the combined action of either a DNA
transforming virus and a retrovrius or a DNA virus and a
chemical or X-ray irradiation, and support a multistep
process for neoplastic conversion.

It has been known that normal human cells in culture
are remarkably resistant to experimentally induced
tumorigenicity.  However, as shown above, normal human
cells could now be transformed into tumorigenic cells.

## Acknowledgements

We would like to acknowledge my main collaborators involved in the different phases of this work:  R. Huebner, P. Arnstein, E. Weisburger, W. Nelson-Rees, G. Jay, K. Sanford, S. A. Aaronson, C. Harris, M. Durst, W. Peterson and S. Reynolds.

## References

1.   E. Farber. _Cancer Res_., 44, 4217 (1984).
2.   G. Klein, E. Klein. _Nature_, 315, 190 (1985).
3.   J. Rhim. _Anticancer Res_., 9, 1345 (1989).
4.   A.J. Girardi, F.C. Jensen, _et al_. _J. Cell Comp. Physiol._, 65, 69 (1965).
5.   F. L. Graham, J. Smiley, _et al_. _J. Gen. Virol_., 36, 59 (1977).
6.   C. Borek. _Nature_, 283, 776 (1980).
7.   G. Milo, J. DiPaolo. _Nature_ (London), 275, 130 (1978).
8.   J.J. McCormick, V.M. Maher. _Mutation Res._, 199, 273 (1988).
9.   W. O'Brien, G. Stenman, _et al_. _Proc. Natl. Acad. Sci. USA_, 83, 8659 (1986).
10.  M. Namba, K. Nishitani, _et al_. _Int. J. Cancer_, 37, 419 (1986).
11.  H. Land, L.V. Parada, et al. _Nature_, 304, 596-602 (1983).
12.  H.E. Ruley. _Nature_, 304, 602-606 (1983).
13.  R.M. McAllister, M.B. Gardner, _et al_. _Cancer_, 27, 397 (1971).
14.  J.S. Rhim, H.Y. Cho, _et al_. _Int. J. Cancer_, 15, 23 (1975).
15.  J.S. Rhim, D.K. Park, _et al_. _Nature_, 256, 751 (1975).
16.  J.S. Rhim, G. Jay, _et al_. _Science_, 227, 1250 (1985).
17.  H.M. Shein, J.F. Enders. _Proc. Natl. Acad. Sci. USA_, 48, 1164 (1962).
18.  H. Koprowski, J.A. Ponten, _et al_. _J. Cell. Comp. Physiol._, 59, 281 (1962).
19.  B.H. Sweet, M.R. Hillman. _Proc. Soc. Exp. Biol. Med._, 105, 420 (1960).
20.  J.S. Rhim, H.Y. Cho, _et al_. In:  Clemmesen, J. and Yohn, D.S. (Eds.):  Comparative Leukemia Research. 1975, Bibl. Haemat., No. 43, Basel, Karger, 84-87 (1976).

21. Y. Bernwald, L. Sachs. J. Natl. Cancer Inst, 35, 641 (1965).
22. C. Heidelberg. In: Klein, G. and Weinhouse, S. (eds), Advances in Cancer Research, New York, Academic Press, Vol. 18, 317-366 (1973).
23. J.A. DiPaolo, P.J. Donovan. Exp. Cell Res., 48, 361-377 (1967).
24. R.S. Leith and L. Hayflick. Proc. Am. Assoc. Cancer Res., 15, 86 (1974).
25. R.R. McAllister, J.E. Filbert, et al. Nature (New Biology), 230, 279-282 (1971).
26. G.J. Todaro, C.A. Meyer. J. Natl. Cancer Inst., 52, 167 (1974).
27. H.Y. Cho, E.C. Cutchins, et al. Science, 194, 951 (1976).
28. H.Y. Cho, P. Arnstein, et al. Int. J. Cancer, 21, 22 (1978).
29. Y.H. Yang, J.S. Rhim, et al. J. Gen. Virol., 43, 477 (1979).
30. G. Cooper. Science, 217, 801 (1982).
31. R.A. Weinberg. Adv. Cancer Res., 36, 149 (1982).
32. H. Zarbl, S. Sukumar, et al. Nature, 315, 382 (1985).
33. C.S. Cooper, D.G. Blair, et al. Cancer Res., 44, 1 (1984).
34. C.S. Cooper, M. Park, et al. Nature, 311, 29 (1984).
35. M. Park, M. Dean, et al. Cell, 45, 895 (1986).
36. M. Dean, M. Park, et al. Nature, 318, 385 (1985).
37. R. White, S. Woodward, et al. Nature, 318, 382 (1985).
38. D.P. Bottaro, J.S. Rubin, et al. Science, 251, 802 (1991).
39. J.S. Rhim, J. Fujita, et al. Carcinogenesis, 8, 1165 (1987).
40. S. Rasheed, J.S. Rhim, et al. Am. J. Hum. Genet., 35, 919 (1983).
41. J.S. Rhim. Proc. Soc. Exp. Biol. Med., 174, 217 (1983).
42. T. Kakunaga. Proc. Natl. Acad. Sci. USA, 75, 1334 (1978).
43. J.J. McCormick, D. Yang, et al. Carcinogenesis, 9, 2073 (1988).
44. M.L. Steinberg, V. Defendi. Proc. Natl. Acad. Sci. USA, 76, 801 (1979).
45. S.P. Banks-Schlegel, P.M. Howley. Cell. Biol., 96, 330 (1983).
46. J.S. Rhim, J. Fujita, et al. Science, 232, 385 (1986).

47. P. Thraves, Z. Salehi, et al. Proc. Natl. Acad. Sci. USA, 87, 1174 (1990).

48. J.S. Rhim, T. Kawakami, et al. Leukemia, 2, 1515 (1988).

49. J.S. Rhim, J.B. Park, et al. Oncogene, 4, 1403 (1989).

50. O. Fasano, D. Birnbaum, et al. Mol. Cell. Biol., 4, 1695 (1984).

51. Y. Yuasa, T. Kaniyama, et al. Oncogene, 5, 589 (1990).

52. P. Thraves, S. Reynolds, et al. Proc. Amer. Assoc. Cancer Res., 32:115 (1991).

53. R.R. Reddel, Y. Ke, et al. Cancer Res., 48, 1904 (1988).

54. J.S. Rhim, R.I. Fox, et al. In: Epstein-Barr Virus and Human Disease 1988, Ablashi, D. V. et al., ed. The Humana Press, Clifton New Jersey, pp 155 (1988).

55. B.J. Scholte, J. Bkjman, et al. Exp. Cell. Res., 182:559 (1989).

56. P.L. Zeitlin, L. Lu, et al. Am. J. Resp. Cell and Mol. Biol., 4, 313 (1991).

57. R. Gantt, K.K. Sanford, et al. Cancer Res., 47, 1390 (1987).

58. R.R. Reddel, Y. Ki, E. Kaigh, et al. Oncogene Res., 3, 401 (1988).

59. M. Durst, D. Gallahan, et al. Virology, 73, 767 (1989).

60. R.F. Newbold, R.W. Overell. Nature, 304, 648 (1983).

61. J.S. Rhim, C.M. Kim, et al. J. Natl. Cancer Inst., 55, 1291 (1975).

62. J.S. Rhim. Proc. Soc. Exp. Biol. Med., 167, 597 (1981).

63. J.S. Rhim, R. Trimmer, et al. Proc. Soc. Exp. Biol. Med., 170, 350 (1982).

64. P. Boukamp, E.J. Stanbridge, et al. Cancer Res., 50, 2840 (1990).

65. P. Amstad, R.R. Reddel, et al. Carcinogenesis, 1, 151 (1988).

66. R. Clark, M.R. Stampfer, et al. Cancer Res., 48, 4689 (1988).

67. K.H. Walen, P. Arnstein. Dev. Biol., 2, 57 (1986).

68. J.A. DiPaolo, C.D. Woodworth, et al. Oncogene, 4, 395 (1989).

69. C.A. Reznikoff, L.J. Loretz, et al. Carcinogenesis, 9, 1427 (1988).

70. B.C. Christian, C. Kao, et al. Proc. Am. Assoc. Cancer Res., 29, 459 (1988).

71. K.E. Cole, A.M.A. Pfeifer, *et al*. Proc. Amer. Assoc. Cancer Res., 31, 19 (1990).
72. A. Haungen, D. Ryberg, *et al*. Int. J. Cancer, 45, 572 (1990).
73. R.D. Cone, M. Platzer, *et al*. Endocrinology, 123, 2067 (1988).
74. N.R. Lemoine, E.S. Mayall, *et al*. Br. J. Cancer, 60, 897 (1989).
75. R.D. Berry, S.C. Powell, *et al*. Br. J. Cancer, 57, 287 (1988).
76. A.C. Williams, S.J. Harper, *et al*. Cancer Res., 50, 4724 (1990).
77. D.P. Chopra, R.L. Shoemaker, *et al*. Unpublished.
78. K. Dutt, M. Scott, *et al*. Oncogene, 5, 195 (1990).
79. G.D. Stoner, M.E. Kaighn, *et al*. Cancer Res., 51:365 (1991).
80. K. Melber, G. Zhu, *et al*. Cancer Res., 49, 3650 (1989).
81. M.E. Kaighn, R.R. Reddel, *et al*. Cancer Res., 49, 3050 (1989).
82. M. Namba, K. Nishitani, *et al*. Mutat. Res., 199, 415 (1988).
83. P.J. Hurlin, V.M. Maher, *et al*. Proc. Natl. Acad. Sci. USA, 86, 187-191 (1989).

# I. Preneoplastic Events

COMPARISON OF HUMAN VERSUS RODENT CELL TRANSFORMATION:

IMPORTANCE OF CELL AGING

J. Carl Barrett

National Institute of Environmental Health
Sciences, Research Triangle Park, NC 27709 USA

Rodent models are used for the identification of
carcinogenic agents and for studies of mechanisms of
carcinogenesis.  An underlying assumption is that the
information gained from animal studies will extend to
humans.  However, a fundamental difference must exist
between human and rodents in terms of neoplastic
development because cancers generally arise in rodents
after a few years whereas the same cancers require decades
in humans.  For example, the spontaneous incidence of
tumors in rodents after two years is approximately equal
to that in humans at 70 years (1).  It is an important
problem in cancer biology to understand this fundamental
difference between rodents and humans.  One approach to
this problem is to elucidate the underlying mechanisms of
neoplastic transformation of cells in culture from
different species by determining the number and type of
genetic events involved.  Cellular and molecular studies
offer the opportunity to examine species differences and
similarities.

Cancer is a multistep process involving multiple
genetic changes.  The difference in time of occurrence of
cancers in humans versus rodents suggests either that
fewer steps (genetic events) are required in rodent tumors
or that the rates of transition between the steps are
slower in humans.

Cell culture models using both human and rodent
cells have been developed to study mechanisms of

neoplastic progression (2). Extensive studies of
neoplastic transformation of rodent cells by chemical
carcinogens, viruses, and activated oncogenes have been
reported (see ref. 2 for review). Fewer studies exist
with human cells in culture due to the greater difficulty
in transforming these cells (2,3). Nonetheless, sufficient literature exists to allow a few generalizations
concerning the similarities and differences between
normal, diploid human and rodent cells in terms of
mechanisms of neoplastic transformation in culture.

Neoplastic conversion of both human and rodent
cells in culture is a multistep process involving both
activation of proto-oncogenes and inactivation of tumor
suppressor genes (2). Cooperation between oncogenes
increases the neoplastic progression of both human and
rodent cells (4,5) and inactivation of multiple tumor
suppressor genes has been shown in human and rodent
tumors (6-8). Despite these similarities, one major
species difference is clear from studies of cell
transformation; the ability of rodent cells in culture to
escape cellular senescence spontaneously or following
carcinogen treatment is significantly greater than for
human cells (2,3).

Both human and rodent cells in culture can be grown
for only a limited, fixed number of cell divisions after
which they exhibit morphological changes and cease
proliferation, a process termed cellular senescence or
cellular aging (9). Diploid, human cells can be grown for
50-60 population doublings before senescence if they are
derived from embryonic or neonatal tissues. Cells from
rodent embryos grow for 20-40 population doublings before
losing proliferative potential. There is a general
correlation between the life span of the species and the
number of population doublings that can be achieved in
culture (9,10). Cells from the Galapagos tortoise, which
has a life span of 175-200 years, can be grown for 90-125
population doublings (9,11). This observation suggests
that aging in culture and aging of the organism may be
related, which is further supported by the findings of an
inverse correlation between doubling potential in culture
and age of the human or rodent donor (9), and decreased
population doublings in vitro of cells derived from
individuals who exhibit premature aging (e.g., progeria
and Werner syndrome) (9,11-13).

The age-specific incidence curves of cancer in humans and rodents are similar if time is expressed as the percentage of life span achieved (1). This implies that the processes that allow a longer life span in humans may also delay the development of cancer in humans. Taken together with the observation that escape from cellular senescence is different in humans versus rodents, this suggests that fundamental differences exist among species in terms of cellular and organismic aging, which are determinants in the cancer process.

Several key questions arise from this hypothesis that can be addressed by studies of cellular aging: What is the molecular and genetic basis for cellular aging? Is escape from cellular aging a rate limiting step in the cancer process? How do rodent and human cells differ in regard to the mechanisms of cellular aging? How is the escape from senescence different in rodent versus human tumor cells?

We have proposed the following hypotheses: Cellular senescence is controlled by genes that are activated or whose functions become manifested at the end of the life span of the cell. Defects in the function of these gene products can allow cells to escape the program of senescence and become immortal. Immortalization relieves one constraint on tumor cell growth, allowing malignant progression.

Escape from cellular senescence is an important step in neoplastic progression of human and rodent cancers (2). Many, but not all, tumor cells can be grown indefinitely in culture and therefore have escaped senescence and are termed immortal. It is not clear whether the failure of some tumor cells to grow in culture is a technical artifact or an indication that escape from senescence is not required for these cancers. Many of these tumors also cannot be grown in vivo in nude mice, which may indicate that only a small growth fraction of cells exists in the tumor. Improvements in cell culture techniques have led to the establishment of many cell lines from most tumor types, suggesting that it is possible to obtain immortal cell lines if the culture conditions are optimal. Since no property of cancer cells is universal, it is not necessary to demonstrate that escape from senescence has occurred in every cancer.

However, in those cancers where this change is evident, it
is probably a critical change based on the following
additional lines of evidence (2).

The observation that treatment of normal cells with
diverse carcinogenic agents (including chemical carcinogens, viruses, and oncogenes) allows cells to escape
senescence indicates that this change is important in
cancer induction.  While immortality is not sufficient for
neoplastic transformation, most immortal cells have an
increased propensity for spontaneous, carcinogen-induced
or oncogene-induced neoplastic progression (2).  Therefore, escape from senescence is a preneoplastic change
that predisposes cells to neoplastic conversion.  Thus,
immortal cells are further along the multistep pathway to
neoplasia than normal cells (2).

Cellular senescence may be one of the mechanisms by
which tumor suppression occurs (2,13).  Tumor suppression
is controlled by a family of normal cellular genes that
must be inactivated, lost, or mutated in cancer cells.
Since cellular senescence limits the growth of cells, it
is reasonable that senescence might be one mechanism by
which tumor suppressor genes operate.  Hayflick has shown
that cells from adults can be grown in culture for 14 to
29 population doublings (9).  If all the changes necessary
for tumorigenic conversion were to accumulate in an adult
cell without loss or gain of life span potential, then
this cell could grow to form a tumor of 16,384 cells (14
doublings or $2^{14}$ cells) to 5.4 x $10^8$ (29 doublings or $2^{29}$
cells).  It is estimated that a tumor formed after 30 cell
doublings would be approximately 1 $cm^2$ in size (14).
Interestingly, Paraskeva and coworkers have shown that
colon adenomas of < 1$cm^2$ in size are rarely capable of
indefinite growth <u>in vitro</u> whereas cells from adenomas of
>1 $cm^2$ are often immortal (15-17), which suggests that
escape from senescence is a requirement for tumor growth
beyond a certain size or cell number and is consistent
with the hypothesis that cell senescence is a constraint
on tumor growth.

Two major theories of cellular senescence have been
proposed for many years (9,18).  One is the error
catastrophe or damage model, which proposes that random
accumulation of damage or mutations in DNA, RNA, or
protein leads to the loss of proliferative capacity.  The

experimental evidence in support of the error accumulation hypothesis has been criticized (18).  A second hypothesis is that senescence is a genetically programmed process, and recent support for a genetic basis for senescence was provided by experiments of Pereira-Smith and Smith (19) and by Sugawara et al. (20).

It is possible to fuse cells of different origins and then to select for the hybrid cells using biochemical markers for drug sensitivity or resistance that differ in the parental cells.  When cells with a finite life span are fused to immortal cells with an indefinite life span, the majority of these hybrids senesce, indicating that senescence is dominant over immortality (19,21).  Even hybridization of two different immortal human cell lines with each other can result in senescence, indicating that different complementation groups exist for the senescence function lost in these cells.  Four complementation groups have been established, suggesting that loss or inactivation of one of multiple genes might allow escape from senescence (19).  If this hypothesis is correct, it should be possible to map the genes involved in cellular senescence.  Recent findings with hamster and human interspecies hybrids have mapped putative senescence genes to specific human chromosomes (20,22,23).

When normal human cells with a finite life span are fused to immortal hamster cells, the hybrids that form exhibit a finite life span characteristic of the normal human cells.  At the end of this life span, the cells display signs of cellular senescence characteristic of the parental human cells at the end of their life span. Criteria for senescence include cellular enlargement and flattening, and cessation of proliferation as measured by the failure to increase cell number in two weeks, failure to subculture, failure to form colonies at clonal density, and lack of significant incorporation of $^3$H-thymidine as measured by labeled nuclei (<2%) following autoradiography (20).

When MRC-5 cells, which are normal human lung fibroblasts with a life span of 60 population doublings, were fused at a population doubling level of 40, the human-hamster hybrids grew for approximately 20 population doublings, i.e., the remaining life span of the parental human cells.  Since the cell hybrids grew extensively

before dying, the cessation of growth was not due to a
toxic effect of the fusion protocol or some other trivial
reason.  Furthermore, when earlier passage MRC-5 cells
were used (population doubling level 30), the hybrids grew
longer, for up to 30 population doublings, again achieving
the life span of the parental cells.  Therefore, the
senescence of the hybrids is an active process dictated by
the senescence program of the normal human cells.  The
limited life span of the hybrids indicates that cellular
senescence is dominant in these hamster-human hybrids.  A
similar conclusion was drawn from studies of intraspecies,
i.e., human-human and hamster-hamster hybrids (19,21).

Although the majority of the hamster-human hybrids
senesced, some of the hybrids ultimately escaped
senescence (Fig. 1).  Senescent cells appeared in all of

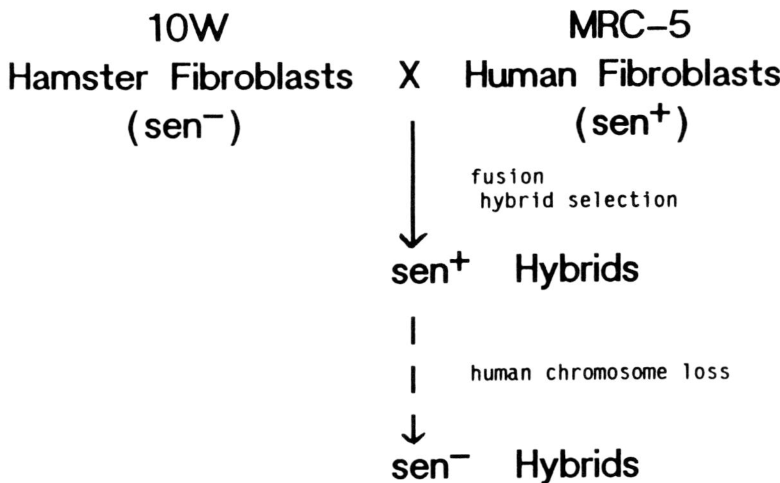


Fig. 1.  Hybrids between immortal (sen⁻) hamster cells and
normal human cells senescence (sen⁺).  Rare variants
escape senescence (sen⁻) after losing human chromosomes.

the hybrid clones after two to three passages. In some of
the clones a few nonsenescent cells persisted and
continued to proliferate, achieved >100 population
doublings, and had high labelling indices and colony
forming efficiencies (20). These results indicated that
these hybrid clones had escaped senescence. Since it is
known that human chromosomes are usually lost in
interspecies hybrids, the possibility that escape from
senescence is due to loss of an essential chromosome or
chromosomes was examined by karyotypic examination of the
hybrids after escape from senescence (approximately 40
population doublings). Since it is possible to
distinguish human and hamster chromosomes, the simple
question was asked whether escape from senescence involved
the loss of any specific human chromosome. Without
exception, all of the human-hamster hybrid clones that
escaped senescence had lost both copies of human
chromosome 1. All other human chromosomes were present in
one or two copies in at least one of the immortal hybrids
(20).

In order to determine whether the loss of chromosome
1 in nonsenescent hybrids was the fortuitous consequence
of human chromosome loss in the hybrid or an indication
that a gene on this chromosome influenced the senescence
process, two additional approaches were undertaken. The
hamster cells used in these experiments lacked HPRT gene
activity (20). Hamster-human hybrid clones were selected
in HAT medium, which requires the cells to retain the HPRT
gene located on the human X chromosome. Karyotypic analysis
confirmed that all immortal hybrids retained a human X
chromosome. Normal human fibroblasts with a translocation
between the human chromosome X and either chromosome 1 or
chromosome 11 were obtained. The translocated portion of
the chromosome contained the HPRT gene located on the long
arm of the X chromosome. Both cell strains had a finite
life span and hybrids between the human cells and hamster
cells senesced. The percentage of senescent hybrids was
40% in the case of fusions between hamster cells and human
cells with a t(X;11) chromosome, similar to the percentage
with normal diploid human MRC-5 and hamster cells. In
contrast, nearly 90% of the cell hybrids between the
hamster cells and human cells with a t(X;1) chromosome
senesced. This increased frequency of senescent hybrids
is consistent with the hypothesis that chromosome 1
contains a gene(s) involved in the senescence process.

The gene(s) must be on the long arm of the chromosome 1
since only this portion of chromosome 1 is present on the
translocated chromosome.  The few hybrids that escaped
senescence were examined karyotypically and no intact
t(X;1) chromosome was observed.  We interpret these
results to indicate that a deletion of the critical
portion of chromosome 1 occurred, which allowed these
hybrids to escape senescence.  Since the cells still grow
in HAT medium, the HPRT gene on chromosome X must be
retained in these cells.

     To further confirm the role of human chromosome 1
in the senescence of hamster cells, transfer of a single
copy of chromosome 1 into immortal hamster cells by the
microcell transfer technique was attempted (20).  Mouse A9
cells containing a single human chromosome 1 or 11 tagged
with a dominant selectable marker (neomycin) were isolated
by techniques previously described (24).  Chromosome 1 or
chromosome 11 was transferred by microcell fusion to
immortal Syrian hamster cell lines and mouse A9 cells.
Numerous colonies were observed following transfer of
chromosome 11 into the hamster cells, and no colonies
senesced.  The frequency of colonies following transfer of
chromosome 1 into the mouse A9 cells was similar to that
observed with chromosome 11, but only one large colony was
observed in 10 experiments with the hamster cell line (the
frequency was reduced by at least two orders of
magnitude).  This clone, however, senesced after 4 weeks
and failed to grow to more than 1000 cells.  Several
small, senescent colonies (8 to 20 cells) were observed
following transfer of chromosome 1 into the hamster cells,
but these colonies ceased proliferating and sometimes
detached from the dish.

     The data presented above suggest that a gene or
genes on human chromosome 1 are involved in the senescence
of hamster-human hybrids.  This conclusion is based on
three experimental approaches: interspecies cell hybrids
with diploid human cells, interspecies cell hybrids with
human cells carrying X;autosomal chromosome translocations, and microcell hybrids with individual human
chromosomes.  Each experimental approach alone is
inconclusive, but taken together, the results strongly
implicate human chromosome 1 in cellular senescence.

     Recently, in collaboration with Dr. Max Costa and

coworkers, we have mapped another senescence gene to
chromosome X (22).  In addition, Ning, Pereira-Smith and
Smith have mapped a senescence gene for HeLa cells to
chromosome 4 (23).  Thus, three senescence genes have now
been mapped (Table 1).

Table 1.  Mapping of Putative Senescence Genes

| Chromosome localization of sen[+] gene | Cell(s) | Reference |
| --- | --- | --- |
| Chromosome 1 | Syrian hamster 10W | Sugawara et al. (20) |
| | Syrian hamster BHK | Annab & Barrett, unpublished |
| | Human endometrial | Yamada et al. (28) |
| Chromnosome 4 | Cervical carcinoma (HeLa) | Ning, Weber et al. (23) |
| Chromosome X | Chinese hamster ($N_i$-2) | Klein et al. (22) |

These results provide support for the hypothesis
that cellular senescence is controlled by genes that are
activated or whose function becomes manifested at the end
of the life span of the cell.  The cloning and
identification of these genes should provide new insights
into the cancer and aging processes.

The significance of these findings with respect to
differences in life span and cancer rates in humans versus
rodents remains to be determined.  The senescence gene on
chromosome 1 appears to operate in both human and hamster
cells, suggesting a commonality between species.  Furthermore, escape from senescence is a multistep process in
both humans and rodents (2,25).  We have postulated that
one mechanism involved in immortalization of hamster cells

is induction of aneuploidy (2,26).  When human and hamster
cells are compared for susceptibility to aneuploidy
inducing chemicals, human cells are less susceptible but
the difference is not sufficient to explain the inability
of chemicals to induce immortalization (26,27).  Therefore, additional research is needed to explain the
differences between human and rodent cells and the
identification of senescence genes and their mechanism(s)
of inactivation in immortal cells may provide new insights
into this problem.


REFERENCES


1.   R. G. Cutler and  I. Semsei. <u>J. Gerontol.</u> 44, 25
     (1989).
2.   J. C. Barrett and W. F. Fletcher. In: J. C. Barrett
     (ed.), Mechanisms of Environmental Carcinognesis:
     Multistep Models of Carcinogenesis, 73-116, CRC Press,
     Boca Raton, Florida (1987).
3.   J. J. McCormick and V. M. Maher. <u>Mutat. Res.</u> 199, 273
     (1988).
4.   R. A. Weinberg. <u>Science</u> 230, 770 (1985).
5.   J. S. Rhim, G. Jay, *et al.* <u>Science</u> 227, 1250 (1985).
6.   E. R. Fearon and B. Vogelstein. Cell 61, 759 (1990).
7.   R. A. Weinberg. <u>Cancer Res.</u> 49, 3713 (1989).
8.   J. A. Boyd and J. C. Barrett. <u>Pharmacol. Ther.</u> 46, 469
     (1990).
9.   L. Hayflick. <u>New Engl. J. Med.</u> 295, 1302 (1976).
10.  V. J. Cristofalo and D. G. Ragona.  In: R. C. Adelman
     and G. S. Roth (eds.), Testing the Theories of Aging,
     201-219, CRC Press, Boca Raton, Florida (1987).
11.  S. Goldstein. <u>Exp. Cell Res.</u> 83, 297 (1974).
12.  S. Goldstein, S. Murano and R. J. S. Reis. <u>J. Gerontol.</u>
     45, B3 (1990).
13.  R. Sager. <u>Cancer Res.</u> 46, 1573 (1986).
14.  V.T. DeVita Jr. <u>J. Natl. Cancer Inst.</u> 82, 1522 (1990).
15.  C. Paraskeva, S. Finerty and S. Powell. <u>Int. J. Cancer</u>
     41, 908 (1988).
16.  C. Paraskeva, S. Finerty, *et al.* <u>Cancer Res.</u> 49, 1282
     (1989).
17.  C. Paraskeva, S. Finerty and S. Powell. <u>Int. J. Cancer</u>
     43, 743 (1989).
18.  A. Macieira-Coelho. In: H. P. von Hang (ed.),
     Interdisciplinary Topics in Gerontology, Vol. 23,
     Karger, Basel (1988).

19.  O. M. Pereira-Smith and J. R. Smith. <u>Proc. Natl. Acad. Sci. USA</u> 85, 6043 (1988).
20.  O. Sugawara, M. Oshimura, *et al.* <u>Science</u> 247, 707 (1990).
21.  M. Koi and J. C. Barrett. <u>Proc. Natl. Acad. Sci. USA</u> 83, 5992 (1986).
22.  C. B. Klein, K. Conway, *et al.* <u>Science</u> 251, 796 (1991).
23.  Y. Ning, J. L. Weber, *et al.* <u>Proc. Natl. Acad. Sci. USA</u>, in press.
24.  M. Koi, H. Morita, *et al.* <u>Molec. Carcinogen.</u> 2, 12 (1989).
25.  D. J. Fitzgerald, H. Kitamura, *et al.* <u>Cancer Res.</u> 46, 4642 (1986).
26.  J. C. Barrett, M. Oshimura, *et al.* In: V. Dellarco, P. E. Voytek and A. Hollaender (eds.), Aneuploidy: Etiology and Mechanisms, 523-538, Plenum Press, New York (1985).
27.  T. Tsutsui, N. Suzuki, *et al.* <u>Mutat. Res.</u> 240, 241 (1990).
28.  H. Yamada, N. Wake, *et al.* <u>Oncogene</u> 5, 1141 (1990).

From: *Neoplastic Transformation in Human Cell Culture,*
Eds.: J. S. Rhim and A. Dritschilo ©1991 The Humana Press Inc., Totowa, NJ

DEFICIENT DNA REPAIR, AN EARLY STEP IN NEOPLASTIC

TRANSFORMATION OF HUMAN CELLS IN CULTURE


K.K. Sanford and R. Parshad

National Cancer Inst., Bethesda, MD 20892 and
Howard Univ., Washington, DC 20059 USA


The following three factors appear to be necessary
for the malignant neoplastic transformation of normal
cells in culture or *in vivo*: 1) DNA damage, 2) deficient
DNA repair during $G_2$ phase of the cell cycle and 3) a
continued proliferative stimulus from activation of proto-
oncogenes or loss of suppressor genes. Continued cell
proliferation alone leads to hyperplasia and benign
growths. Deficient repair of DNA damage provides the
genomic instability that can result in production of new
genetic variants characterizing malignant neoplasia.

Exposure of human cells in culture to DNA-damaging
agents such as radiation (x-rays, near- UV visible light,
UV) or chemicals (alkylating agents, radiomimetic drugs)
during $G_2$ phase of the cell cycle, *i.e.*, just before
mitosis, produces several DNA lesions including strand
breaks and base damage. Additional DNA strand breaks may
also develop during repair of base damage (1). Unrepaired
strand breaks can be quantified as chromatid breaks and
gaps at the first posttreatment metaphase (Fig. 1).
Because each chromatid contains one continuous molecule of
double-stranded DNA (Fig. 2), chromatid breaks represent
unrepaired DNA double-strand breaks. Chromatid breaks
show a discontinuity with displacement of the broken
segment. Chromatid gaps show a discontinuity but no
displacement, and were scored in our studies only if the
discontinuity was longer than the chromatid width (Fig.
3). These are sometimes referred to as non-displaced
breaks that may represent unrepaired DNA single- or

double-strand breaks (4).  Frequencies of chromatid breaks
and gaps in metaphase cells examined at short intervals
after $G_2$ phase DNA damage thus provide a measure of
unrepaired DNA strand breaks.

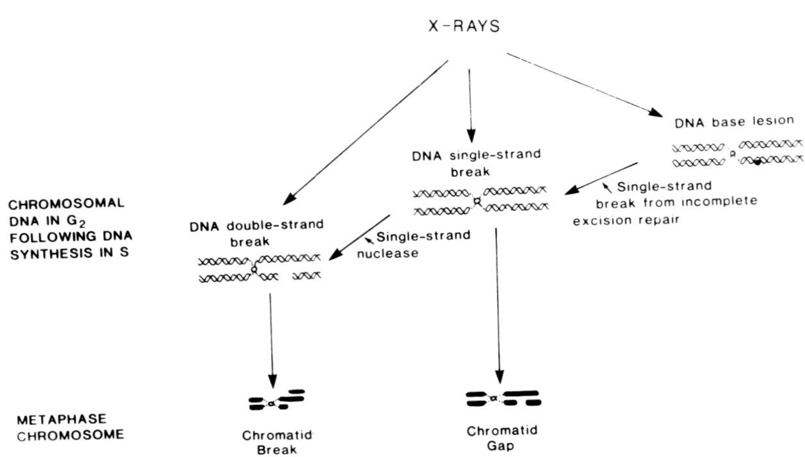


Fig. 1.  Schematic origin of radiation-induced chromatid
breaks and gaps.  These develop from unrepaired DNA strand
breaks during chromatin condensation to form the metaphase
chromosome.  Each chromatid is formed from condensation
through coiling and folding of a chromatin fiber
containing a single continuous molecule of double-stranded
DNA (see Fig. 2).  Chromatid breaks with displacement of
the broken segment, therefore, represent unrepaired DNA
double-strand breaks (DSB's) produced directly by
irradiation or indirectly from single-strand breaks
(SSB's) processed by SS nuclease (2, 3).  SSB's can be
produced directly by irradiation or indirectly during
repair of base damage if excision repair is incomplete
after endonuclease incision at the damaged site.  During
prophase, condensation of a chromatin fiber with DNA
strand break would lead to displacement of the broken
fragment and result in a chromatid break seen at
metaphase.  The SSB, as such, or if converted to a DSB at
a late stage of condensation during prophase would appear
as a chromatid gap at metaphase.

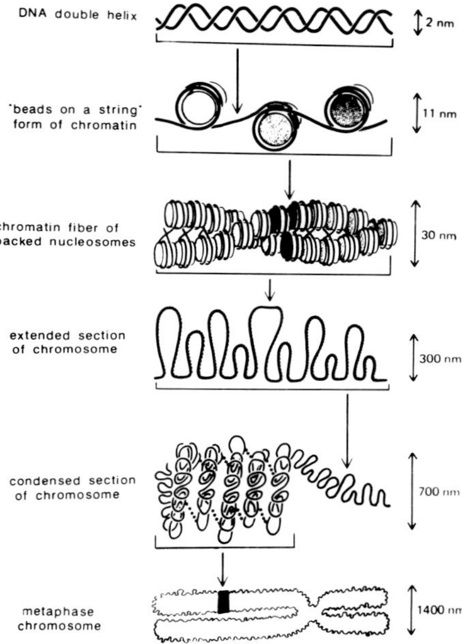


Fig. 2. Schematic illustration of the many orders of chromatin packing postulated to give rise to the highly condensed metaphase chromosome. The chromatin fiber contains a single continuous molecule of double-stranded DNA wrapped around cores of histone proteins. Courtesy of B. Alberts *et al.*, Molecular Biology of the Cell, Garland Publishing, Inc. NY 1989.

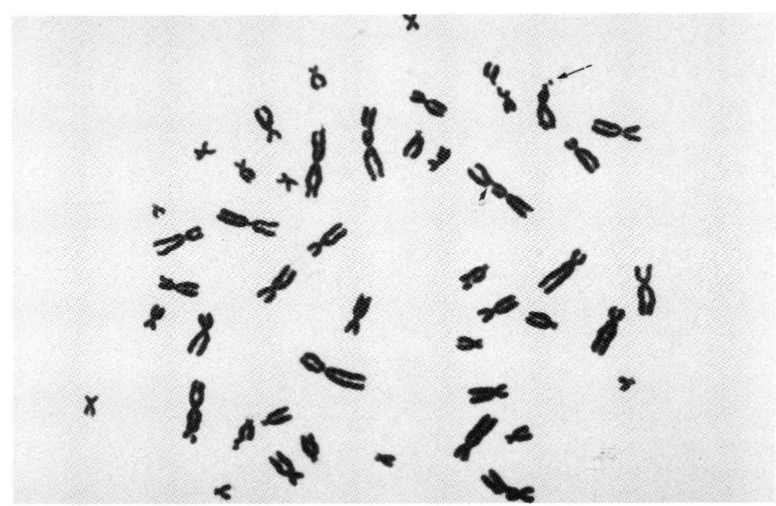

Fig. 3.  Metaphase spread of a human cell to show
chromatid break with displacement of the broken segment
(arrow) and chromatid gap with no displacement (arrow
head) X1024.


*$G_2$ DNA repair deficiency and cancer*

     Several genetic disorders manifesting widely
different clinical symptoms predispose the affected
individual to a high risk of cancer.  These include, among
others, ataxia telangiectasia, Bloom syndrome, familial
polyposis, Fanconi anemia, Gardner syndrome, and xeroderma
pigmentosum (5).  Skin fibroblasts from affected
individuals or individuals with a family history of
cancer, compared to cells from clinically normal controls,
with few exceptions, showed at least a two- to four-fold
higher frequency of chromatid breaks and gaps when
arrested by colcemid 0.5 to 1.5 hr after $G_2$ phase x-
irradiation (6-8) (Fig. 4).  This difference in response
between cancer-prone and normal cells was minimal in
metaphase cells arrested during the first 30 min after x-
irradiation, but increased significantly during the
subsequent incubation period when the level in normal
cells decreased precipitously (7).  Chromatid aberrations
in cancer-prone cells, on the other hand, increased during
the same postirradiation period.  During this period the
rates at which cancer-prone and normal cells entered
metaphase relative to unirradiated controls were almost

identical (7). The increase in aberrations in cancer-
prone cells presumably resulted from accumulation of DNA
strand breaks developed during repair of the radiation-
induced DNA damage. A low level of persistent chromatid
damage (<60 breaks and gaps per 100 cells) thus
characterizes normal DNA repair-efficient human cells. In
contrast a high level (at least 2-3 fold higher)
characterizes DNA repair-deficient cells (6). It appears
that deficient DNA repair during $G_2$ phase is associated
with genetic susceptibility to cancer (6, 11). Furthermore, this abnormal response to x-irradiation was also
observed in all human tumor cells examined to date
regardless of tissue of origin or histopathology (10).

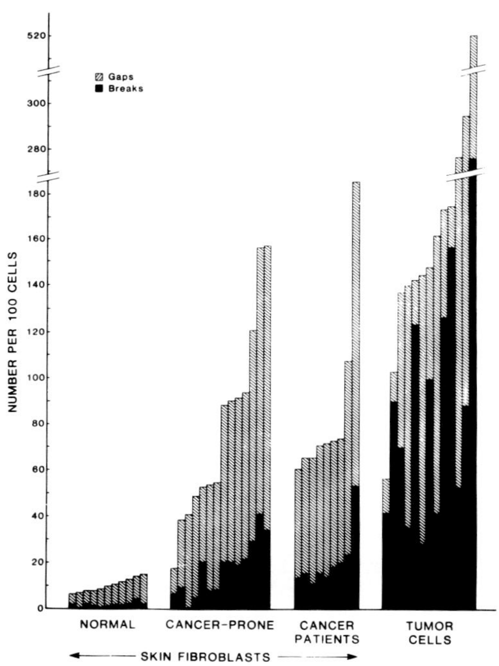


Fig. 4. Comparison of chromatid damage in skin
fibroblasts from normal donors (a) skin fibroblasts from
individuals with a genetic disorder predisposing to cancer
(b) skin fibroblasts from familial cancer patients (c) and
human tumor cells (d). Metaphase cells were arrested by
colcemid from 0.5 to 1.5 hr after x-irradiation (68R)
during $G_2$ phase; and all assays were carried out blind on

coded preparations. Results on skin fibroblasts from
normal donors is representative of more than 50 assays to-
date only 2 of which (4%) showed the high level of damage.
The genetic disorders represented, in order of increasing
chromatid damage, were xeroderma pigmentosum variant.
Gardner syndrome (GS), xeroderma pigmentosum,
complementation group E (XP-E), GS, Bloom syndrome, XP-C,
familial polyposis, ataxia telangiectasia heterozygotes
(five individuals) and homozygotes (two individuals) (7,
9). The tumor cells were from malignancies of diverse
tissues of orgin and histopathology (10).

The $G_2$ phase DNA repair deficiency associated with
human cancer has a genetic basis. Addition of a single
human chromosome 11 (ch 11) from normal fibroblasts by
microcell fusion to cells from cervical carcinoma, two
renal carcinomas and lung adenocarcinoma, and addition of
the long arm (isochromosome) only of ch 11 to embryonal
rhabdomyosarcoma resulted in efficient repair of the DNA
damage to the level in normal cells. Furthermore, a
single copy of human t(x;11) chromosome (11pter
>11q23::xq26 >xqter) added to Wilms tumor cell line, G401-
6TG, also resulted in efficient repair of the radiation-
induced DNA damage. In four of the six tumor lines
restoration of DNA repair by ch 11 was associated with
tumor suppression (12). These results show that genes on
ch 11 are associated with repair of radiation-induced DNA
damage and tumorigenicity. In at least one tumor, the
putative repair gene is located on the long arm of ch 11.
Addition of t(x;11) chromosome to Wilms tumor cells
further localizes this gene to the segment between
centromere and q23 of ch 11. A tumor-suppressor gene for
HeLa cells has been localized to region 11q 13-23 (13).
The ataxia-telangiectasia (A-T) gene which predisposes to
a high risk of cancer, both in homozygous and heterozygous
state, has also been localized to 11q22-23 (14). The A-T
gene is associated with cellular hypersensitivity to
killing by ionizing radiation (15) and deficient DNA
repair manifest as persistent chromatid breaks and gaps
after $G_1$ or $G_2$ phase x-irradiation (16, 17). Whether the
same or different genes are involved in DNA repair and
tumor suppression remains to be established.

*$G_2$ DNA repair deficiency and neoplastic transformation of
human epithelial cells in culture*

To evaluate the role of DNA repair capacity in
malignant neoplastic transformation of cells in culture,

three continuous lines of human skin keratinocytes and two
lines of mammary epithelial cells were examined before and
after introduction of *ras* oncogene.

The three lines of skin keratinocytes had maintained
the repair-efficient phenotype when examined at passage
18, 20 and 66 respectively.  Introduction of *ras* oncogene,
either by infection with KiMSV or transfection with the
plasmid pSV2 *ras* DNA, significantly modified the cellular
response to ionizing radiation when cells were first
examined 3 to 8 passages after ras treatment (18, 19).
This modification consisted of a 4.8 to 8.8-fold increase
in chromatid breaks and 3.4 to 6.0-fold increase in
chromatid gaps in metaphase cells harvested from 0.5 to
1.5 hrs postirradiation.  This difference in cytogenetic
response to irradiation associated with introduction of
*ras* oncogene was statistically significant in all three
lines ($P<1.5 \times 10^{-4}$).  When implanted in nude mice 3 to 8
passages after introduction of *ras* oncogene, cells from
all repair-deficient lines grew as carcinomas.  The
repair-efficient cells when tested in nude mice at
passages 20 and 62 were non-tumorigenic.  In two of the
three lines, cells had acquired the repair-deficient
phenotype spontaneously when examined at passage 25 and 28
respectively or after MNNG (N-methyl-N'-nitro-N-
nitrosoguanidine) exposure.  Of the two carcinogen (MNNG)-
treated repair-deficient lines, only one grew as a
carcinoma in nude mice.

Two continuous cell lines, 184A1 and 184B5 were
established from normal mammoplasty tissue by repeated
treatments of primary cultures with benzo($\alpha$)pyrene (20).
Line 184 A1 and its sublines had maintained the repair-
efficient phenotype when examined at passages 34, 44 and
50 or even after treatment with N-ethyl-N-nitrosourea
(ENU) at passage 36 and examined at passage 45.  A
subline, A1N4, however when examined at passage 47 had
acquired the repair deficient phenotype.  A subline of
A1N4, treated with SV40 T antigen and HaMSV, when assayed
13 passages after virus treatment, was repair-deficient
and grew as undifferentiated carcinomas in nude mice (21).
In contrast to sublines of 184A1, the sublines of 184B5
were repair-deficient when first tested at passage 25.
Cells of line 184B5 treated with KiMSV produced a tumor in
nude mice.  The cells of this tumor maintained the repair-
deficient phenotype when grown in culture.

SUMMARY AND CONCLUSIONS

1.     A genetic deficiency in DNA repair, manifest as
persistent chromatid damage after $G_2$ phase exposure to
DNA-damaging agents, was observed in all human tumor cells
examined and could be complemented by addition of normal
chromosome 11 to cells of six different tumor lines.

2.     The repair deficiency characterizes cells from
individuals with any one of the diverse genetic disorders
predisposing to cancer or from individuals with familial
cancer.

3.     The repair deficiency can be acquired spontaneously
or induced by *ras* oncogene in continuous lines of human
epithelial cells in culture prior to or in association
with their malignant neoplastic transformation.  The *ras*
oncogene thus satisfies two requirements for neoplastic
transformation: 1) a proliferative stimulus from the
encoded p21 protein and 2) induction of deficient $G_2$ phase
DNA repair.

4.     Since the repair deficiency is manifest when DNA
damage is sustained during $G_2$, increased rates of cell
cycling from activation of tissue-specific genes
controlling proliferation (such as oncogenes) increases
genomic instability essential for malignant neoplastic
development.

5.     DNA strand breaks leading to chromatid breaks can
result in deletions of acentric fragments during the
subsequent mitosis; unrepaired "open" chromatid breaks
persisting from $G_2$ into mitosis and $G_1$ phase can rejoin to
form chromatid interchanges, inversions, duplications and
translocations with consequent gene rearrangements.  The
$G_2$ repair deficiency thus provides a mechanism for the
genetic and chromosomal alterations (such as gene
mutations, chromosomal translocations and deletions of
suppressor genes) known to be associated with the genesis
of human cancer.

REFERENCES


1.     P. C. Hanawalt, P. K. Cooper, *et al.*  Ann. Rev.
       Biochem. 48, 783 (1979).
2.     A. T. Natarajan, G. Obe, *et al.* Mutat. Res. 69, 293
       (1980).
3.     R. J. Preston.  Mutat. Res. 69, 71 (1980).

4. K. K. Sanford, R. Parshad, *et al.* <u>Critical Rev. in Oncogenesis</u> 1, 323 (1989).
5. R. B. Setlow. <u>Nature</u> 271, 713 (1978).
6. K. K. Sanford, R. Parshad, *et al.* <u>Int. J. Radiat. Biol.</u> 55, 963 (1989).
7. R. Parshad, K. K. Sanford, *et al.* <u>Proc. Natl. Acad. Sci. USA</u> 80, 5612 (1983).
8. R. Parshad, K. K. Sanford, *et al.* <u>Proc. Natl. Acad. Sci. USA</u> 82, 5400 (1985).
9. R. Parshad, K. K. Sanford, *et al.* <u>Cancer Genet.</u> Cytogenet. 14, 163 (1985).
10. R. Parshad, R. Gantt, *et al.* <u>Cancer Res</u>. 44, 5577 (1984).
11. R. Gantt, R. Parshad, *et al.* <u>Radiat. Res</u>. 108, 117 (1986).
12. R. Parshad, F. M. Price, *et al.* Submitted for publication.
13. B. C. Misra, E. S. Srivatsan. <u>Am. J. Human Genet</u>. 45, 565 (1989).
14. R. A. Gatti, I. Berkel, *et al.* <u>Nature</u> 336, 577 (1988).
15. H. Nagasawa, S. A. Latt, *et al.* <u>Mutat. Res</u>. 148, 71 (1985).
16. K. K. Sanford, R. Parshad, *et al.* <u>J. Natl. cancer Inst</u>. 82, 1050 (1990).
17. M. N. Cornforth and J. S. Bedford. <u>Science</u> 227, 1589 (1985).
18. R. Gantt, K. K. Sanford, *et al.* Cancer Res. 47, 1390 (1987).
19. R. Parshad, F. M. Price, *et al.* In preparation.
20. M. Hosobuchi and M. R. Stampfer. <u>In Vitro</u> 25, 705 (1989).
21. R. Clark, M. R. Stampfer. <u>Cancer Res</u>. 48, 4689 (1988).



The authors are grateful to Dr. E.M. Valvarius formerly of the Laboratory of Tumor Immunology and Biology of the National Cancer Institute and to Dr. R. Clark of Cetus Corporation, Emeryville, CA for cultures of the subline of AIN4 virus-treated and untreated.

USE OF IMMORTALIZED HUMAN KERATINOCYTES FOR THE STUDY OF SQUAMOUS DIFFERENTIATION AND MUTAGENESIS

B. Lynn Allen-Hoffmann[1], Nader Sheibani[1],
Jill S. Hatfield[1] and Johng S. Rhim[2]

[1]Department of Pathology, University of Wisconsin,
Madison, WI 53706 and [2]Laboratory of Cellular and
Molecular Biology, NCI, Bethesda, MD 20892

We have used human keratinocyte (HK) multistep models
of neoplastic transformation developed by Rhim, Durst and
coworkers to:  1) develop an epithelial system for
quantification of DNA damage at a defined genetic locus and
2) determine new epithelial-specific phenotypes associated
with malignant conversion.   HK lines RHEK-1 and HPK-1A
were established by immortalization by a hybrid of
adenovirus 12 and simian virus 40 (Ad12-SV40) (1) or human
papillomavirus type 16 DNA (HPV 16) (3), respectively.
Malignant conversion was achieved by transfection with an
activated <u>ras</u> oncogene (2,4).   RHEK-1 and HPK-1A are
immortal but nontumorigenic, whereas RHEK-1/ras and HPK-
1A/ras produce aggressively growing tumors in nude mice
(Table 1).

TABLE 1. Human epidermal keratinocyte lines and strains

| Cell Line | Immortalizing Agent | Transforming Agent | Tumor Formation | Reference |
|---|---|---|---|---|
| RHEK-1 | Ad12-SV40 virus | - | - | 1. |
| RHEK-1/ras | Ad12-SV40 virus | H-ras | + | 2. |
| HPK-1A | HPV 16 DNA | - | - | 3. |
| HPK-1A/ras | HPV 16 DNA | H-ras | + | 4. |
| Normal keratinocytes | - | - | - | |

**Use of Immortalized Human Keratinocytes for the Quantification of DNA Damage at a Defined Genetic Locus**

The availability of immortalized keratinocyte lines has allowed us to address questions concerning the genotoxic effect of environmental carcinogens on human stratified epithelia. Previously, these studies were restricted to either normal diploid keratinocytes or a near-diploid, tumorigenic, human squamous cell carcinoma cell line (SCC-13Y) (5). We have recently used the RHEK-1 cell line to measure chemically-induced mutation at the hypoxanthine phosphoribosyltransferase (HPRT) locus. RHEK-1 cells have a high colony forming efficiency (50 - 80%), do not require a 3T3 feeder layer for serial cultivation at high density, and are not tumorigenic. An additional advantage of this cell line for mutagenicity testing is the low amount (<15%) of contact- or cross-feeding of toxic thioguanine (TG) nucleotide by wild-type RHEK-1 cells to hprt⁻ mutants. Cross-feeding results in a decreased recovery of induced thioguanine-resistant (TG$^r$) mutants from high-density cultures. In a direct replating assay, two polycyclic aromatic hydrocarbons known to induce skin tumors in rodents, dimethylbenzanthracene (DMBA) and benzo[a]pyrene (BP), induced a 30 to 40-fold increase in mutation frequency over control cultures. TG$^r$ mutants were isolated from DMBA-treated cultures of RHEK-1 cells. All clones were resistant to TG at 10 $\mu$g/ml, were aminopterin-sensitive, and possessed no HPRT activity. Identification of TG$^r$ colonies was unambiguous. Wild-type RHEK-1 colonies detach from the dish during the selection process and mutant colonies are easily identified (Fig. 1). This human epithelial mutation system should be useful in assessing and screening the mutagenicity of other classes of environmental agents that are in contact with external epithelia.


**Epithelial-Specific Phenotypes Associated with Malignant Conversion**

We have used normal human keratinocytes, HPV 16- (3) or Ad12-SV40-immortalized human keratinocytes (1), and the corresponding _ras_ transfected cell lines (2,4) to identify new phenotypes associate with malignant conversion of human keratinocytes. These keratinocyte lines are unique

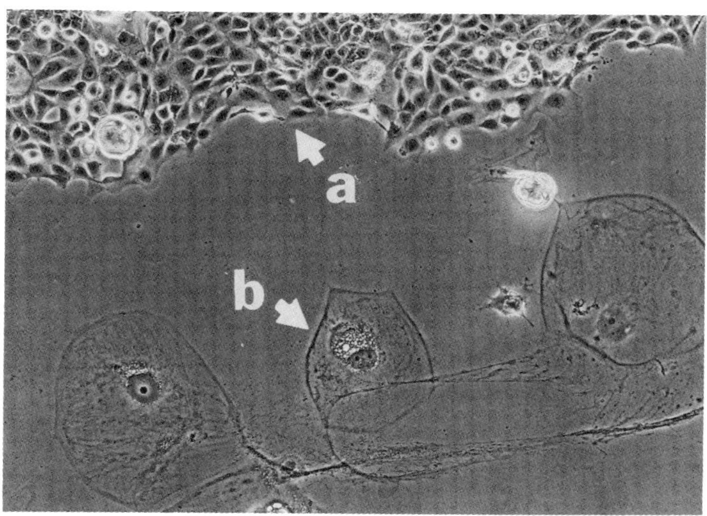


Fig. 1. TG$^r$ mutant clone of RHEK-1 after 3 weeks in TG-containing selection medium. Vigorous mutant clone of closely packed TG$^r$ RHEK-1 cells (arrow a). Note abortive TG-sensitive RHEK-1 wild type cells (arrow b).


cellular reagents representing discrete stages of the transformation process: immortalization and malignant conversion.

For our studies normal keratinocytes were established from newborn human foreskin and cultured in the presence of a mitomycin C-treated 3T3 feeder cells as described by Allen-Hoffmann and Rheinwald (5) with the following modifications. The culture medium was composed of a mixture of Ham's F12:Dulbecco's modified Eagle medium (DME) (3:1, 0.66 mM $Ca^{2+}$) supplemented with 2.5% fetal calf serum, 0.4 $\mu$g/ml hydrocortisone, 10 ng/ml choleratoxin, 5 $\mu$g ml insulin, 24 $\mu$g/ml adenine and 10 ng/ml EGF. All transformed keratinocyte lines were cultured in the same medium as the normal keratinocytes with the exceptions that these cells require neither EGF nor a 3T3 feeder layer when passaged at high density. Normal keratinocytes were used for experiments prior to passage 4. Transformed keratinocytes were passaged 1:10 every 4-5 days. For experiments using low $Ca^{2+}$-containing medium, $Ca^{2+}$-free

Ham's F12 and $Ca^{2+}$-free DME were mixed (3:1) and $CaCl_2$ was added to a final concentration of 0.05 mM.

We found that malignantly converted HK cells exhibit an enhanced ability to synthesize a fibronectin-containing extracellular matrix. Increased production of soluble and cell surface-associated fibronectin was observed in both HPV 16- and Ad12-SV40-immortalized keratinocytes malignantly converted with ras. The soluble fibronectin content of medium conditioned by normal HK and the transformed HK lines was determined by a competitive immunosorbent assay for human fibronectin. Immuno-fluorescence staining with anti-human plasma fibronectin revealed that, relative to normal keratinocytes, RHEK-1 cells exhibited increased numbers of short, stitch-like fibronectin fibrils (Fig. 2, A and C). The tumorigenic RHEK-1/ras cells, however, organized and deposited a dense fibronectin-containing extracellular matrix (Fig. 2, E and G). We found that relative to RHEK-1 cells the tumorigenic RHEK-1/ras keratinocytes incorporated increased levels of fibronectin into their matrices regardless of the calcium concentration of the medium (Fig. 2, E and G). Similar results were observed with HPK-1A/ras tumorigenic keratinocytes (6).

To determine if fibronectin mRNA levels were enhanced in RHEK-1 transformed cell lines we isolated poly $A^+$ mRNA from populations of early passage RHEK-1 and RHEK-1/ras cells. For comparison, we also isolated poly $A^+$ mRNA from cultures of HPK-1A and HPK-1A/ras cells. We examined the steady state mRNA levels for several extracellular matrix glycoproteins, namely; fibronectin, thrombospondin and types I and IV procollagen. Densitometric scanning of the autoradiogram showed that RHEK-1/ras cells contained at least 10-fold more fibronectin mRNA as compared to immortalized RHEK-1 cells. Similar results were obtained with keratinocytes immortalized by HPV 16 DNA and malignantly converted with activated ras. This was in agreement with the observed elevated levels of soluble and matrix-associated fibronectin. We probed the same RNA blot with cDNA probes specific for human thrombospondin and type I procollagen. In addition to fibronectin, the malignantly converted keratinocytes exhibited an increase in the steady state mRNA levels for thrombospondin when compared to normal keratinocytes or the immortal RHEK-1 cells.

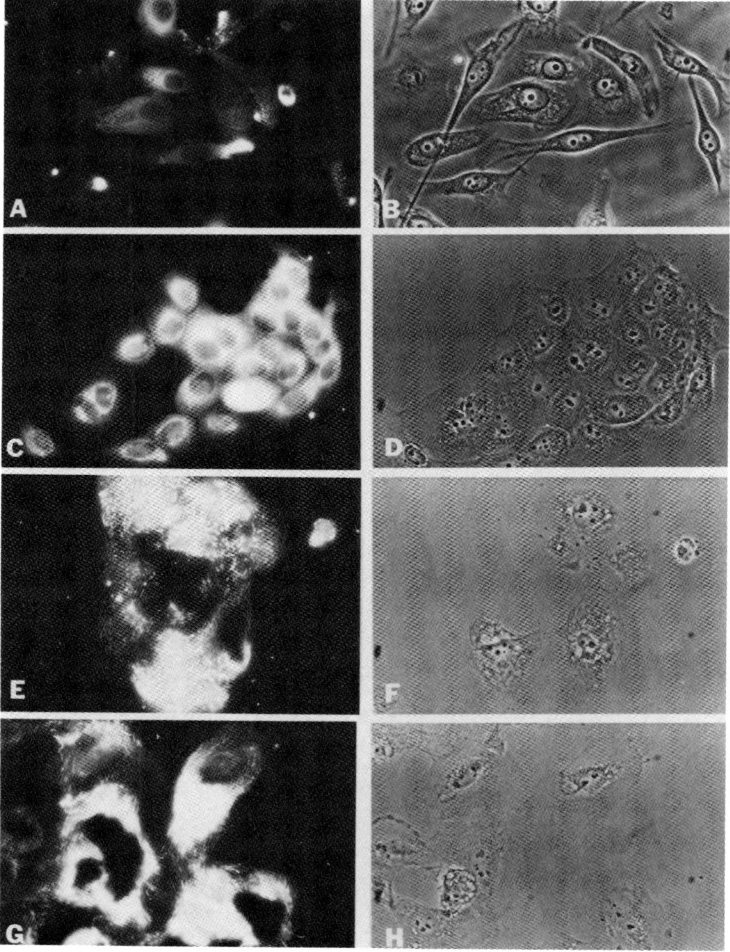

Fig 2.  **Extracellular matrix fibronectin content of Ad12-SV40-transformed keratinocytes.**  Indirect immuno-fluorescence staining of preconfluent keratinocytes with a rabbit polyclonal antibody to human plasma fibronectin followed by fluorescein-conjugated goat anti-rabbit IgG was performed: A and B, RHEK-1 (0.05 mM $Ca^{++}$); C and D, RHEK-1 (0.66 mM $Ca^{++}$); E and F, RHEK-1/ras (0.05 mM $Ca^{++}$); G and H, RHEK-1/ras (0.66 mM $Ca^{++}$).

Thrombospondin is a large, multifunctional glycoprotein
secreted by growing cells (7).   The RHEK-1/ras cells also
produced high levels of type (I) procollagen mRNA.  Unlike
the tumorigenic RHEK-1/ras keratinocytes, there was no
detectable difference in the level of type (I) procollagen
mRNA in normal, RHEK-1 or HPK-1A cells.   Type (I)
procollagen mRNA was only modestly elevated in the
HPK-1A/ras cells.  We did not detect changes in α1 type
(IV) collagen mRNA levels in any of the keratinocyte lines.

To further investigate the mechanisms of loss of growth
control and enhanced expression of extracellular matrix
molecules we examined the steady state mRNA levels for
transforming growth factors type-α (TGF-α) and type-ß (TGF-
ß) in normal keratinocytes and the keratinocyte lines at
different stages of neoplastic transformation.  Normal
human keratinocytes produce and respond to these growth
factors.  TGF-ß1 has been shown to enhance production of
fibronectin, thrombospondin, and type (I) collagen in
variety of cell lines (8-11).  We reasoned that the altered
pattern of extracellular matrix glycoprotein expression
might be a response to altered production of growth
factors, particularly the members of the TGF-ß family.  The
mRNA steady state levels for TGF-α and TGF-ß1 were analyzed
by Northern blot analysis.  Neither the HPV 16-immortalized
nor the HPV 16 tumorigenic cells produced increased levels
of TGF-α or TGF-ß1 mRNA.  However, the tumorigenic RHEK-
1/ras cells exhibited an increase in the steady state mRNA
levels for both these growth factors.  The increased
production of TGF-ß1 is consistent with the enhanced
procollagen type (I) mRNA production seen specifically in
these cells.

To find out more about mechanisms contributing to
altered differentiation during epithelial carcinogenesis,
we compared the ability of normal HK and transformed HK
lines to differentiate in response to loss of adherence.
Cornified envelopes (CE) and involucrin expression were
used as measures of squamous differentiation.  Since
increased expression of fibronectin and thrombospondin was
a consistent characteristic of malignantly converted
keratinocytes, we asked whether these extracellular matrix
glycoproteins possibly contributed to the <u>in vitro</u>
differentiation characteristics of the keratinocyte lines
at different stages of neoplastic transformation.

Interaction of these glycoproteins with their cognate cell
surface receptors appear to be important events during
terminal differentiation of stratified squamous epithelia
(12,13).

Both the HPV 16 and Ad12-SV40-immortalized and
malignantly converted keratinocytes exhibited aberrant
suspension-induced differentiation.  Less than 10% of the
HPV-transformed cells produced CE after suspension-induced
differentiation compared to 70% of normal keratinocytes.
RHEK-1 cells do not produce detectable CE even after three
days in suspension (Fig. 3).  RHEK-1 and HPK-1A cells

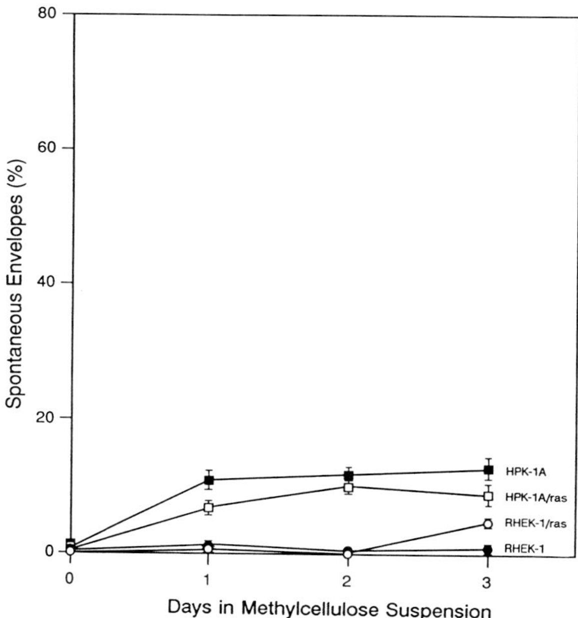


Fig. 3.  **Ability of immortalized and tumorigenic
keratinocytes to produce cornified envelopes.**  Normal human
keratinocytes, HPV 16- and Ad12-SV40-immortalized
keratinocytes and the corresponding tumorigenic cells were
signaled to differentiate by removal from substrata and
suspension in methylcellulose-containing medium.  Following
suspension for varying times, cells were recovered from
methylcellulose, washed, and the percentages of cells
producing cornified envelope were determined.

produced 40- and 8-fold less involucrin protein, respectively, when compared to preconfluent normal keratinocytes. The decreased production of involucrin protein is reflected in decreased steady state levels of involucrin mRNA. Malignant conversion further attenuated involucrin protein as well as mRNA levels. Immortalization alone was sufficient to confer a differentiation-defective phenotype. Therefore, poor differentiation potential is associated with the immortalization stage _in vitro_ and occurs prior to changes in production of keratinocyte fibronectin. We have also found that release from substrata attachment increases the steady state levels of TGF-ß1 mRNA in normal HK cells (Allen-Hoffman, et al., unpublished observations). However, loss of substrate attachment does not alter TGF-ß1 mRNA levels in the tumorigenic Ad12-SV40 and HPV 16 transformed HK lines.

From our studies it appears that virally induced alterations in the expression of fibronectin and thrombospondin and perhaps their cognate cell surface receptors may contribute to the acquisition or maintenance of malignant phenotypes in stratified squamous epithelia. For example, HPV types 16, 18, 31 and 33 are associated with development of cervical cancer (reviewed in 14). In preliminary screening of human cervical biopsies our _in vitro_ observations of increased fibronectin and thrombospondin expression have _in vivo_ correlates (Desouky and Allen-Hoffmann, unpublished observations). Our purpose is to determine whether changes in extracellular matrix molecules or their cognate cell surface receptors are consistently observed in cervical samples from patients with confirmed condylomata or cervical intraepithelial neoplasia (CIN grades I-III).

## Summary

1. We have detected and isolated rare hypoxanthine phosphoribosyltransferase-deficient mutants of the immortalized human keratinocyte line, RHEK-1.

2. Both immortal and malignantly converted keratinocyte lines exhibit an altered response to suspension-induced differentiation.

3. Unlike either normal or immortalized keratinocytes, malignantly converted keratinocyte lines produce increased amount of certain extracellular matrix glycoproteins, such as fibronectin and thrombospondin.

4. Altered terminal differentiation <u>in vitro</u> is associated with immortalization events and occurs prior to changes in production of fibronectin and thrombospondin.

5. Overproduction of the autocrine growth factors, TGF-$\alpha$ or TGF-ß1, is not a consistent characteristic of malignantly converted human keratinocytes.

This work was supported by grant R29 AR40284 (to B.L.A.-H.); N.S. is a trainee on grant HD07118 from the National Institutes of Health.

## REFERENCES


1.  J.S. Rhim, G. Jay, P. Arnstein, F.M. Price, K. K. Sanford, and S.A. Aaronson. <u>Science</u>, 227, 1250-1252, (1985).

2.  J.S. Rhim, J.B. Park, and G. Jay. <u>Oncogene</u> 4, 1403-1409 (1989).

3.  M. Durst, R.T. Dzarlieva-Petrusevska, P. Boukamp, N.E. Fusenig, and L. Gissmann. <u>Oncogene</u> 1, 251-256, (1987).

4.  M. Durst, D. Gallahan, G. Jay, and J.S. Rhim. <u>Virology</u> 173, 767-771 (1989).

5.  B.L. Allen-Hoffmann and J.G. Rheinwald. <u>Proc. Natl. Acad. Sci. USA</u> 81, 7802-7806 (1984).

6.  N. Sheibani, J.S. Rhim, and B.L. Allen-Hoffmann. Submitted to <u>Cancer Res.</u>, 1991.

7.  W.A. Frazier. <u>J. Cell Biol.</u> 105, 625-32 (1987).

8.  B.L. Allen-Hoffmann, C.L. Crankshaw, and D.F. Mosher. <u>Mol. Cell. Biol.</u> 8, 4234-4242 (1988).

9.  R.A. Ignotz, and J. Massague. <u>J. Biol. Chem.</u> 261, 4337-4345 (1986).

10.  R.A. Ignotz, T. Endo, and J. Massague. <u>J. Biol. Chem.</u> 262, 6443-6446 (1987).

11.  R.P. Penttinen, S. Kobayashi, and P. Bornstein. <u>Proc. Natl. Acad. Sci. USA.</u>, 85, 1105-1108 (1988).

12.  J.C. Adams and F.M. Watt. <u>Nature</u> 340, 307-309 (1989).

13.  J.C. Adams and F.M. Watt. <u>Cell</u> 63, 425-435 (1990).

14.  H. Zur Hausen. <u>Cancer Res.</u> 49:4677-4681 (1989).



From: *Neoplastic Transformation in Human Cell Culture,*
Eds.: J. S. Rhim and A. Dritschilo ©1991 The Humana Press Inc., Totowa, NJ

# STUDIES OF MUTAGEN-ACTIVATED GENES WHICH CONFER ANCHORAGE-INDEPENDENCE: THE c-*sis* GENE AS A MODEL

William E. Fahl, William H. Brondyk,
Hua-Ming Jin, Craig W. Stevens,
Carsten-Peter Carstens, Gregory C. Kujoth
and Helen L. Ng

McArdle Laboratory for Cancer Research,
University of Wisconsin, Madison,
Wisconsin  53706

The majority of human tumor cells, and particularly those of mesenchymal origin, have the ability to grow in semi-solid medium (i.e., anchorage-independent growth; refs. 1-5), a phenotype, which aside from some hematopoeitic cells, is rarely observed in nonneoplastic human cells.  Treatment of rodent or human fibroblasts with mutagens has been shown to induce anchorage-independent growth at frequencies consistent with mutation at a single, dominant-acting gene (6,7), or perhaps pool of genes, any locus of which is permissive for the phenotype in its mutant form. Mutagen-induced acquisition of anchorage-independent growth in many aneuploid, immortal rodent cell lines has been shown to correlate well with acquisition of tumorigenic growth (8), whereas with diploid human fibroblasts, mutagen treatment has been shown to induce anchorage-independent cell populations that do not yield progressively growing tumors (9), and, consistent with this, the anchorage-independent cell clones senesce at passage levels similar to non-anchorage-independent cell clones (6). When neoplastic transformation is viewed in the context of a multiple-step transition from normal to neoplastic cell (10), mutagen-induced anchorage-independence is likely to represent one of these discrete steps, where this acquired phenotype is related mechanistically to the final tumorigenic state.

By designing experiments which allow us to
identify and isolate genes which can dominantly confer
this growth phenotype, a phenotype which is largely
peculiar to <u>neoplastic</u> mammalian cells, we are identify-
ing genes and their activating mutations which are
intimately involved in why tumor cells grow as tumor
cells.  The assumption in this approach is that those
aberrant genes which enable cells to overcome the selective pressure of an artificially-constructed agar culture are the same genes which help the tumor cells to
colonize in an animal.  To date, nobody knows what the
selective pressures are in agar or methylcellulose culture, nor why growth in this medium is well correlated
with tumor growth in an animal.

A second focus of our studies on genes which confer anchorage-independence, involves study of the c-*sis*
gene and the product which it encodes, platelet-derived
growth factor (PDGF-BB). Because this cellular protooncogene is transcriptionally activated in a large percentage of human mesenchymal neoplasms (11), which contain both $\alpha$ and $\beta$ form PDGF receptors, and because we
have shown that this activated oncogene can confer the
anchorage-independent phenotype to human fibroblasts
(12), we have chosen to study this gene focussing upon
two simple questions: i) is the presence of an activated
c-*sis* gene, which has been repeatedly observed in a
large percentage of human tumors, in part responsible
for those cells being tumorigenic, often metastatic cancer cells, or is it a chance genetic change that simply
occurs during the 30-35 cell generations of genetically
unstable tumor cell expansion that precedes a patient's
clinical symptoms; and ii) why is the c-*sis* protooncogene, which is transcriptionally quiescent in the
large majority of normal human cells, frequently found
to be actively transcribed, encoding the mitogenic
growth factor PDGF, in a large percentage of human tumor
cells of mesenchymal origin (i.e. containing PDGF receptors) as well as human tumor cells of epithelial origin.

This fundamental interest in human genes which
confer anchorage-independent growth, as well as an evolutionary focus of our work upon one gene, the c-*sis*
oncogene, will be the subject of the work described in
this brief chapter.

## MUTATION ACTIVATES DOMINANT ANCHORAGE-INDEPENDENCE GENES IN DIPLOID HUMAN FIBROBLASTS

Our first objective in these experiments was to quantitatively determine the relationship between frequencies for the induction of anchorage-independent colonies and for the induction of mutations at the single *hprt* locus in diploid, human foreskin fibroblasts. Secondly, we asked whether the anchorage-independent phenotype was heritable and genetically stable during clonal expansion, a characteristic which would be required of a phenotype resulting from a mutation.

In order to answer these questions, early passage, human, foreskin fibroblasts were exposed to a mutagen, benzo(a)pyrene *anti* diol-epoxide, and surviving cells were scored either for the dose-dependent frequency of mutations at the *hprt* gene or for the frequency with which anchorage-independent clones developed (Fig. 1A), clones which showed a recurrent morphology (Fig. 1B). As can be seen, the dose-dependent frequencies for appearance of the two phenotypes closely paralleled each other, and within error, they were the same (1-10 X $10^{-4}$). This result, alone, suggests a common mechanism for the induction of these two phenotypes. The observation that the anchorage-independent phenotype was stable for at least 20 generations of clonal expansion (Fig. 1C) reinforced the notion that this phenotype resulted from a stable, heritable mutation. Two additional, notable points from these experiments were that at least one stably anchorage-independent clone (BO-J, Fig. 1C) was found to have arisen spontaneously, and that none of the anchorage-independent clones showed life-spans longer than the 30-60 doublings seen for normal foreskin fibroblasts (6).

In aggregate, these results, particularly the frequency for mutagen induction of anchorage-independent clones ($10^{-4}$ - $10^{-3}$), suggested that there was one or a few human genes, which upon mutagen activation of only one cellular copy, could dominantly confer anchorage-independent growth.

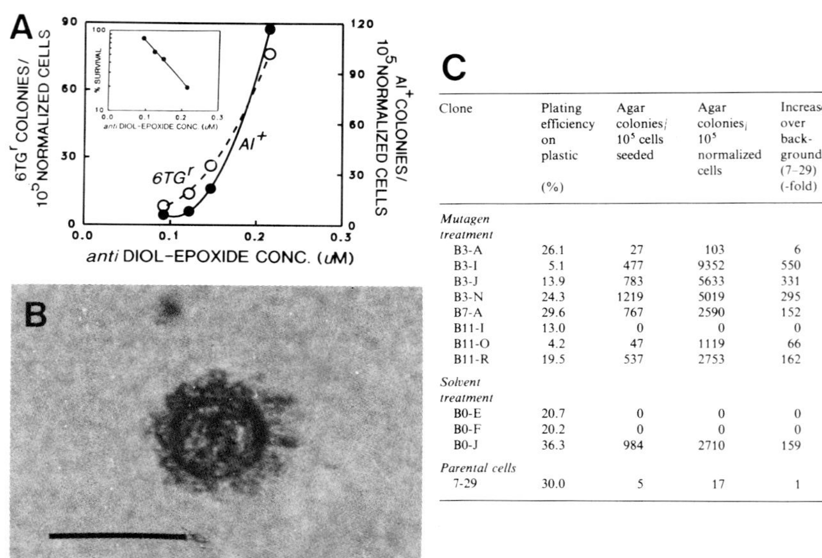



| Clone | Plating efficiency on plastic (%) | Agar colonies/ 10$^5$ cells seeded | Agar colonies/ 10$^5$ normalized cells | Increase over back-ground (7-29) (-fold) |
|---|---|---|---|---|
| *Mutagen treatment* | | | | |
| B3-A | 26.1 | 27 | 103 | 6 |
| B3-I | 5.1 | 477 | 9352 | 550 |
| B3-J | 13.9 | 783 | 5633 | 331 |
| B3-N | 24.3 | 1219 | 5019 | 295 |
| B7-A | 29.6 | 767 | 2590 | 152 |
| B11-I | 13.0 | 0 | 0 | 0 |
| B11-O | 4.2 | 47 | 1119 | 66 |
| B11-R | 19.5 | 537 | 2753 | 162 |
| *Solvent treatment* | | | | |
| B0-E | 20.7 | 0 | 0 | 0 |
| B0-F | 20.2 | 0 | 0 | 0 |
| B0-J | 36.3 | 984 | 2710 | 159 |
| *Parental cells* | | | | |
| 7-29 | 30.0 | 5 | 17 | 1 |

**Fig. 1.** (A) Quantification of anchorage-independence (AI) and *hprt* mutation (6TG$^r$) frequencies for BP *anti* diol-epoxide-treated human fibroblasts. (B) Photomicrograph of representative agar (i.e., anchorage-independent) colony consisting of 40-70 cells; *bar* represents 100 μm. (C) Stable retention of anchorage-independent phenotype upon re-seeding of expanded clones into agar; 7-29 is the parental strain of normal human fibroblasts (see ref. 6 for details of these experiments).

## IDENTIFICATION, ANALYSIS AND CLONING OF DOMINANT ANCHORAGE-INDEPENDENCE GENES

One interest here was to determine whether mutagen-induced soft agar growth could be assigned to an activating mutation of a specific human gene. In early work (6) 162 anchorage-independent colonies were picked and expanded, and for 17 representative colonies, DNA and RNA were purified and examined for amplification, rearrangement or over-expression of any one or more of 15 cellular oncogenes which might explain the anchorage-independent phenotype; no changes were observed. In a subsequent approach (13), genomic DNAs from the same 17 expanded, anchorage-independent colonies were independently co-transfected with pSV2neo into NIH3T3 cells, and G418-resistant cells were found to induce tumors in nude mice in 11 of 17 groups where no tumors were observed in negative controls (Fig. 2A). In two tumor groups (i.e., groups where NIH3T3 tumors arose from NIH3T3 cells originally transfected with genomic DNA

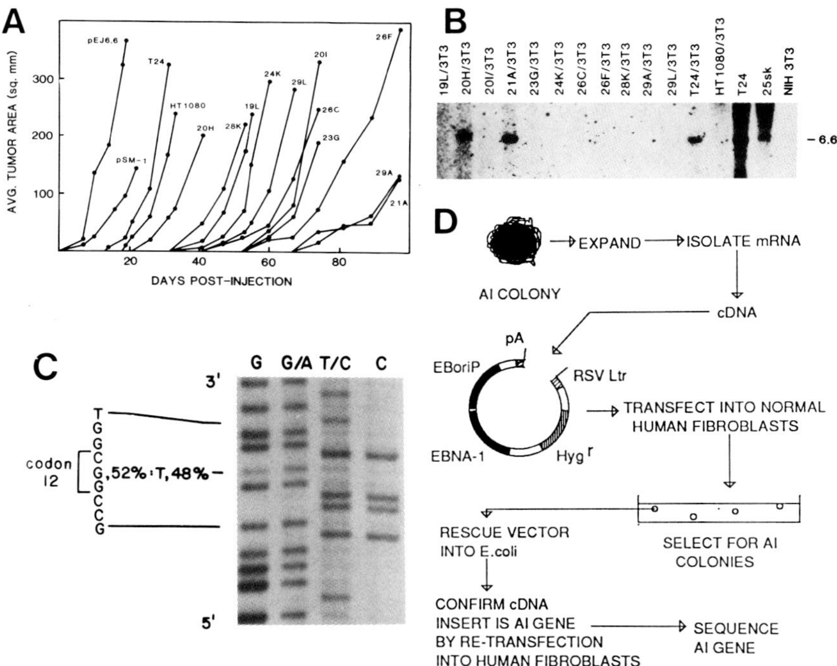


**Fig. 2.** (A) Growth of NIH3T3 tumors in nude mice induced by transfection with known oncogenes or with DNA isolated from *anti* diol-epoxide-induced anchorage-independent human fibroblast clones. (B) Southern blot analysis of genomic DNA from NIH3T3 tumors using a probe to identify the presence of an intact (6.6 kb) human Ha-*ras* gene. (C) Nucleotide sequence of Ha-*ras* codon 12 and flanking codons in PCR-amplified DNA from human anchorage-independent clone 21A (see ref. 13 for details of these experiments). (D) Cloning strategy for isolation of mutagen-activated, dominant anchorage-independence (AI) gene using episomally-replicating EBV vector.

                                                    *Fahl et al.*

from human anchorage-independent colonies 21A or 20H),
intact, human Ha-*ras* genes were detected (Fig. 2B) in
the DNA isolated from the NIH3T3 tumors.  When exon 1 of
the human Ha-*ras* gene was PCR-amplified from the genomic
DNA of anchorage-independent clone 21A and sequenced
(Fig. 2C), an activating, codon 12 GC → TA (Gly → Val)
transversion mutation in one of the two Ha-*ras* gene
copies was observed.  The notable message from this
experiment was that diploid, foreskin fibroblasts from a
baby born on April 25, 1984 (i.e., 25sk), when exposed
to a ubiquitous environmental carcinogen, yielded cells
with an anchorage-independent phenotype, a phenotype
which is common in human cancer cells, and the basis for
this phenotype was an activating codon 12 point mutation
in one Ha-*ras* gene.  This result provides a straightfor-
ward experimental explanation for an event which is
routinely observed in clinical tumor specimens (14).

Which gene or genes are responsible for the majority of cases (9 of 11, Fig. 2B) of mutagen-induced
anchorage-independence is presently unknown.  From our
initial efforts, we have concluded that we will not be
able to identify or isolate these anchorage-independence
genes using NIH3T3 as reporter cells.  Therefore, we
have developed a cloning vector and strategy (Fig. 2D)
that will rely upon preparing cDNA libraries from
anchorage-independent cells and expressing these cDNAs
in normal human fibroblasts by using an episomally
maintained EBoriP/EBNA-1 vector.  Following electroporation of the expression library into normal human fibroblasts, rare, anchorage-independent colonies induced by
the expressed anchorage-independence gene, will be
picked, expanded and the plasmid-encoded cDNA will be
analyzed to identify the dominant-acting anchorage-independence gene.

## c-*sis* GENE IS EXPRESSED IN HUMAN CANCER CELLS;
## IMPLICATIONS FOR ANCHORAGE-INDEPENDENCE

Expression of c-*sis* oncogene mRNA, as well as production of mitogenic proteins which are immunoprecipitable using anti-PDGF antibodies, have been shown to
occur in the majority of human tumors, tumors of both
mesenchymal and epithelial origin (15,16) (Fig. 3A).
Normal, human cell controls (e.g., pieces of normal

human tissue or human fibroblast cultures, 7-29 cells,
Fig. 3A) do not produce detectable levels of c-*sis* mRNA
(11).  Many human tumor cell types which were reported
to be c-*sis* expressors were separately reported to be
anchorage-independent.  This correlation, as well as
other observations, led us to wonder whether an
expressed (i.e., activated) c-*sis* oncogene played a
functional role in conferring anchorage-independence to
human fibroblasts, and if it did, whether the c-*cis* gene
played a broader role in supporting the tumorigenic
phenotype in human mesenchymal tumors.

## Is c-*sis* Expression in Part Responsible for Human Cells Being Cancer Cells?

In our first experiments, the goal has been to
express a human c-*sis* cDNA in normal human fibroblasts
to the same level as that found in human tumors and then
determine whether this single event would induce any of
the phenotypes which are commonly observed in human
mesenchymal tumors.  Following co-electroporation of a
recombinant $CMV_{ie}$ promoter: c-*sis* cDNA construct with
pSV2neo, and G418-selection, PDGF-B producing clones
(41 kDa dimeric PDGF-BB protein, Fig. 3B) were identified by immunoprecipitation and also shown to colonize
at greatly increased (95-210 fold) frequencies (Fig. 3C)
when seeded into soft agarose cultures.

A separate, $\alpha_2$(I)collagen promoter: c-*sis* cDNA
construct (Fig. 3D) has been constructed and injected
into fertilized FVB mouse eggs, and at least two founder
mice containing this transgene have now been identified
(Fig. 3D).  Mouse 731 which contains the intact transgene at less than one copy per haploid genome (i.e., is
mosaic) is being bred to see if an F1 animal and subsequent stable mouse line will emerge.  The fact that we
have so far identified only two animals with either a
mosaic (#731) or mosaic, rearranged (#746) transgene
(Fig. 3D) raises the possibility that this fibro-
blast-directed transgene may be developmentally lethal,
a possibility under study.

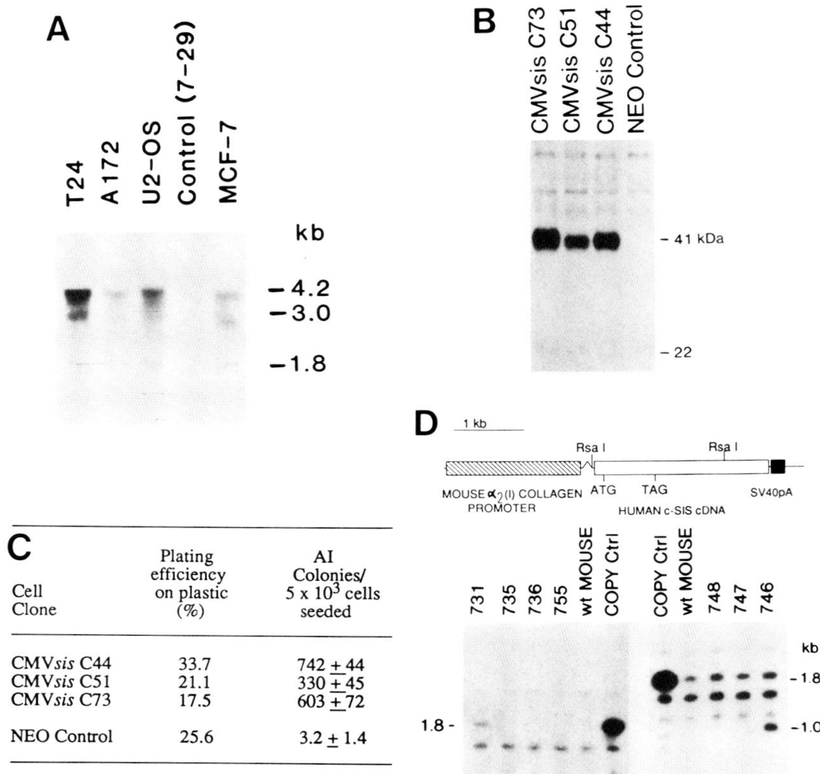



| C Cell Clone | Plating efficiency on plastic (%) | AI Colonies/ 5 x $10^3$ cells seeded |
|---|---|---|
| CMV*sis* C44 | 33.7 | 742 $\pm$ 44 |
| CMV*sis* C51 | 21.1 | 330 $\pm$ 45 |
| CMV*sis* C73 | 17.5 | 603 $\pm$ 72 |
| NEO Control | 25.6 | 3.2 $\pm$ 1.4 |

**Fig. 3.** (A) Northern blot analysis of c-*sis* mRNA (4.2 kb) level in 50 μg of total cellular RNA isolated from the indicated human mesenchymal (A172, U2-OS) and epithelial (T24, MCF-7) tumor cell lines or normal human fibroblasts (7-29). (B) Immunoprecipitation from culture medium of dimeric (41 kDa) or monomeric (22 kDa) PDGF-B proteins from human fibroblast clones expressing a recombinant c-*sis* expression vector; cells were exposed to suramin during radiolabeling. (C) Increased anchorage-independent colony formation in human fibroblast clones expressing PDGF-BB. (D) Southern blot analysis of RsaI-digested mouse genomic DNA (25 μg/lane) to identify presence of intact (i.e., 1.8 kb) α coll: *sis* transgene. Different probes were used in left and right panels, hence different endogenous bands. For copy control, 40 pg (approx. 1 copy transgene/cell equivalent) of RsaI-digested plasmid was added to 25 μg of wild-type (wt) mouse genomic DNA.

## Why is the c-*sis* Gene Transcriptionally-Activated in a Large Percentage of Human Cancers?

Since *sis*-specific mRNA was first detected in 1982 in human tumor cells (11) by using a v-*sis* probe, people have found c-*sis* mRNA in a wide variety of human tumor types (15,16), where generally, c-*sis* was not detectably expressed in the nonneoplastic cell control. Although effects upon c-*sis* mRNA levels have been described for treatments with molecules such as forskolin (17) and TGF-$\beta$ (18), and consensus sequences for certain transcriptional effectors have been identified in the c-*sis* 5' flanking region (19), no comprehensive understanding has emerged to explain how c-*sis* transcription is normally regulated, and how it goes awry in human cancer cells.

Our efforts to understand c-*sis* gene activation led us to isolate the entire c-*sis* gene (~20 kb, Fig. 4A) from a human genomic library, including 4 kb of DNA which lies 5' to the previously mapped (19) c-*sis* mRNA cap site. Portions of this 4 kb region, including a 400 bp region (Fig. 4A) have been inserted into vectors containing either the firefly luciferase or bacterial CAT reporter genes. Known effectors (both TGF-$\beta$, + and forskolin/cAMP, -) of endogenous c-*sis* mRNA production (Fig. 4B) have been shown by us to modulate reporter gene expression using transient transfection assays. In addition, by using nuclear run-on analyses (Fig. 4B, 4C and data not shown), we have shown that the inducing effect of TGF-$\beta$ can be explained by a direct effect upon c-*sis* transcription. Currently, high resolution deletion mutations of the 400 bp 5' region are being used to map the DNA sites responsible for the transcriptional effects of TGF-$\beta$ and cAMP.

The results in Fig. 4D illustrate that when T24 tumor cells (*sis* mRNA[+], Fig. 3A and 4D, inset) are fused to normal human fibroblasts (7-23 strain, *sis* mRNA[-]) the large majority of hybrid clones contain no detectable c-*sis* mRNA (Fig. 4D, dot blot and northern (inset) results). What the gene product is in human fibroblasts that can totally suppress c-*sis* transcription in T24 tumor cells is unknown. Likewise, it is also unknown whether random loss of a suppressor protein may provide a global explanation for the c-*sis* gene activation seen in human cancers. These topics are under study.

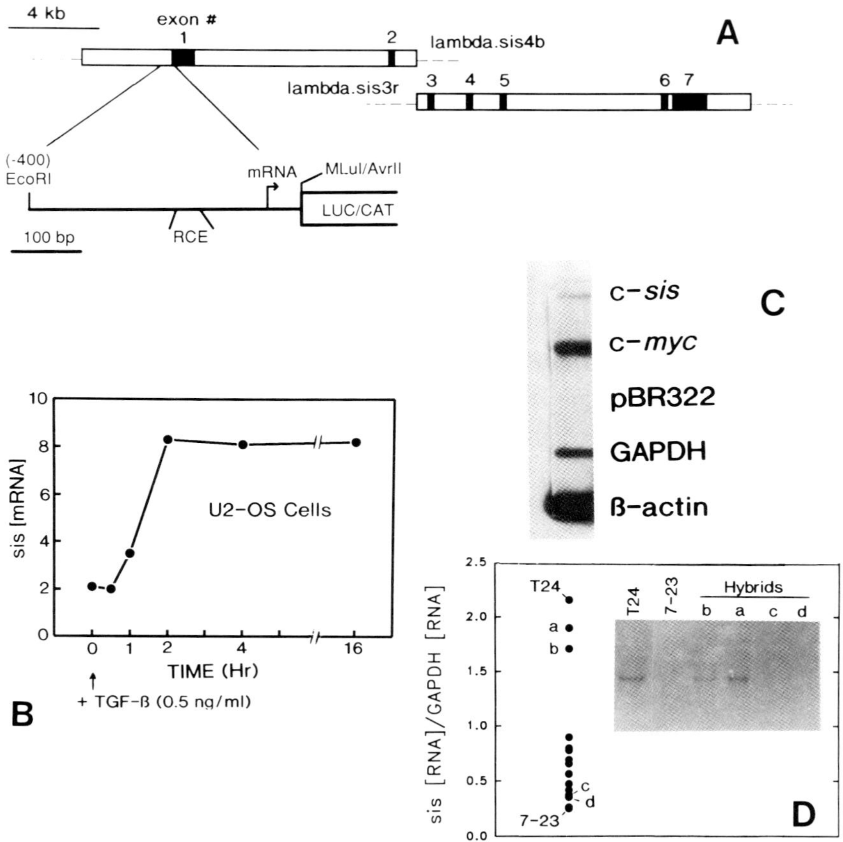


**Fig. 4.** (A) Phage lambda clones containing separate
halves (all 7 exons) of the human c-*sis* gene; 400 bp of
5' flanking region containing mRNA cap site and a putative retinoblastoma control element (RCE, ref. 20) was
inserted into luciferase or CAT expression vectors.
(B) Time-course for stimulation of c-*sis* mRNA production
in U2-0S cells following exposure to TGF-β. (C) Nuclear
run-on analysis of initiated transcription complexes for
the indicated genes using labeled nuclei from U2-0S
cells. (D) Abundance of *sis* mRNA relative to GAPDH mRNA
internal standard in parental T24 (human bladder carcinoma) and 7-23 (normal human fibroblast) as well as
hybrid fusion clones following minimal expansion of the
clones. (Inset), representative northern blot of *sis*
mRNA species in parental cells and indicated hybrid
clones.

## CONCLUDING THOUGHTS

As we and others identify mutagen-activated genes which can dominantly confer anchorage-independent growth, many or all of which are presently identified as oncogenes, one then wonders how these disparate regulatory genes (e.g. genes encoding tyrosine kinases, G-proteins, etc.) can all induce the human cells to assemble a matrix that allows for this uncharacteristic growth phenotype. Does it occur through multiple, independent pathways in a cell, or perhaps more likely, does it occur through a common final pathway into which several different signals in a cell converge where they can exert influence when their normal regulatory functions have been distorted, either by mutation or by introduction of a mutant form of the gene into the cell via a vector such as an RNA or DNA tumor virus.

One interesting, and speculative, ramification of this latter hypothesis is that there is a common *in vivo* process in anchorage-independent human tumors through which they assemble the extracellular matrix necessary for their tumor cell-specific, aberrant growth which is a potential target for therapeutic intervention. And, one would predict, this aberrant growth characteristic would be a common target for therapy in cancer cells, irrespective of the number or type of activated oncogenes which were responsible for the phenotype.

## ACKNOWLEDGEMENTS

This work was supported by grants R37-CA42024 and P30-CA07175 from the National Cancer Institute.

## REFERENCES

1.   A. W. Hamburger and S. E. Salmon. <u>Science</u> 197, 461-463 (1977).
2.   Z. P. Pavelic, H. K. Slocum, *et al.* <u>Cancer Res.</u> 40, 2160-2164 (1980).
3.   Z. P. Pavelic, H. K. Slocum, *et al.* <u>Cancer Res.</u> 40, 4151-4158 (1980).
4.   R. F. Ozols, J. K. Willson, *et al.* <u>Cancer Res.</u> 40, 2743-2747 (1980).

5.    D. N. Carney, A. F. Gazdar, and J. D. Minna. <u>Cancer Res.</u> 40, 1820–1823 (1980).

6.    C. W. Stevens, W. H. Brondyk, and W. E. Fahl. <u>J. Cancer Res. Clin. Oncol.</u> 115, 118–128 (1989).

7.    V. M. Maher, L. A. Rowan, *et al.* <u>Proc. Natl. Acad. Sci., U.S.A.</u> 79, 2613–2617 (1982).

8.    J. C. Barrett, B. D. Crawford, *et al.* <u>Cancer Res.</u> 39, 1504–1510 (1979).

9.    R. J. Zimmerman and J. B. Little. <u>Cancer Res.</u> 43, 2183–2189 (1983).

10.   J. C. Barrett, B. D. Crawford, and P. O. P. T'so. In: N. Mishra, V. Dunkel, and M. Mehlman (eds.), Mammalian Cell Transformation by Chemical Carcinogens, 467–500, Senate, New Jersey.

11.   A. Eva, K. C. Robbins, *et al.* <u>Nature</u> 295, 116–119 (1982).

12.   C. W. Stevens, W. H. Brondyk, *et al.* <u>Mol. Cell. Biol.</u> 8, 2089–2096 (1988).

13.   C. W. Stevens, T. H. Manoharan, and W. E. Fahl. <u>Proc. Natl. Acad. Sci., U.S.A.</u> 85, 3875–3879 (1988).

14.   J. L. Bos, E. R. Fearon, *et al.* <u>Nature</u> 327, 293–297 (1987).

15.   H. Igarashi, C. Rao, *et al.* <u>Oncogene</u> 1, 79 (1987).

16.   C. Betsholtz, A. Johnsson, *et al.* <u>Nature</u> 320, 695–699 (1986).

17.   G. R. Harsh, W. M. Kavanaugh, *et al.* <u>Oncogene Res.</u> 4, 65–73 (1989).

18.   E. B. Leof, J. A. Proper, *et al.* <u>Proc. Natl. Acad. Sci., U.S.A.</u> 83, 2453–2457 (1986).

19.   M. Pech, C. D. Rao, *et al.* <u>Mol. Cell Biol.</u> 9, 396–405 (1989).

20.   P. D. Robbins, J. M. Horowitz, and R. C. Mulligan. <u>Nature</u> 346, 668–671 (1990).



From: *Neoplastic Transformation in Human Cell Culture,*
Eds.: J. S. Rhim and A. Dritschilo ©1991 The Humana Press Inc., Totowa, NJ

# CYTOSKELETAL CHANGES IN HUMAN TRANSFORMED CELLS: STUDIES ON HOS CELLS


C. Chandra Kumar*, Cecile Chang[+] and Johng Rhim[++]

*Dept. of Tumor Biology, Schering-Plough Research, Bloomfield, NJ 07003, [+]Cold Spring Harbor Laboratory, Cold Spring Harbor, NY 11724, [++]National Cancer Research Institute, Bethesda, MD 20892


The cytoskeleton is the network of filaments mainly responsible for controlling and maintaining cellular morphology and motility. Three major filaments constitute the cytoskeleton and these are 1) acitn and myosin based microfilaments, 2) tubulin based microtubules and 3) intermediate filaments composed of proteins which are specific to different cell types. Since neoplastic transformation is associated with characteristic changes in cell morphology and motility, it is conceivable that there are important changes in the synthesis and organization of the cytoskeletal proteins following transformation. Indeed, microfilaments, also known as actin cables or stress fibers are known to be reorganized from a bundle state in normal cells into randomly interwoven meshwork in many transformed cells (1,2). This phenomenon, commonly referred to as diffusion of actin cable network, has been found to be a characteristic of many transformed cell lines. The mechanisms involved in the rearrangement of actin cable network are not clearly understood. However, analysis of protein differences between normal and transformed cells using quantitative two-dimensional gel electrophoretic technique has shown that the synthesis of several cytoskeletal proteins such as vimentin, tropomyosin, and $\alpha$-actin is repressed in transformed cells (3-5). The fact that these cytoskeletal changes may be critical for the establishment of the transformed phenotype is underscored by the discovery of oncogenes such as v-fgr and trk which are fusions of a tyrosine kinase with $\gamma$-actin and tropomyosin genes respectively (6-11). Mutations affecting the cytosketal components such as ß and $\gamma$ actin, tubulin and tropomyosins have also been observed in certain cancers (9).

A number of studies indicate that changes in cytoskeletal proteins, observed in transformed cells, are specific to the transforming agent and not an inevitable consequence of transformation. For example, Cooper et al. (10), have shown that transformation of NIH 3T3 cells by papovaviruses such as SV40 and polyoma virus caused no suppression of synthesis of specific tropomyosin isoforms, whereas suppression did occur in retrovirus transformed 3T3 cells.

Detailed two-dimensional gel studies of rat REF 52 cells led to a similar conclusion that changes seen in different tropomyosin isoforms are specific to the transforming agent (11). Our studies on human smooth muscle (sm) specific myosin light chain-2 (MLC-2) expression in different transformed cell lines support this general conclusion (12).

In order to systematically investigate the role of different oncogenes on cytoskeletal changes, we have chosen to work with human osteosarcoma derived fibroblasts, known as HOS cells (TE-85, clone F5, ATCC CRL 1543). HOS cells exhibit flat morphology and are non-tumorigenic in nude mice (13). Recent studies indicate that HOS cells contain a mutant form of p53 gene and appear to have lost the wild type allele (14). The mutant form of p53 protein was found to be stable, being associated with heat shock protein (hsp) 70 and also defective for association with large T antigen (15, 16). These results suggest that the mutant p53 gene may be responsible for the immortalization of HOS cells and its susceptibility to transformation by retroviruses. HOS cells can undergo morphological transformation following treatment with chemical carcinogens such as MNNG (N-methyl-N-nitro-N-nitrosoguanidine), DMBA (Dimethylbenzathracene) and 3-MC (3-Methyl cholanthrene) or also following infection with retroviruses such as Kirsten murine sarcoma virus, Rous sarcoma virus (RSV) etc. (17-21). The transformed HOS sublines such as MNNG-HOS (MNNG-transformed), K-HOS (Kirsten murine sarcoma virus transformed), HOS-RSV (RSV transformed), and HOS-FeLV (Feline leukemia virus transformed) (28) are tumorigenic in nude mice.

Two revertants of K-HOS, known as K-HOS (240S) and K-HOS (312H) that lack the viral genome have been isolated (22). Another series of revertants which still retain the viral genome and express elevated levels of ras p21 protein have also been characterized (23). HOS cells are also susceptible to transformation by cloned oncogene DNAs, as the murine NIH 3T3 cells (24). The HOS family of cell lines is therefore a system in which the phenotypic changes following transformation and their subsequent reversion to normal phenotype can be analyzed.

## MLC-2 GENE EXPRESSION IN HOS CELL LINES

MLC-2 is a 20 KDa protein associated with Myosin heavy chain (MHC) and phosphorylated by the enzyme MLC Kinase (25). Phosphorylation of MLC-2 by MLC kinase in the presence of calcium and calmodulin is known to regulate contraction in smooth and non-muscle cells. Phosphorylation of MLC-2 increases actin activated myosin ATPase activity which is necessary for the assembly of myosin into ordered bipolar filaments (26). We have recently characterized human smooth muscle (sm) specific MLC-2 cDNA from an umbilical artery library and shown that this isoform is expressed in a number of non-muscle cell lines such as fibroblasts and epithelial cells but not in haemopoietic cell lines (27). Northern blot analysis of RNAs derived from HOS, K-HOS, MNNG-HOS and K-HOS (240S) showed that smMLC-2 mRNA is completely repressed in transformed K-HOS and MNNG-HOS cells, whereas the revertant cell line (K-

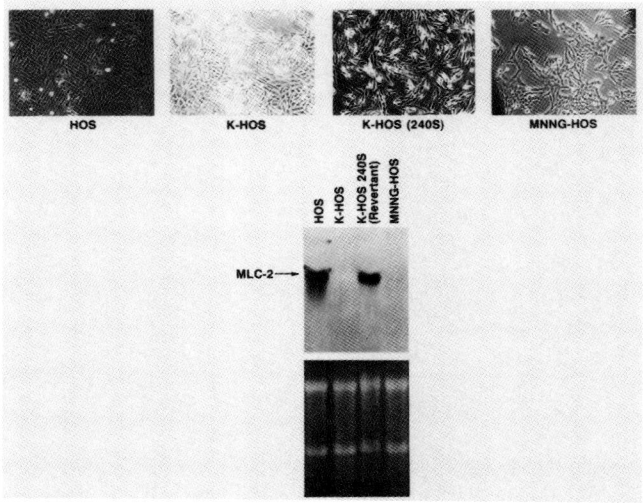


Fig. 1     Sm MLC-2 mRNA levels in different HOS cells detected by Northern blot analysis using human sm MLC-2 cDNA Probe.  The ethidium bromide staining pattern of RNAs is shown below the autoradiogram to indicate that equal mounts of RNA were loaded in the gel.

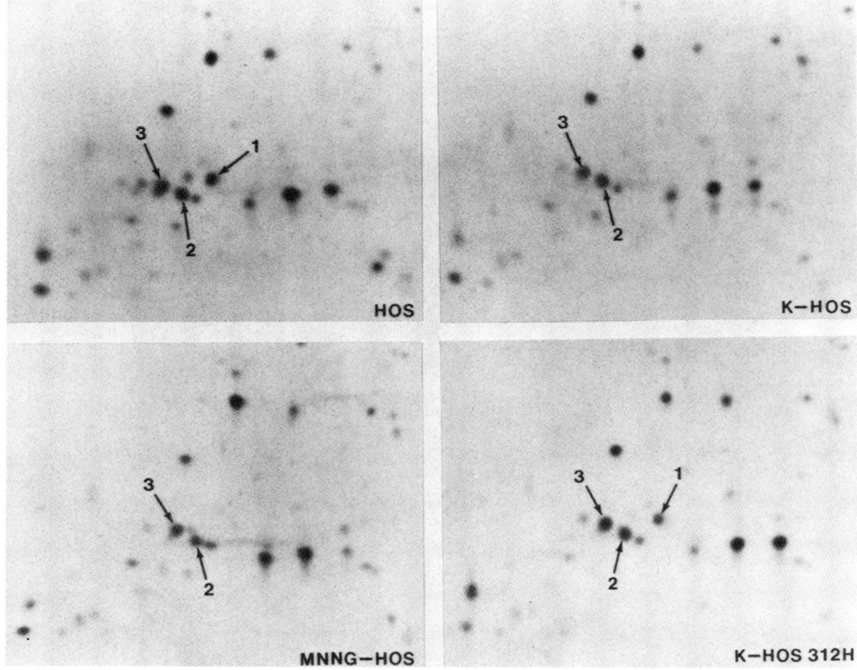


Fig. 2    Quantitative two-dimensional gel electrophoretic analysis of MLC-2 isoform levels in different HOS cell lines.  Total [$^{35}$S]-methionine labeled protein extracts of different HOS cells were resolved by the two-dimensional gel system. Labeling of cells was a period of 2 hours and equal amounts of TCA precipitable radioactive counts were loaded in each case and gels were processed for fluorography and exposed to Kodak x-ray film for 4 weeks.

HOS (240S) cells expressed normal levels of the MLC-2 mRNA as the HOS cells (Fig. 1). Transformation of HOS cells by Ha-ras oncogene sequences either by retroviral infection or by transfection followed by selection for tumorigenic cells in nude mice also results in complete repression of smMLC-2 mRNA level (12). Using antibodies raised against purified chicken gizzard MLC-2, we have shown that HOS cells synthesize three MLC-2 isoforms resolved by the two-dimensional gel electrophoretic system (27). The identity of the smMLC-2 isoform was established by co-electrophoresis of the *in vitro* synthesized MLC-2 protein, corresponding to the cloned cDNA, in the two-dimensional gel system along with total [$^{35}$S] methionine labeled HOS cell proteins. Quantitative two-dimensional gel electrophoretic analysis of MLC-2 isoforms in different HOS cells indicates that the synthesis of smMLC-2 isoform (designated as 1 in Fig. 2) is specifically repressed to an undetectable level in transformed K-HOS and MNNG-HOS cells, whereas the two non-muscle MLC-2 isoforms (designated 2 of 3) are relatively unaffected (Fig. 2). We have extended this analysis to the other transformed HOS cell lines such as HOS-RSV, HOS-FeLV and HOS-MC. The results shown in Fig. 3 indicate that, whereas smMLC-2 is repressed in K-HOS, MNNG-HOS and HOS- MC cells, its level is only partially repressed in HOS-RSV cells and is unchanged in transformed HOS-FeLV (28) cells containing a defective Moloney murine sarcoma virus (MO-MSV) genome (Fig. 3). These results support the previous observations by others (10, 11) that the cytoskeletal changes, associated with cellular transformation, are not an inevitable consequence of transformation but are specific to the transforming agent. These studies also indicate that smooth muscle specific contractile proteins such as smMLC-2 and smα-actin are  sensitive to repression by transformation and the non-muscle isoforms of MLC-2 and actin (ß and γ) are unaffected by transformation.

## **TUMOR PROMOTING AGENTS DOWN REGULATE MLC-2 GENE EXPRESSION IN HOS CELLS**

Rifkin et al. (29) first showed that treatment of chick embryo fibroblasts with 12-0-tetradecanoyl-phorbol-13-acetate (TPA) induces rapid dissolution of stress fibers. These changes are similar to those observed following transformation by oncogenic viruses. Hence, tumor promoters are considered to be a good tool to study cytoskeletal changes that are associated with cellular transformation. We have observed that treatment of HOS cells with TPA, results in a reduction in the level of smMLC-2 mRNA by about 24 hours (Fig. 4). Quantitative two-dimensional gel electrophoretic analysis, again indicates that smMLC-2 isoform level is specifically repressed following treatment with TPA whereas the non-muscle MLC-2 isoforms are unaffected (Fig. 5). Other tumor promoting agents such as Bryostatin II and Teleocidin have similar effect on MLC-2 mRNA level, whereas A23187, a Ca$^{++}$ ionophore has no effect  (unpublished observations).

TPA is known to induce a highly pleiotropic response including changes in cell morphology, proliferation and differentiation and transient mimicry of the transformed phenotype (30). TPA induces the transcription of several mitogen responsive genes such as c-myc, c-fos, actin, etc. and also inhibit the

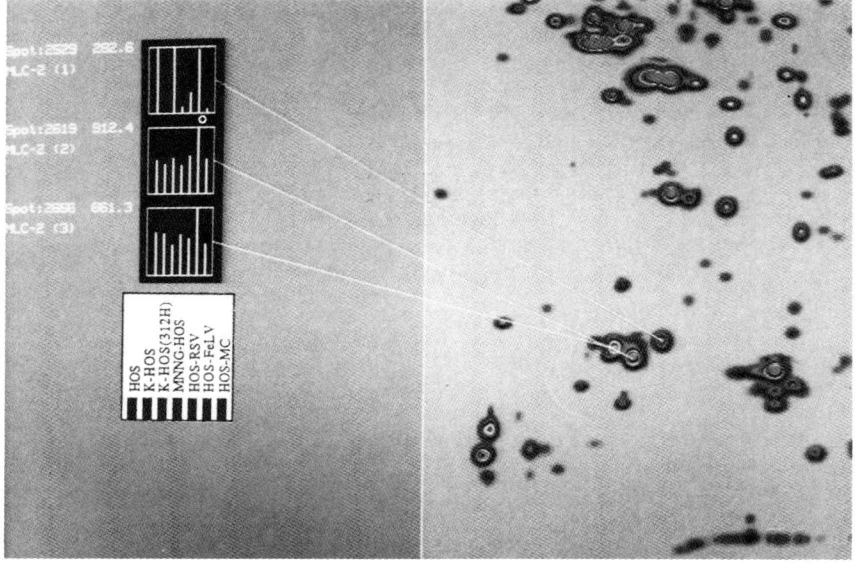


Fig. 3      Quantitative data for MLC-2 isoforms in different HOS cell lines - spot graph analysis.  Shown on the right half is a portion of a gel for HOS cells showing the three MLC-2 isoforms.  The spot graphs in the upper left present quantitative data for three MLC-2 isoforms in different HOS cells.  Each bar represents the intensity of MLC-2 isoform in one cell line and the order of different HOS cells analyzed is shown below the spot graph.

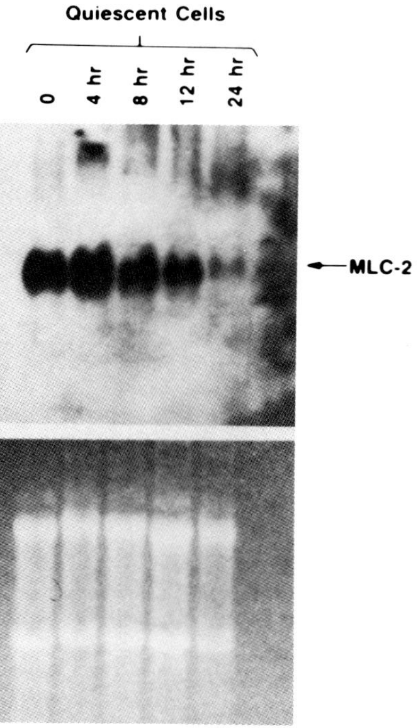



Fig. 4     Time course of changes in sm MLC-2 mRNA level following TPA treatment of HOS cells.  HOS cells were treated with TPA (100 ng/ml) and at various times total RNA was isolated and analyzed as described in the legend for Fig. 1.

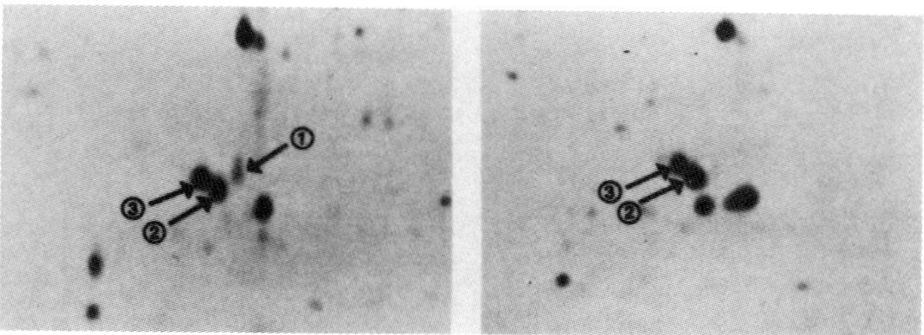



Fig. 5     Two-dimensional gel electrophoretic analysis of MLC-2 isoforms in control (DMSO) and TPA treated HOS cells.  HOS cells were treated with either DMSO or TPA (100 ng/ml) for 22 hrs and [$^{35}$S]-methionine   (500 µCi/ml) was added to the medium and labeling continued for 2 hrs.  Cell lysates were electrophoresed on the two-dimensional system.

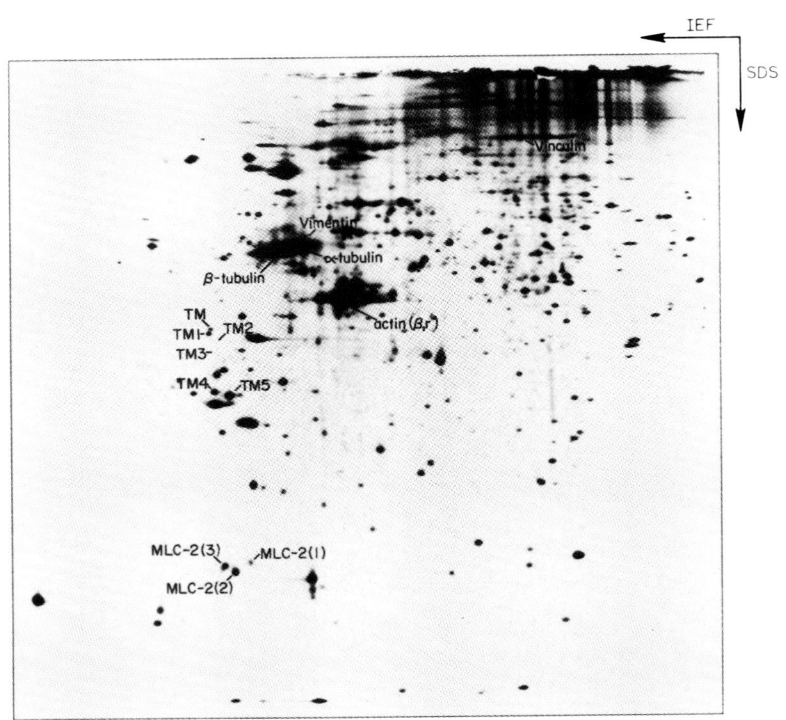



Fig. 6     The reference map for HOS cell data base showing the location of some of the known cytoskeletal proteins.

expression of certain other genes such as collagen, and glycophorin (31).  TPA is known to bind to and activate Protein Kinase C,a $ca^{++}$ activated phospholipid dependent enzyme.  Protein Kinase C is a key component of the signal transduction process that operates in response to external stimuli and is involved in the control of normal cell proliferation and tumor promotion (32).

## HOS CELL DATABASE

We have initiated a systematic, quantitative analysis of proteins in HOS cells and its transformed derivatives.  HOS cell line is well suited for these studies because  1) it is one of the well characterized human immortalized cell line,  2) it does not give rise to spontaneous transformants, and  3) a series of transformants are already available.  A typical two-dimensional gel pattern of HOS cell proteins with the location of some of the known cytoskeletal proteins is shown in Fig. 6.  A system for quantitative analysis of at least 1600 proteins in the two-dimensional gel patterns and for construction of protein data bases has been developed (33, 34).  This system has already been used to establish a protein data base for rat REF 52 cells.  A protein data base allows quantitative data from many different experiments to be compared and correlated.  So far we have concentrated on analyzing MLC-2 changes in various HOS cells.  The data base provides the means to store and compare quantitative data for up to 2000 proteins.  As more of the known proteins become identified on the two-dimensional gel patterns, we can hope to obtain a more complete understanding of the protein changes that occur as human cells are transformed through the action of known transforming agents.

## ACKNOWLEDGEMENTS

We thank Drs. Joseph J. Catino and Claude Nash for support and encouragement.  We also thank Ms Rita J. Cunniff for typing this manuscript.

## REFERENCES

1.  Pollack, R., Osborn, M. and Weber, K. (1975) Pro. Natl. Acad. Sci. USA 72:994-998.
2.  Shin, S. L., et al., (1975) Proc. Natl. Acad. Sci. USA 72:4435-4439.
3.  Leavitt, J. (1989) in George Milo (ed.), Human Fibroblast Transformation.  CRC Press, Inc. pp 1-28.
4.  Garrels, J. I. and Frenza, B. R., Jr. (1989) J. Biol. Chem. 264:5299-5312.
5.  Bravo, R. and Celis, J. E. (1982) Clin. Chem. 28:949-954.
6.  Rasheed, et al., (1974) Cancer Res. 33:1027-1033.
7.  Naharro, et al., (1984) Science 226:63-66.
8.  Martin-Zancar, et al., (1986) Nature 319:743-748.
9.  Chow, et al., (1987) Proc. Natl. Acad. Sci. USA 84:2575-2579.

10.     Cooper, M. L., et al., (1985) Mol. Cell. Biol. 5:972-983.
11.     Matsumura, et al., (1983) J. Biol. Chem. 258:13954-13964.
12.     Chandra Kumar, C., et al., (1991) Manuscript in Preparation.
13.     McAllister, et al., (1971) Cancer 27:397-402.
14.     Romano, J. W., et al., (1989) Oncogene 4:1483-1488.
15.     Ehrhart, J. C., et al., (1988) Oncogene 3: 595-603.
16.     Van Roy, F., et al., (1990) Oncogene 5, 207-218.
17.     Rhim, J. S., et al., (1975) Nature 256:751-753.
18.     Rhim, J. S., et al., (1975) J. Natl. Cancer Inst. 55:1291-1294.
19.     Rhim, J. S., et al., (1975) Int. J. Cancer 15:23-29.
20.     Rhim, J. S., et al., (1982) Proc. Soc. Exp. Biol. Med. 170:350-358.
21.     Cho, H. Y., et al., (1978) Int. J. Cancer 21:22-26.
22.     Cho. H. Y., et al., (1976) Science 194:951-953.
23.     Bassin, R. H. and Benade, L. E. (1990) in "Tumor Suppressor
        Genes", ed by George Klein, Marcell-Dekker Publ. New York.
        p 15-47.
24.     Tainsky, M. A., et al., (1987) Mol. Cell. Biol. 7:1280-1284.
25.     Adelstein, R. A. and Eisenberg, E. A. (1980) Ann. Rev. Biochem.
        49:921-956.
26.     Scholey, J. M., et al., (1980) Nature  287:233-235.
27.     Chandra Kumar, C., et al., (1989) Biochemistry 28:4027-4035.
28.     Rhim, J. S. (1981) Proc. Soc, Exp. Biol. Med. 167:597-606.
29..    Rifkin, D. B., et al., (1979) Cell 18:361-368.
30.     Weinstein, I. B., et al., (1979) J. Supramol. Struct. 12:195-208.
31.     Angel, P., et al., (1986) Mol. Cell. Biol. 6:1760-1766.
32.     Nishizuka, Y. (1986) Science 233:305-312.
33.     Garrels, J. I. (1989) J. Biol. Chem. 264:5269-5282.
34.     Garrels, J. I. and Franza, B. R. (1989) J. Biol. Chem. 264:5283-5298.

Polyamine Metabolism in Human Epidermal Keratinocytes
Transformed with AD12-SV40, HPV16-DNA and K-*ras* Oncogene.

S. Beninati[1,2], S.C. Park[2]. M. Piacentini[1],
J.S. Rhim[3] and S.I. Chung[2*].

[1]Department of Biology, 2nd University of
Rome Tor Vergata, Italy, [2]National
Institute of Dental Research, NIH,
[3]National Cancer Institute, NIH, Bethesda,
MD 20892.

The intracellular concentration of the polyamines,
spermidine and spermine, and their precursor, putrescine,
vary with the growth rate of the cell. Although the
specific role of these amines is still not well understood
at the molecular level, recent studies have shown that
their concentration is highly regulated and that polyamines
are necessary for normal cell growth and differentiation
(see reviews 1 - 3). The pathway of polyamine biosynthesis
from ornithine and methionine in mammalian tissues is well
char-acterized (4). Biosynthesis is modulated by rapid
induction of both ornithine decarboxylase (ODC) and S-
adenosylmethionine decarboxylase (AdoMetDC) both of which
are present in very small amounts in quiescent cells and
both of which have very short time turnovers (5,6).
Exposure of resting cells to growth-promoting stimuli
results in a rapid rise in ODC activity which thereafter
parallels the proliferation response. In addition to the
possibility of rapidly changing their rate of polyamine
synthesis, cells are equipped with an effective pathway for
degradation of spermidine and spermine. The first, and
rate-limiting, step in this degradation is an acetylation
of the polyamines, which is catalyzed by the inducible
enzyme, spermidine/ spermine N[1]-acetyltransferase (7).
This enzyme also has an extremely short half-life (8), is
rapidly induced by various polyamines (9) and appears to
play a role in cellular protection against the deleterious
effects of too high intracellular polyamine concentrations.

Clinical and experimental observations have suggested
that cancer is a multiple-step process (see reviews, 10-
12). The increased rate of polyamine biosynthesis and
transport associated with neoplastic tissues relative to
their normal controls (13,14), and the decrease in c-myc
expression in human colon carcinoma cells accompanying
polyamine depletion (15) suggested a possible involvement
of polyamines in the neoplastic conversion process.  In
this study, we have examined polyamine interconversions and
polyamine involve- ment in the posttranslational
modification of proteins during neoplastic transformation
of human epidermal keratinocytes by  AD12-SV40, HPV-16 DNA
and K-*ras* oncogene in order to elucidate the possible
mechanism of polyamine effects on cellular events
associated with virally-induced neoplastic conversion.

Methods:


RHEK-1 cells were established from primary human foreskin
epithelial cells following infection with AD12-SV40 as
described earlier (11).  Transfection of primary human
epidermal cells with human papilloma virus 16 (HPV-16 DNA)
resulted in a continued proliferative cells in culture
without the concomitant acquisition of the neoplastic
phenotype (HPK-1A)(16, 17). Infection of HPK-1A cells with
Kirsten murine sarcoma virus induced the cells become
tumorigenic (K-*ras*/HPK-1A).  RHEK-1 cells transfected with
human EJ *ras* oncogene induced morphological alterations
associated with the acquisition of malignant conversion
(pSV$_2$-*ras*)(18).

Polyamine Determination: the cells were grown to confluency
and continued in culture for three days in the presence of
[$^3$H]putrescine.  In order to measure the free polyamines in
the cells, washed cells were scraped into phosphate
buffered saline and an equal volume of cold 20%
trichloroacetic acid was added.  After centrifugation for
15 min at 5,000 x g, the supernatant was collected and the
pellet was washed twice with 5% trichloroacetic acid.  The
supernatant and washes were combined and polyamines in
aliquotes were measured by means of an ion exchange
chromatographic procedure carried out on a Durrum D-400
amino acid analyzer equipped with 4 x 80 mm column packed
with Dionex DC 6A resin.  A three-buffer system for elution
and o-phthal- aldehyde for detection were employed as
described previously (19).

An aliquot of the acid insoluble fraction was hydrolyzed in 6 N HCl for 18 h at 110°C; other aliquots were
digested with proteases employing Pronase, aminopeptidase M
and carboxypeptidase A and B as outlined earlier (19). The
digestion was continued for an additional 8 h period after
addition of carboxypeptidase Y at a level of 0.01 mg/mg
protein of the sample. Amino acids were determined with an
automated amino acid analyzer (Beckman) using ninhydrin for
detection.  For detection of γ-glutamyl amines, the digests
were first separated on the Dionex DC 6A column without
mixing with o-phthalaldehyde (OPA) and γ-glutamyl amines in
the eluted fractions were derivatized with OPA and determined by reverse-phase HPLC as described (20).

Results and Discussion:

Both RHEK-1 and HPK-1 cells are non-tumorigenic
immortalized cells and additional infection with viral p21
ras oncogene resulted in malignant transformation. In order
to determine the possible role of polyamines in the
processes of neoplastic transformation, the *ras* transformed
human keratinocytes were examined for their ability to
incorporate and metabolize polyamines. The cells were

cultured for 72 hours in the presence of [³H]putrescine and polyamine metabolites were measured.

<u>Polyamine Biosynthesis</u>: In all mammalian cells, putrescine is synthesized from ornithine by the catalytic action of ornithine decarboxylase (ODC), which is a pyridoxal phosphate-dependent enzyme. To convert putrescine to spermidine

### Table I

### Enzyme Activity in Human Keratinocytes

Ornithine decarboxylase activity was determined by measuring the liberation of [$^{14}$C]CO$_2$ from D,L-[1-$^{14}$C]ornithine (56 mCi/mmol; NEN, Boston) (21). S-adenosyl methionine decarboxylase activity was assayed by measuring the liberation of [$^{14}$C]CO$_2$ from S-adenosyl-L-[1-$^{14}$C]methionine (54 mCi/mmol; Amersham, Arlington Heights, IL) (22). Polyamine oxidase activity was assayed by measuring the amount of [$^{14}$C]spermidine formed from [$^{14}$C]spermine (110 mCi/mmol; Amersham)(23). One unit of enzyme activity is defined as the amount of enzyme catalyzing the formation of 1 nmol of spermidine per minute from spermine.

| Cells | ODC | AdoMetDC | PAO |
|---|---|---|---|
| | nmol [$^{14}$C]CO$_2$/h/mg | nmol [$^{14}$C]CO$_2$/h/mg | units/mg |
| HEK | 0.3 | 2.3 | 2.5 |
| RHEK-1 | 1.8 | 12.2 | 0.03 |
| HPK-1A | 1.0 | 6.0 | 0.04 |
| pSV$_2$*ras*/RHEK-1 | 15.8 | 25.8 | 0.04 |
| K-*ras*/HPK-1A | 13.6 | 32.0 | 0.10 |

an aminopropyl group must be added. This aminopropyl moiety is derived from methionine which is first converted into S-adenosyl methionine (AdoMet) and is then decarboxylated by S-adenosylmethionine decarboxylase (AdoMetDC). The resulting decarboxylated S-adenosylmethionine is then used as an aminopropyl donor in a reaction catalyzed by spermidine synthetase. Another aminopropyl group from AdoMet is needed to convert spermidine into spermine. As shown in Table 1, polyamine biosynthesis in the four cell lines was affected by virally induced transformation of keratinocytes. Both ODC and AdoMetDC were increased several fold in the

immortalized RHEK-1 and HPK-1 cells and the level of enzyme
activities was further increased in the tumorigenic pSV$_2$-
*ras*/RHEK-1 and K-*ras*/HPK-1A cells (Table I).  The end
results of the increased ODC and AdoMetDC in these cells are
reflected in the rise of the levels of unconjugated polyamines found in the 5% TCA soluble fractions (see Fig. 1).
In organs and tissues as well as in epidermis, spermidine
was found to be 1.4 to 2.5 fold higher than spermine (1).
However, cultured keratinocytes showed slightly higher
spermine than spermidine levels.  In the transformed cells,
the total level of polyamines was increased more than ten
fold over the parent keratinocytes; of these increased
polyamines, spermine represents the greatest percentage (60
to 90 %) of the increase in polyamines.

Spermine can be converted to spermidine by the sequential action of two enzyme systems: spermine-N$^1$-acetyltrans-
ferase and polyamine oxidase. The former enzyme uses acetyl
CoA to convert spermine into N$^1$-acetylspermine and this
derivative then becomes a substrate for polyamine oxidase
which cleaves at the internal nitrogen to yield N-acetyl-
propionaldehyde and spermidine (23).  However, polyamine
oxidase can cleave spermine directly in the presence of
aldehyde activators (24).  A 90 % decrease of "polyamine
oxidase", as measured here (Table I) is reflected in the
unusually high level of spermine in these cells (Fig. I).
This finding is consistent with earlier reports of spermine
as a predominant polyamine in human colon carcinoma HT29/219
cells and low activities of polyamine oxidation in 48 hr
cultures of all human breast epithelial carcinoma cells
ZR-75-1 and colorectal epithelial carcinoma HT29/219 cells
(25).
<u>Polyamine conjugated into proteins</u>:  The posttranslational
modification of proteins involving structural elements of
polyamines occurs by two separate metabolic pathways. One
results in the formation of hypusine [N$^\epsilon$-(4-amino-2-hydr-
oxybutyl)lysine] (review 26, 27).  In this case, the butyl-
amine residue derived from spermidine is transferred to the
$\epsilon$-amino group of peptide-bound lysine and subsequently
hydroxylated.  Hypusine is found in only one cellular protein, translation initiation factor eIF-5A (formerly known
as eIF-4D)(27, 28). Interestingly, the level of hypusine was
increased three to four fold in the transformed cells (see
Table II).  When differentiation of mouse epidermal cells
was induced by high Ca$^{++}$ ion or 12-0-tetradecanoylphorbol-
13-acetate, the hypusine was rapidly reduced to undetectable
levels (29).  The increase in the hypusine level in the
transformed cells seen here may reflect requirements of
eIF-5A in the hyperproliferative state of cells.

The other posttranslational modification involving polyamines is their covalent attachment through amide linkage to
the γ-carboxyl groups of glutamyl residues of proteins.
Formation of these protein components through exchange of a
polyamine for ammonia at the carboxamide groups of glutamyl
residues is catalyzed by transglutaminases (30, 31).  It is
known that polyamines are excellent substrates for transg-

lutaminases *in vitro and in vivo* (19).  In the transformed
cells, the level of transglutaminase activity is decreased
significantly. In K-*ras*/HPK-1A cells, the enzyme level was
only 10 to 15% of that of the parent keratinocytes (Fig. 2).
Although the levels of polyamines were elevated in these
transformed cells, polyamines conjugated into proteins were
significantly decreased in comparison with those of the
parent cells.  In K-*ras*/HPK-1A cells which contained the
lowest cellular transglutaminase activity, the polyamines
conjugated into proteins were much lower.

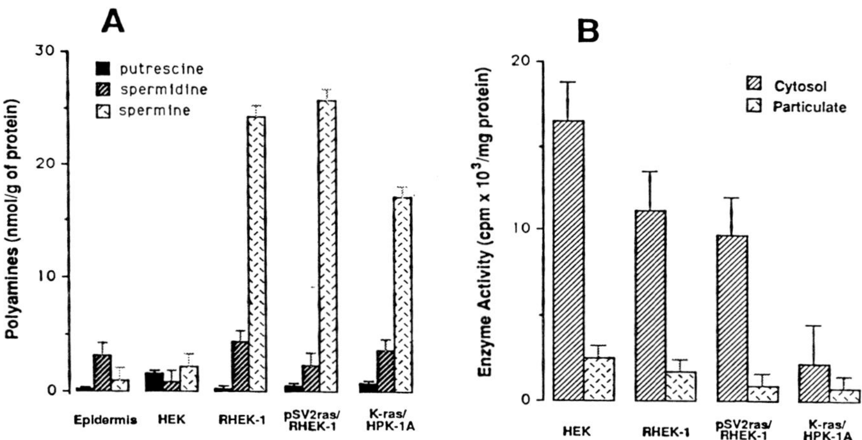


Fig. 1  A. Polyamine levels in keratinocytes. Free putrescine, spermidine and spermine present in the cells and
epidermis.  B. Transglutaminase activity in keratinocytes.
Transglutaminase activity was assayed as described (30). To
400 $\mu$l reaction mixture of 0.1 M Tris acetate buffer, pH
8.0, containing 10 mM $CaCl_2$, 1 mM EDTA, 0.5% Lubrol, 0.15 M
NaCl, 1% succinylated casein, 5 mM DTT, and 0.5 $\mu$Ci of
[$^{14}$C]putrescine, 50- to 200 $\mu$l portions of samples to be
assayed were added.  The reactions were conducted at 37° C
for 1 h and stopped by addition of 2 ml portions of cold 10%
TCA.  The precipitates were washed twice with cold 5% TCA
and collected on glass filters (Whatmann GF/A), and the
radioactivity was measured.

$N^1$,$N^8$-Bis($\gamma$-glutamyl)spermidine, which represents 70 to 80%
of the total polyamine conjugated into protein in the HEK
cells, is decreased more than 90 % in the transfected cells
(see Table II).  On the other hand, N-($\gamma$-glutamyl)spermine
which is not detectable in the HEK cells, represented 60 to

70 % of the total polyamine conjugated into proteins in
transfected cells.

Previous studies have shown a temporal association between new polyamine biosynthesis and the expression of c-myc
(31). Celano et al. (15) provided evidence that there might
be a direct requirement of polyamines for the expression of
the protooncogene, c-myc. Our findings of the increase in
polyamine synthesis upon the expression of p21 (11) in human
keratinocytes further support the close association of the
oncogenic protein with polyamine synthesis.

### Table II

Levels of the products of the posttranslational modification
of protein by polyamines in human keratinocytes

The amounts were calculated using the specific radioactivi-
ties of the component polyamines (data not shown). For
hypusine calculation the specific activity of the immediate
precursor of hypusine, spermidine was used. The data are
means of 4 determination differing by less than 15%. Ptc:
putrescine, Spd: spermidine and Spm: spermine.

| Derivatives | HEK | RHEK-1A | HPK-1A | pSV$_2$ras /RHEK-1 | K-ras /HPK-1A |
|---|---|---|---|---|---|
| | | | nmol/g of protein | | |
| Hypusine | 51.1 | 160.0 | 150.4 | 98.0 | 86.0 |
| N-($\gamma$-Glutamyl)Ptc | 0.21 | 0.22 | 0.53 | 0.12 | 0.23 |
| N$^1$,N$^4$-Bis($\gamma$-glutamyl)Ptc | 0.22 | 0.44 | 0.55 | 0.32 | 0.25 |
| N$^1$($\gamma$-Glutamyl)Spd N$^8$($\gamma$-Glutamyl)Spd | 0.71 | 0.1 | 0.25 | 0.09 | nd |
| N$^1$,N$^8$-Bis($\gamma$-glutamyl)Spd | 5.31 | 0.52 | 0.23 | 0.21 | nd |
| N-($\gamma$-Glutamyl)Spm | nd | 3.86 | 2.93 | 2.96 | 1.41 |
| N$^1$,N$^{12}$-Bis($\gamma$-glutamyl)Spm | nd | nd | nd | 0.097 | 0.11 |

nd: not detectable.

These findings clearly indicate that neoplastic transformation induced by oncogene in human keratinocytes results in
significant changes in the expression of the enzymes
involved in polyamine metabolism; these changes may play a

role in hyper-proliferation of transformed keratinocytes and
also in the perturbation of terminal differentiation of
keratinocytes, thus leading to an improper transglutaminase-
dependent assembly of cornified envelope.

Summary:

Human foreskin keratinocytes (HEK) were used to
examine polyamine metabolism and polyamine involvement in
the posttranslational modification of proteins during the
process of virally-induced neoplastic transformation.
Cellular levels of putrescine, spermidine and spermine in
HEK cells were found in the range of 1 to 2 nmol/mg protein.
Transfection of HEK cells with SV40 T-antigen or with DNA of
human papilloma virus type 16, which induced immortalization
of the cells (RHEK-1, HPK-1A), resulted in a 3 to 6 fold
increase in the levels of both ODC and AdoMetDC activities
and a significant decrease in the level of polyamine oxidase
activity. After incubation of cells with[$^3$H]putrescine,
analysis of the labeled polyamines in the TCA-soluble fraction of RHEK-1 or HPK-1A cells showed decrease in labeled
putrescine and a 10 to 12 fold increase in labeled spermine
compared to HEK cells. Transformation of RHEK-1 with pSV$_2$-
*ras* oncogene (pSV$_2$*ras*/RHEK-1) or HPK-1 with K-*ras* virus
(Ki/HPK-1A) which caused additional increases in the levels
of ODC and AdoMetDC activities. In the TCA-insoluble cellular fraction labeled polyamines were found conjugated to
protein through transglutaminase (TGase) actions. N$^1$ or N$^8$-
(γ-Glutamyl)-spermidine (0.5 to 1 nmol/g) and N$^1$,N$^8$-bis(glutamyl)spermidine (1 to 1.4 nmol/g) were identified in the
digests of cellular protein of HEK cells. In RHEK-1 cells, a
significantly decreased level of N$^1$,N$^8$,-bis(γ-glutamyl)s-
permidine (0.15 nmol/g) and a relatively high level of N$^1$-
(γ-glutamyl)spermine (3.8 nmol/g) were found. In both
transformed cells, TGase activity was significantly decreased and this change was reflected in the much lower levels
of protein-conjugated polyamines. The polyamine-derived
amino acid, hypusine [N$^e$-(4-amino-2-hydroxybutyl)lysine]
which was also identified in digests of cellular protein,
increased from 51.1 nmol/g in HEK cells to 160 nmol/g in
both RHEK-1 or HPK-1A cells following viral transfection.

* To whom correspondence should be addressed: Laboratory of
Cellular Development and Oncology, National Institute of
Dental Research, Bldg. 30, Rm 211, Bethesda, MD 20892.

References:

1.   A. E. Pegg and P. P. McCann. Am J. Physiol. 243
     (Cell Physiol. 12), C212 (1982).
2.   M. A. Grillo. Int. J. Biochem. 17, 943 (1985).
3.   A. E. Pegg. Biochem. J. 234, 249 (1986).
4.   P. P. MaCann. In: Polyamines in Biomedical Research,
     ed by J. M. Gaugas. New York, Wiley, pp. 109 (1980).
5.   J. Jänne, H. Pösö, et al. Biochim. Biophys. Acta 473,
     241 (1978).
6.   A. E. Pegg, H. Hibasami, et al. Adv. Enzyme Reg. 19,

427 (1981).

7. I. Matsui, L. Wiegand, et al. J. Biol. Chem. 256, 2454 (1981).

8. L. Persson and A. E. Pegg. J. Biol. Chem. 259, 12364 (1984).

9. A. E. Pegg and B. G. Erwin. Biochem. J. 231, 285 (1985).

10. J. D. Minna. Chest 96(1 Suppl), 17S (1989).

11. J. S. Rhim, G. Jay, et al. Science 227, 1250 (1985).

12. G. M. Cooper. Oncogenes, Jones and Bartlett Publishers Boston, MA pp. 3 (1990).

13. A. N. Kingsnorth, A. B. Lumdsen, et al. Br. J. Surg. 71, 791 (1984).

14. A. E. Pegg. Cancer Res. 48, 759 (1988).

15. P. Celano, S. B. Baylin, et al. J. Biol. Chem. 263, 5491 (1988).

16. M. Dürst, R. T. Dzarlieva-Petrusevska, et al. Oncogene 1, 251 (1987).

17. M. Dürst, D. Gallahan, et al. Virology 173, 767 (1989).

18. J. S. Rhim, J. B. Park, et al. Oncogene 4, 1403, (1989).

19. J. E. Folk, M. H. Park, et al. J. Biol. Chem. 255, 3695 (1980).

20. S. Beninati, N. Martinet, et al. J. of Chromatography 443, 329 (1988).

21. D. H. Russell and S. H. Snyder. Proc. Natl. Acad. Sci., USA 60, 1422 (1968).

22. A. E. Pegg, H. Polso, et al. Biochem. J. 202, 519 (1982).

23. E. Höltta. Methods in Enzymology 94, 306 (1983).

24. E. Höltta. Biochemistry 16, 91 (1977).

25. H. M. Wallace, M. E. Nuttall, et al. In: Progress in polyamine research: Novel biochemical, pharmacological, and clinical aspects, eds V. Zappia and A. E. Pegg pp.331 (1988).

26. M. H. Park, H. L. Cooper, et al. Proc. Natl. Acad. Sci. USA 78, 2869 (1981).

27. M. H. Park, E. C. Wolff, et al. In: Progress in Polyamine Research: novel biochemical, pharmacological and clinical aspects. eds V. Zappia and A. E. Pegg, Plenum Press, New York pp. 435 (1988).

28. H. L. Cooper, M. H. Park, et al. Proc. Natl. Acad. Sci. USA 80, 1854 (1983).

29. M. Piacentini, M. G. Farrace, et al. J. Invest. Dermatol. 94, 694 (1990).

30. J. E. Folk and S. I. Chung. Methods in Enzymology 113, 358 (1985).

31. S. I. Chung. Ann. N. Y. Acad. Sci. 202, 240 (1972).

32. A. Katz and C. Kahana. Mol. Cell. Biol. 7, 2641 (1987).

From: *Neoplastic Transformation in Human Cell Culture,*
Eds.: J. S. Rhim and A. Dritschilo ©1991 The Humana Press Inc., Totowa, NJ

# II. Radiation Transformation
and Oncogenes

TRANSFORMATION OF HUMAN DIPLOID FIBROBLASTS

BY RADIATION AND ONCOGENES

J.B. Little, L.-N. Su and Y. Kano

Department of Cancer Biology, Harvard
School of Public Health, Boston, MA 02115
USA


Most human cancers appear to be clonal in
origin; that is, they are derived from a single cell
that has apparently undergone the process of malignant
transformation *in vivo*. Whether the progeny of this
cell will eventually give rise to an invasive,
malignant tumor depends upon a number of host and
tissue factors. The malignant transformation of cells
*in vitro* is also a complex, multi-step process by
which normal cells acquire the various phenotypic
characteristics of cancer cells. Three major steps
appear to be involved: the development of morphologic
transformation, immortality, and tumorigenicity.
Although rodent cells will readily undergo immortalization *in vitro* either spontaneously or in response to
treatment with chemical or physical carcinogens,
immortalization appears to be the rate-limiting step
in the transformation of human diploid cells (1).

In contrast to cells derived from tumors, normal
human diploid fibroblasts have a limited proliferative
capacity *in vitro*. After subcultivation for several
months, the cells gradually assume a senescent morphology and proliferation ceases after about 50 mean
population doublings. Although treatment of these
cells with physical or chemical carcinogens can result
in phenotypic changes associated with morphologic
transformation, such as conversion to anchorage-
independent growth, this phenomenon is rarely

associated with the development of immortalized cells
(2,3).  The genetic basis for escape from the
commitment to senescence in human cells has not been
examined systematically.  Although numerous attempts
to achieve complete transformation of human fibroblasts by radiation or chemical carcinogens have
generally proven unsuccessful, immortalization can be
achieved in cells transfected with certain viral
sequences.

In this report, we describe two approaches to
gaining a better understanding of factors involved in
the immortalization of human diploid fibroblasts.  In
the first, cells were treated with single or multiple
doses of x-rays and followed throughout their lifespan
*in vitro*.  Our aim was to establish a technique
whereby diploid cells could be systematically
transformed to immortality by x-rays, and to correlate
this process with the development of specific
karyotypic changes.  In the second approach, cells
were transfected with SV40 early region containing the
large T-antigen.  The appearance of changes in cell
growth, chromosomal abnormalities, and frequency of
spontaneous mutations were correlated with the
emergence of immortalized cells in order to gain
information concerning the genetic basis for this
phenomenon.  Finally, we examined the influence of
transfection with SV40-T and immortalization on
cellular radiosensitivity.

## MATERIALS AND METHODS

Normal human diploid fibroblast cell strains
were obtained from the Human Genetic Mutant Cell
Repository, Camden, NJ.  They were grown and
maintained by standard techniques in Eagle's Minimal
Essential Medium supplemented with 10% fetal bovine
serum as described elsewhere (4).  Early passage
cultures were x-irradiated or transfected with SV40-T,
then continuously passaged by subcultivation at a 1:4
dilution at approximately weekly intervals throughout
their lifespan *in vitro*.  When the cells reached
senescence or "crisis", they were maintained in the
incubator for several months with regular medium

changes to monitor the emergence of immortalized cells.

For radiation experiments, cells were exposed to single doses of 400 or 600 rads, or from 3 to 15 multiple doses of 200-600 rads at sequential passages. The various radiation groups and protocols are described in detail elsewhere (5). In one case, cells were exposed to daily doses of 25 rads for 100 consecutive days. At regular intervals during passaging, the cell population was examined for stable and unstable chromosomal aberrations as well as for the appearance of marker chromosomes as previously described (4).

For studies with SV40-T, we used a plasmid (pSV3neo) containing the SV40 early region and encoding the T antigen. Transfection was carried out either by calcium phosphate precipitation or electroporation, and the cells selected for neo-resistance with G418 prior to serial subcultivation. In some experiments, the cells were x-irradiated one or two passages prior to SV40-T transfection. At regular intervals after transfection, the cell population was examined for cloning efficiency, saturation density at confluence, the frequency of spontaneous mutations to 6-thioguanine resistance (hprt locus) and chromosomal aberrations including dicentrics, rings, fragments, exchanges and breaks (6). Integration of SV40-T in transformed cell lines was confirmed by Southern blot analysis. The measurements of cellular radiosensitivity in wild-type and transfected cell strains was carried out by standard techniques.

## RESULTS

### Lack of Immortalization by X-irradiation

Exposure of human diploid cells to single or multiple doses of x-rays induced both unstable chromosomal aberrations (such as rings, dicentrics and fragments) as well as stable aberrations (particularly

translocations).  Unstable aberrations were rapidly
lost from the cultures with serial passaging, whereas
the frequency of induced translocations remained
essentially constant throughout the lifespan of the
cells.  Thus, persistent genetic changes occurred in
cells surviving radiation exposure.

The appearance of abnormal clones, characterized
by marker chromosomes, was observed in a number of
irradiated cultures.  These appeared as soon as 6
passages or approximately 12 mean population doublings
(MPD) after irradiation and often expanded to include
30-80% of the population.  Evidence of clonal
succession was observed in some cultures; that is, the
successive appearance of several different abnormal
clones.  These abnormal clones senesced and
disappeared from the cell population in most cases.
Sometimes, however, they emerged as the terminal cell
population.  Two of these terminal clones showed a
markedly prolonged lifespan (104 and 114 MPD) as
compared with the mass cultures which senesced at
approximately 50 MPD.  Eventually, however, these
clones also senesced.  Thus, the emergence of
immortalized cells was never observed in a total of 46
different experiments in which cells were irradiated
with single or multiple doses of x-rays and followed
throughout their lifespan *in vitro*.

The effect of irradiation on mean lifespan of
the cultures in these experiments is shown in Figure
1.  The two cultures described above in which terminal
cell clones emerged with greatly prolonged lifespans
are not included in these data.  As can be seen, the
mean lifespan of irradiated cultures was slightly
prolonged over that of non-irradiated cells; this
difference is significant in the case of cells exposed
to multiple radiation doses.

Characteristics of Immortalization by SV40-T

Transfection of cells with SV40-T significantly
prolonged their lifespan prior to becoming senescent
or entering a "crisis" phase.  This result is also
shown in Figure 1.  Lifespan was not significantly
altered, however, if the cells were irradiated prior

to transfection.  Prior to crisis, SV40-T transfected cells entered a period of genetic instability marked by the appearance of high frequencies of spontaneous chromosomal aberrations and specific gene mutations, as well as a decline in saturation density and cloning efficiency.  These results are shown in Figures 2 and 3.  As can be seen in Figure 2, a precipitous decline occurred in cloning efficiency and saturation density as the cells reached the crisis phase.  This was associated with a marked increase in the hprt mutant fraction and the frequency of chromosomal aberrations occurring over the 20-30 population doublings prior to crisis (Figure 3).

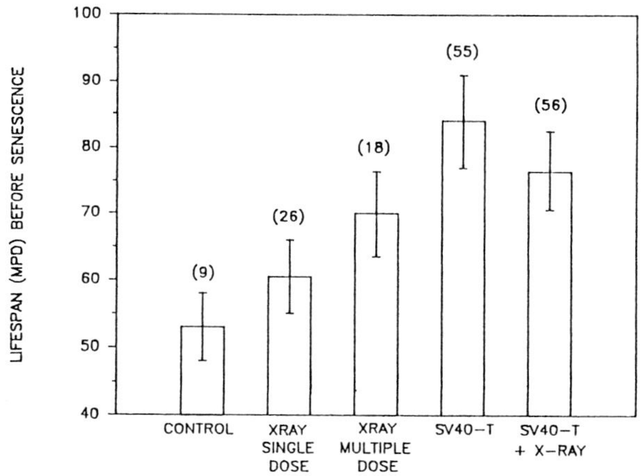


Figure 1.  Lifespan (mean population doublings) from establishment in culture until the cells became senescent or entered crisis for human diploid fibroblast strain AG1522 derived from a newborn foreskin.  Error bars represent one standard deviation of the mean for the number of separate experiments shown in parentheses.  Two experiments in which terminal cell clones emerged with greatly prolonged lifespans (104 and 114 MPD) are not included in the x-ray results shown.  Cultures in the last column were treated with either two doses of 600 rads each at sequential passages, or 100 daily doses of 25 rads each prior to transfection with SV40-T.

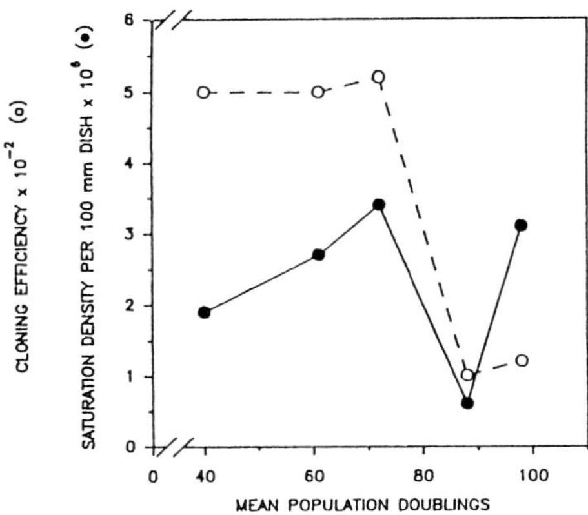


Figure 2. Changes in the cloning efficiency (O) and saturation density at confluence (O) following SV40-T transfection. The cell population in this experiment reached crisis at 88 MPD, after approximately 180 days in culture.

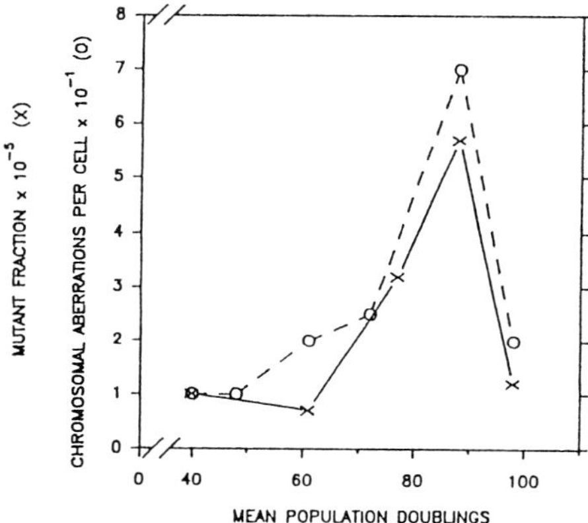


Figure 3. Changes in the hprt mutant fraction (X) and the frequency of gross chromosomal aberrations (O) following SV40-T transfection. These results from the same experiment as those shown in Figure 2. The frequency of mutations and chromosomal aberrations rose progressively during the 20-30 MPD prior to crisis, but fell to background levels in the post-crisis immortalized cell line.

Interestingly, the frequencies of mutations and chromosomal aberrations returned to background levels in the immortalized cell population. Thus, SV40-T transfection appears to prolong the lifespan of human diploid fibroblasts, but this prolongation is associated with the appearance of genetic instability. It is tempting to speculate that this instability characterized by an enhanced frequency of karyotypic changes and specific gene mutations is associated with the emergence of immortalized cell lines during crisis.

During the course of these experiments, we observed that transfection with SV40-T led to a very high frequency of immortalization in two different cell strains each with a partial deletion of the short arm of chromosome 11 (11p14) (6). As is shown in Table 1, 100% of 32 cultures of these two cell lines transfected with SV40-T yielded immortalized cell lines. This compares with a 15% immortalization rate in control cell line AG1522. In addition, however, the 11p deletion cell strains became immortalized with no recognizable crisis phase. These results raise the question whether a gene associated with senescence might be located in this region of chromosome 11.

Table 1. Clonally-derived cultures following SV40-T transfection yielding immortal cell lines.

| Cell strain | Total number cultures | Number immortal-ized | Percent immortal-ized |
|---|---|---|---|
| 1522 (normal) | 48 | 7 | 15% |
| 1522 (normal + x-irradiation) | 56 | 5 | 9% |
| 6938 (11p⁻) | 18 | 18 | 100% |
| 3808 (11p⁻) | 14 | 14 | 100% |

## Other Characteristics of Transformation

Radiation alone induced a dose-dependent increase in the frequency of cells capable of growing under anchorage independent conditions.  However, there was no association between growth in soft agar and the appearance of specific chromosomal abnormalities or longevity.  Neither cells isolated from soft agar colonies nor those which showed an increased lifespan in vitro formed progressively growing, invasive tumors upon injection into nude mice.  Small nodules up to 1 cm in diameter did form in some cases, but these eventually regressed.  When these nodules were excised, and their cells placed into culture, they were diploid, of fibroblastic morphology and senesced rapidly.

Likewise, cells transfected with SV40-T alone were not tumorigenic in nude mice.  This was true for cells tested prior to crisis as well as for post-crisis immortalized cell lines.  Cells transfected with the activated T24 ras oncogene underwent certain morphologic changes including an enhanced frequency of growth in soft agar; however, they did not become immortalized nor was their lifespan significantly prolonged *in vitro*.  The results of preliminary experiments, however, suggest that immortalized cell lines that develop from cultures transfected with activated ras followed by SV40-T transfection may be tumorigenic in nude mice.  These findings suggest that immortalized, tumorigenic cell lines do develop when T-antigen transfection is preceded by transfection with an activated ras oncogene.

## Radiosensitivity of Transfected Cells

There have been sporadic though conflicting reports that transfection with or expression of certain oncogenes may be associated with changes in the radiosensitivity of rodent cells.  In order to test this hypothesis systematically in human cells, experiments were carried out in parallel with those described above to examine the effects of transfection with either SV40-T or activated ras on the sensitivity

of normal diploid fibroblasts.  The results of some of
these experiments are summarized in Figure 4, and will
be described in detail elsewhere.

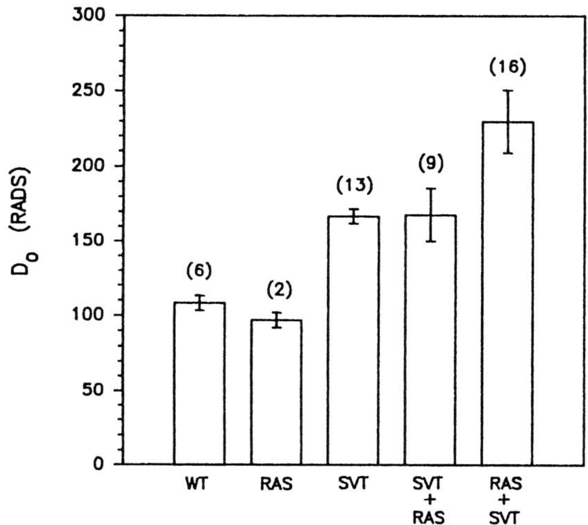


Figure 4.  Radiosensitivity of normal human diploid
fibroblast cell strain AG1522 after transfection with
T24 *ras* or SV40-T.  WT = normal, wild-type cells.
Error bars represent one standard deviation of the
mean of results from the number of clones examined
shown in parenthesis.  Three separate, multi-dose
survival experiments were carried out for each clone.
Radiosensitivity is expressed in terms of the $D_0$
(inverse of the slope of the survival curve), but
other parameters such as the $D_{10}$ showed similar
results.

In these experiments, a number of clonally
derived cell populations were examined for each
treatment condition.  The results shown in Figure 4
represent the mean ± 1 standard deviation of the
results of the indicated number of clones examined. As
can be seen in Figure 4, transfection with activated
T24 ras had no influence on radiosensitivity; a
similar result has been observed in two other strains

of normal human diploid fibroblasts.  SV40-T transfection, however, produced a significant enhancement
in radioresistance in all cell strains examined.  In
strain GM2149 (Figure 4), prior transfection with T24
*ras* further enhanced radioresistance, whereas transfection with ras following SV40-T had no effect.
However, this enhancement by prior transfection with
ras was not a consistent finding in all cell strains
examined.

Resistance to the cytotoxic effects of x-rays
persisted in immortalized cell lines which arose after
SV40-T transfection.  This is in contradistinction to
the findings shown in Figure 3 for chromosomal
aberrations and mutations.  These results suggest that
the change in radiosensitivity following SV40-T
transfection is independent of the transient genetic
instability observed in pre-crisis cells.


## DISCUSSION

Namba and his co-workers (7) reported the
successful immortalization of human diploid
fibroblasts by exposure to multiple doses of x-
irradiation.  However, this was a rare occurrence;
only 2 immortalized cell lines arose in a large series
of experiments.  To our knowledge, this is the only
case in which human diploid cells have been
successfully immortalized by exposure to physical or
chemical carcinogens.  In a total of 46 separate
experiments with human diploid fibroblast strain
AG1522 reported herein, as well as a number of similar
experiments with other cell strains, we have been
unable to induce immortalization by exposure to single
or multiple doses of x-irradiation.  These and other
findings (1) lead us to conclude that immortalization
is a rate-limiting step in transformation of human
diploid cells.

Radiation did induce persistent genetic changes
in surviving cells, characterized by chromosomal
rearrangements which were transmitted to progeny cells
over many generations of replication.  The cells
possessing such rearrangements sometimes gained a

selective growth advantage and emerged as abnormal
clones which included a significant fraction of the
population.  Some abnormal clones showed a markedly
increased lifespan, but none became immortal.
Unstable chromosomal abnormalities, such as rings,
dicentrics and fragments, disappeared rapidly from the
cultures within the first two passages after
irradiation.  Thus, the genetic changes observed
following radiation exposure differed from those seen
in cells transfected with SV40-T.

SV40-T transfected cells showed an increased
lifespan prior to becoming senescent or entering a
crisis phase.  This period was characterized by
genetic instability with high frequencies of
spontaneous unstable chromosomal aberrations and
specific gene mutations.  Immortal cell lines
occasionally emerged from the crisis phase; however,
these cells showed normal levels of aberrations and
mutations.  It is tempting to speculate that this
period of genetic instability facilitated the
generation of several independent events, such as
mutations in specific oncogenes and loss of
heterozygosity at suppressor gene loci, that may be
necessary for the development of immortality.  The
genetic changes produced by irradiation alone appeared
to be rarely if ever sufficient in themselves to
produce the required series of events.  A similar
phenomena of genetic instability was observed by Ray
et al (8) in human diploid fibroblasts transfected
with SV40 T antigen only in a plasmid construct
lacking the small t-antigen and SV40 origin of
replication.  Thus, the T-antigen protein alone is
sufficient to generate the genetic hypervariability
that appears to lead to neoplastic transformation.

It is of interest that cell strains with an 11p
deletion were immortalized with much higher frequency
by SV40-T, with no recognizable crisis phase.  This
finding is of interest in light of the recent report
by Garcia et al (9) that human milk epithelial cells
immortalized by microinjection of SV40 DNA showed a
systematic deletion in the same region of the short
arm of chromosome 11.  This region includes the Ha-ras
and beta-globin genes.  These results suggest that a

locus involved in the control of senescence or in malignant progression of human cells may be located in this region.

SV40-T immortalized cell lines were not tumorigenic in nude mice, whereas preliminary data indicate that cells co-transfected with SV40-T and an activated ras oncogene prior to crisis give rise to tumorigenic cell lines. These findings are consistent with those of a number of investigators indicating that complete transformation *in vitro* indeed requires several distinct events often involving "cooperating" oncogenes, and that cells rendered immortal by transfection with viral sequences can readily be made tumorigenic by exposure to physical or chemical carcinogens or by transfection with known oncogenes.

Finally, the significance of and mechanism for the effect of SV40-T transfection on radiosensitivity remains to be elucidated. It does not appear to be directly related to the genetic instability observed in pre-crisis cells, as enhanced radioresistance persists in immortalized cell lines that emerge following crisis. Neither does it appear to be related to the transfection procedure nor to transformation *per se*. Transfection with an activated *ras* oncogene had no effect on radiosensitivity in three different human diploid fibroblast cell strains. While some human tumor cell lines are very resistant to radiation, there is marked variability in the response of human tumor cells to irradiation, and cells from some tumor types are unusually radiosensitive.

## ACKNOWLEDGEMENTS

Supported by Outstanding Investigator Grant CA-47542, Training Grant CA-09078 and Center Grant ES-00002 from the U.S. National Institutes of Health.

## REFERENCES


1. R. Cox and J.B. Little. In: <u>Advances in Radiation Biology</u>, O.F. Nygaard, W.K. Sinclair and J.T. Lett, eds., Vol. 15, Academic Press, New York, 1991.
2. R.J. Zimmerman and J.B. Little, *Cancer Res.* 43, 2183-2189 (1983).
3. J.J. McCormick and V.M. Maher, *Mutation Res.* 199, 273 (1988).
4. Y. Kano and J.B. Little, *Cancer Res.* 45, 2550-2555 (1985).
5. Y. Kano and J.B. Little, *Int. J. Cancer* 36, 407-413 (1985).
6. Y. Kano and J.B. Little, *Molecular Carcinogenesis* 2, 314-321 (1989).
7. M. Namba, K. Hyodoh, et al., *Int. J. Cancer* 35, 275-280 (1985).
8. F.A. Ray, D.S. Peabody, et al., *J. Cell Biochem.* 42, 13-31 (1990).
9. I. Garcia, D. Brandt, et al., *Cancer Res.* 51, 294-300 (1991).


From: *Neoplastic Transformation in Human Cell Culture,*
Eds.: J. S. Rhim and A. Dritschilo ©1991 The Humana Press Inc., Totowa, NJ

# IONIZING RADIATION-MEDIATED PROTEIN KINASE C ACTIVATION AND GENE EXPRESSION


Dennis E. Hallahan, Matthew L. Sherman, Donald Kufe and Ralph R. Weichselbaum

Department of Radiation and Cellular Oncology, University of Chicago and Pritzker School of Medicine, Chicago, IL 60637 and Laboratory of Clinical Pharmacology, Dana-Farber Cancer Institute, Boston, MA 02115



Work supported by NCI Grant CA41068


## ABSTRACT


Ionizing radiation-induced neoplastic transformation is postulated to occur as a consequence of an initial common event followed by a rare second event. Genes encoding transcription factors are expressed immediately after x-ray exposure in the absence of de novo protein synthesis. c-*jun*, c-*fos* and Egr-1 are expressed following irradiation of human normal tissue cells and tumor cell lines. Radiation-mediated expression of these immediate early genes is attenuated by protein kinase inhibitors and abrogated when protein kinase C (PKC) is down regulated or when PKC-mediated signal transduction is deficient. PKC is the target for the tumor promoter phorbol esters. This enzyme has been implicated to play a role in neoplastic transformation and in cellular proliferation following mitogenic stimulation. PKC is also, activated rapidly following ionizing radiation exposure. Radiation-mediated PKC activation and immediate early gene induction may represent initial common events which are then followed by rare presumably mutational processes which result in neoplastic transformation. The potential importance of this finding is demonstrated by the recent report that PKC inhibitors partially suppress neoplastic transformation following x-irradiation. The production of growth factors and cytokines within irradiated tissues may also contribute to tumor promotion or progression. This discussion addresses the molecular processes that occur within a cell following x-irradiation and their potential role in neoplastic transformation.

# INTRODUCTION

Neoplastic transformation induced by ionizing radiation or chemical agents is a progressive, multistage process.  Normal cells acquire the phenotypic characteristics of malignant cells through at least three discernable stages of neoplastic transformation (initiation, promotion and progression) which occur over an extended latent period.  An initiating agent is defined as a chemical, physical or biological agent  that can directly and irreversibly alter the native molecular  structure of DNA (1) (reviewed in (2)).  Promoting agents alter the expression of genetic information of the cell but do not necessarily react directly with the DNA.  Most known carcinogenic agents, including ionizing radiation, can both initiate and promote neoplastic transformation and are therefore termed "complete carcinogens".  Little et. al have demonstrated that ionizing radiation causes an initial common event followed by a second rare event resulting in neoplastic transformation (reviewed in (3)).  Radiation- induced neoplastic transformation is thought to be related to DNA damage.  However, the molecular processes and sequence of events preceding tumor promotion following ionizing radiation exposure are presently unknown.

## Protein Kinase C Activation by Ionizing Radiation

PKC-mediated signal transduction from cell surface receptors to the nucleus participates in the cellular response to external stimuli such as serum and growth factors (4) (5).  One of the initial steps in this process is receptor-mediated activation of phospholipase C  which results in the hydrolysis of membrane phospholipids to diacylglycerol and inisitol triphosphate (IP3) (Figure 1) (5) (6).  Diacylglycerol (DAG) may also be formed by hydrolysis of phosphatidyl-choline and subsequently activates members of the phospholipid-dependent, serine/threonine-specific protein kinases C (PKC) family (4).  IP3, in turn, initiates calcium release from intracellular stores.  PKC plays a pivotal role in the regulation of the molecular response to growth factors and mitogens which controls cell proliferation and differentiation (7) (8).  The participation of PKC in radiation-mediated gene induction has been suggested in recent studies. Down-regulation of PKC following prolonged TPA stimulation or PKC inhibition each result in attenuation of x-ray-mediated expression of transcription factor genes jun/AP-1 and Egr-1/zif-268 (9).  In addition, x-ray-mediated transcriptional activation of the long terminal repeat of the Maloney murine sarcoma virus is also abrogated by these approaches (10). To determine directly whether PKC is activated by ionizing radiation, we measured the phosphorylation capacity of PKC in gamma- irradiated human tumor cell lines.  The  synthetic peptide, Gln-Lys-Arg-Pro-Ser(8)-

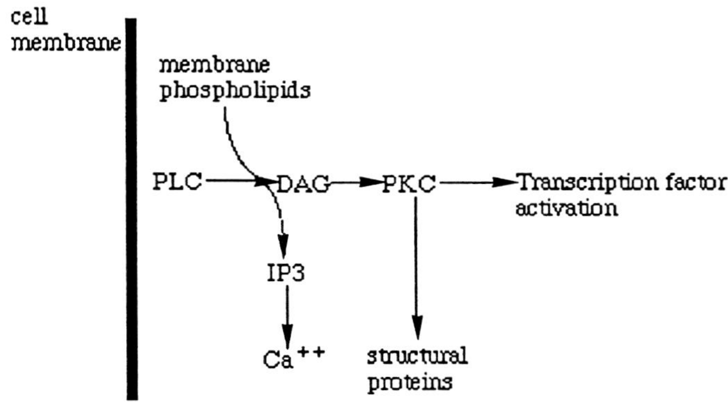


**Figure 1.** The protein kinase C (PKC) mediated signal transduction pathway.

Gln-Arg-Ser-Lys-Tyr-Leu  which is the major site of PKC phosphorylation on myelin basic protein,  has been shown to be a specific substrate for PKC (11) (12).   We utilized this substrate for in vitro assaysof the phosphorylation capacity of PKC.   HL-60 cells were pelleted and irradiated with 20 Gy (320 cGy/sec) and total cellular protein was extracted at 15 second intervals. The  increase in PKC activity  in gamma-irradiated cells was compared to control cells treated under otherwise identical conditions.  The first protein extraction, performed 15  seconds following gamma- irradiation, was found to have PKC activity which was 4.5 fold greater than that of control, while peak PKC activity was 4.7 fold greater at 30 seconds and returned to basal levels by 60 seconds (13).   To further document the participation of this enzyme in the cellular response to ionizing radiation, we analyzed protein phosphorylation using two-dimensional gel electrophoresis (13).   The 80kD "MARCKS" protein which is thought to be a PKC specific substrate (14) was phosphorylated at 45 seconds following gamma-irradiation and the phosphorylation returned to basal levels at 60 seconds.   Thus in vivo phosphorylation of a PKC specific substrate occurs during peak enzymatic activity.

## Proposed  mechanisms  of  PKC  activation  by  ionizing  radiation

In mammalian cells, DNA damage initiates the UV-response which can be modified by the addition of protein kinase inhibitors.   These findings have implicated a reverse signal transduction pathway (10)(15).   This may involve nuclear  signals which are  activated following  DNA damage and then

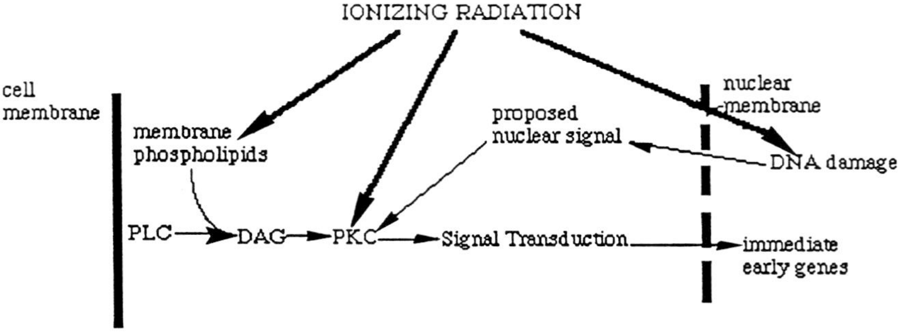


**Figure 2.** Proposed mechanisms of PKC activation by ionizing radiation include oxidation of membrane phospholipids, PKC itself, and/or reverse signal transduction from the nucleus following DNA damage.

transduced to the cytoplasm (Figure 2).  DNA damage may also be an initiating event during radiation-mediated PKC activation.  Alternative mechanisms may involve oxidation of cellular components other than DNA. In this context, ionizing radiation causes free radical production and subsequent oxidative damage within the cell  (16) (17).  Highly reactive hydroxyl radicals produced within the irradiated cell can cause lipid peroxidation  (16) (17) and therefore, one potential mechanism of PKC activation by ionizing radiation  may involve degradation products of oxidized membrane phospholipids (Figure 2).  These phospholipids are hydrolyzed to form fatty acid byproducts such as arachidonate, diacylglycerol and inositol triphosphate (18).  Alternatively,  oxidation of sulfhydryl groups within the regulatory domain of PKC has been proposed as a mechanism of PKC activation by superoxide (19).  Therefore,  potential mechanisms of PKC activation by x-rays include  direct activation of the enzyme following oxidation, or through second messengers originating in the cell membrane, cytoplasm or nucleus.

### Signal Transduction in Mammalian Cells Following Ionizing Radiation Exposure.

Activation of PKC by ionizing radiation may lead to phosphorylation of cytoplasmic proteins which subsequently enter the nucleus to initiate

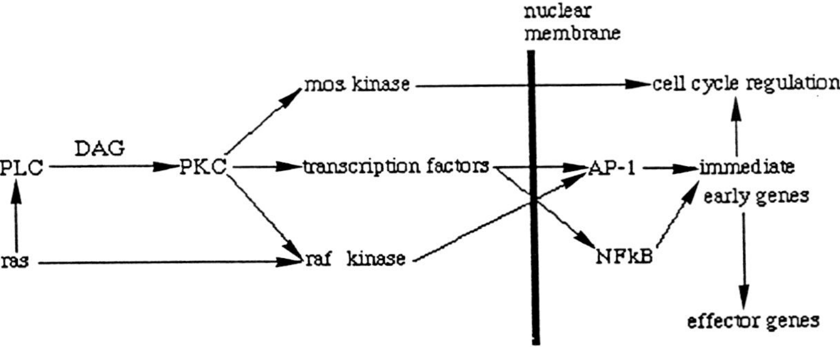


**Figure 3.** Protein kinase C-mediated signal transduction results in cell cycle regulation and transcription of effector genes such as cytokines and growth factors

transcription. Recent studies have demonstrated a 40-kD DNA binding protein which is located within the cytoplasm of untreated cells and is translocated into the nucleus of lymphoblastoid cells following x-irradiation. The activated protein binds to the enhancer region of simian virus 40 (20). Further support for activation of a PKC-dependent pathway by ionizing radiation is the recent observation that PKC inhibition and down-regulation result in attenuation of x-ray-mediated expression of immediate early genes jun/AP-1 and Egr-1/zif-268 (9). In addition, x-ray-mediated transcriptional activation of the long terminal repeat of the Maloney murine sarcoma virus is also abrogated by these approaches (10). This proposed mechanism of signal transduction is analogous to that observed following TPA-induced activation of NF-kB in human lymphoblasts (21). NF-kB is located in the cytoplasm in an inactivate form bound to IkB. IkB is phosphorylated by PKC and NF-kB is translocated into the nucleus to initiate transcription (Figure 3). The activation of NF-kB following DNA damage by UV-irradiation is abrogated by protein kinase inhibitors but not inhibitors of protein synthesis (15). Moreover, we have found that NF-kB is activated in cells exposed to ionizing radiation (unpublished observation). Further evidence supporting cytoplasmic activation of transcription factors is demonstrated by the posttranslational modification of cytoplasmic Jun and Fos which results in translocation into the nucleus. These factors then activate AP-1 sites in promoter regions (Figure 3). The signal transduction pathway initiated following x-ray-mediated activation of PKC may thus involve posttranslational modification and activation of transcription factors.

PKC activates the gene products of raf and mos protooncogenes (22). Raf kinase activity is associated with tumor promotion induced by TPA. These findings have implicated raf in the PKC-mediated signal transduction pathway (23) (Figure 3). The *c-mos* gene product has also been recently found to act as a signal transducer in the PKC pathway (24) (Figure 3). Moreover, ras transformants have recently been demonstrated to have elevated PKC levels (25). PKC expression is also increased following x-irradiation (26). Of potential relevance is the finding that elevated expression of this enzyme increases susceptibility to neoplastic transformation after ras transfection (27). X-ray-mediated signal transduction may therefore participate in signal transduction pathways that include the products of the ras, mos and raf protooncogenes (Figure 3). Moreover, x-ray mediated PKC gene expression may lead to increased frequency of neoplastic transformation.

## Radiation-Mediated Immediate Early Gene Expression

Several families of genes which encode transcription factors are rapidly and transiently expressed following mitogenic stimulation. These include the jun, fos and Egr-1/zif268 gene families. To determine whether these families of growth related genes are expressed following ionizing radiation exposure, we analyzed RNA from irradiated human fibroblasts, myeloid leukemia and epithelial tumor cell lines for the expression of c-jun, Egr-1 and c-fos. We found that each of these transcription factors is induced by ionizing radiation (28), (9). The increase in c-jun transcripts by ionizing radiation was time- and dose-dependent as determined by Northern blot analysis. Transcriptional run-on analysis demonstrated that ionizing radiation increases the rate of c-jun gene transcription in myeloid cell lines. Furthermore, the half-life of c-jun RNA was prolonged in the absence of protein synthesis. These findings indicate that the increase in c-jun RNA observed after x-irradiation is regulated by transcriptional and post-transcriptional mechanisms. Ionizing radiation also increases levels of c-fos transcripts as well as that of jun-B (another member of the jun family) in myeloid cell lines.

We also irradiated the human epithelial tumor cell line SQ-20B, normal human fibroblasts (AG1522) and the virally transformed human kidney epithelial cell line 293 to determine whether the Egr-1, and c-jun genes participate in the response of various cell types to radiation (9). These cell lines have low but detectable levels of Egr-1 and c-jun transcripts prior to stimulation. A time-dependent increase in Egr-1 and c-jun mRNA levels was detected at 3 to 6 hours after irradition of AG1522 and 293 cells. In contrast,

SQ-20B cells demonstrated increased Egr-1 and c-jun expression within 30 minutes after x-irradiation and declined to baseline within 3 hours. Egr-1 expression increased in a dose dependent manner. Levels were low but detectable after 3 and 5 Gy and increased after 10 to 20 Gy. To determine whether Egr-1 and c-jun participate as immediate early genes after x-irradiation, the effects of protein synthesis inhibition were studied in cell lines 293 and SQ-20B. Cells pretreated with cycloheximide and then x-rays demonstrated superinduction of Egr-1 and c-jun mRNA. These findings indicate that de novo protein synthesis is not required for induction of these genes.

PKC is down-regulated when cells are stimulated with micromolar concentrations of phorbol esters for 24 hours (29). Radiation-mediated Egr-1 and c-jun expression was attenuated in cells following prolonged TPA stimulation. Although these findings suggested that PKC may be involved in the induction of gene expression by x-rays, other studies were performed with the isoquinoline sulfonamide inhibitors of protein kinases. H7 is a potent inhibitor of both PKC and the cyclic nucleotide dependent protein kinases (PKA and PKG), whereas HA1004 is a more selective inhibitor of PKA and PKG and has much less affinity for PKC (30)(31). Cells pretreated with H7 had no detectable radiation-mediated Egr-1 and c-jun expression (Figure 3) (9). In contrast, HA1004, had no effect on radiation-induced immediate early gene expression. These data support the notion that PKC dependent signal transduction is required for radiation-mediated Egr-1 and c-jun induction.

*c-jun* is expressed during cell transition from $G_0$ to $G_1$ following mitogenic stimulation (32) and is transcriptionally induced following stimulation with TPA (33-35). Tumor promotion has been associated with expression of the *c-jun* protooncogene (33, 35, 36). Moreover, *c-jun* may play an essential role in neoplastic transformation in other cells (37). In this context, a defect in TPA-induced c-jun expression results in a promotion-resistant variant of JB6 mouse epidermal cells which fail to become tumorigenic following stimulation by this tumor promoter. Taken together, these findings indicate that expression of the *c-jun* gene is requiredfor neoplastic transformation in some cell lines following stimulation by tumor promoters.

## Radiation-mediated immediate early gene induction may be an initial common event preceding x-ray induced neoplastic transformation.

Radiation-mediated *c-jun* expression is in part dependent upon PKC activation. PKC dependent activation of *cis*-regulatory elements in the c-*jun* promoter has been demonstrated during stimulation with TPA (38). Moreover, *c-jun* transcription is positively autoregulated by it's own product Jun/AP-1 (38). Positive autoregulation may result in sustained stimulation.

Therefore, we hypothesize that PKC-mediated *c-jun* activation following ionizing radiation exposure may represent an initial common event during radiation-induced neoplastic transformation.  In this regard, Borek et al. have shown that PKC inhibitors suppress x-ray induced transformation (39).  Therefore, c-jun induction following x-ray-induced activation of PKC may represent an early common event preceding radiation-induced neoplastic transformation.

Recent studies have demonstrated an association between protein kinase C and cell cycle regulation.  PKC deficient yeast mutants are unable to exit from G2 to M suggesting a PKC requirement for this transition (40).  Furthermore, the PKC inhibitor staurosporin produces a G2 block in mammalian cells (41) (42).  In addition to these findings, PKC-mediated signal transduction results in the transcriptional induction of immediate early genes Egr-1 and c-*jun* (43).  These genes are expressed during the G1/S phase transition.  Under physiologic conditions, these processes may lead to cellular proliferation.  However, they may also contribute to carcinogenesis following persistant gene expression or if mutagenic damage is "fixed" during progression through the cell cycle.  Thus transcription factor activation may represent an initial common event preceding radiation-induced neoplastic transformation.  However, a second rare event may  involve mutations which inactivate tumor suppressor genes such as p53 and the retinoblastoma susceptibility gene (Rb) or which activate "dominant" oncogenes such as ras which are known to be associated with radiation carcinogenesis when mutated (44).

## The role of growth factors and cytokines in x-ray-mediated tumor progression

One consequence of PKC activation by x-rays is radiation-mediated tumor necrosis factor-alpha (TNF) gene expression.    The level of TNF in the medium from irradiated cells is elevated over that of nonirradiated cells when analyzed by  ELISA (45).  Several sarcoma cell lines demon-strated this increase,while human fibroblasts and epithelial tumor cell lines did not.  Moreover, a monoclonal antibody to TNF reversed the cytotoxic effects of the medium from irradiated cells.  Increased levels of TNF mRNA were detected in sarcoma cell lines STSAR-13 and STSAR-48 at 3 to 6 hours after exposure to 500 cGy as compared to unirradiated controls.  We have further demonstrated that radiation-induced TNF transcription  is not specific for sarcomas, since TNF expression is increased in HL-60 (human promyelo-cytic leukemia) and U-937 (human monocytic leukemia) cell lines  exposed to ionizing radiation (46).  Radiation-mediated TNF expression in  HL-60 cells is diminished by pretreatment with protein kinase inhibitors and down-regulation of PKC by prolonged TPA treatment.    Consistent with these results, no detectable induction of TNF expression is observed following x-irradiation in the HL-60 variant deficient in PKC-mediated signal transduction.  TNF acts to stimulate growth in fibroblasts suggesting the potential for tumor progression in these tissues.  TNF is also cytotoxic to some cell types.  The cytotoxicity produced by TNF is associated with the production of free radicals and DNA fragmentation which may initiate neoplastic transformation .

Fibroblast growth factor (FGF) and platelet derived growth factor (PDGF) are produced by endothelial cells following irradiation (47).  In addition to growth promotion within irradiated tissues, these growth factors may also induce angiogenesis required for tumor growth.  The resulting induction of proliferation may participate in tumor progression.  Thus a diverse system of protooncogenes and growth factors allow for tissue regeneration after radiation injury under physiologic conditions.  However, these processes  may also contribute to neoplastic transformation.


## SUMMARY

Ionizing radiation is a complete carcinogen since both initiation and promotion of neoplastic transformation occur following x-irradiation.  The finding that radiation exposure is associated with activation of protein kinase C and induction of c-jun protooncogene expression has suggested that these events may contribute to x-ray-induced carcinogenesis.  The time course of enzymatic activation and gene induction following ionizing radiation exposure is illustrated in Figure 4.   These early processes could contribute to late events such as carcinogenesis.  In this context, PKC inhibitors have been shown to attenuate radiation-induced neoplastic transformation (39).  Promotion may involve genes which are associated with cellular proliferation and are expressed following x-irradiation such as jun, Egr-1 and PKC.  Consistant with this model is that ionizing radiation is a complete carcinogen since both initiation and promotion occur during radiation-induced neoplastic trans-formation.  Furthermore, the induction of growth factor and cytokine gene expression by ionizing radiation may contribute to the process of tumor promotion.  Radiation therefore activates a complex of molecular pathways which may interact to result in neoplastic transformation.

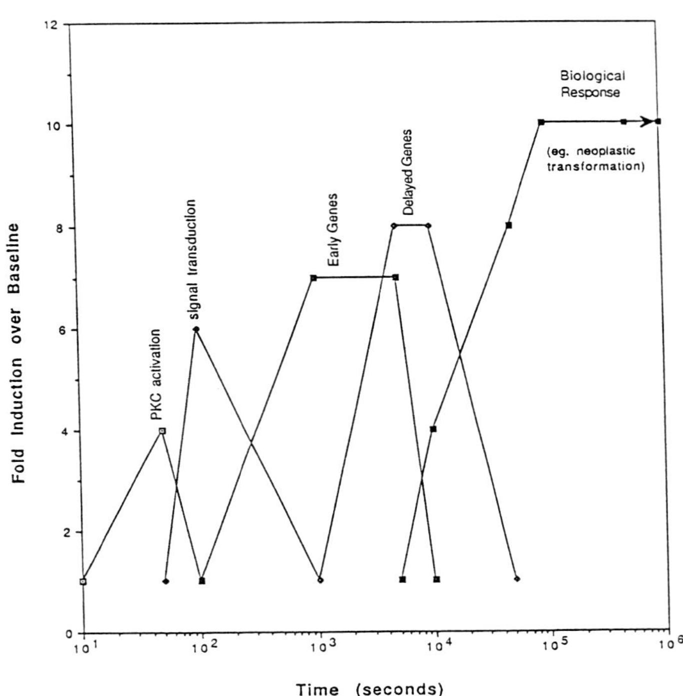



**Figure 4.** Ionizing radiation causes the activation of protein kinase C (PKC) which initializes signal transduction and gene expression.

# Reference


1.  Boutwell, R. K. *Crit. Rev. Toxicol.* 2: 419 (1974).
2.  Pitot, H. C., *Principles of cancer biology: Chemical carcinogenesis* Lippincott, Philadelphia, (1989).
3.  Little, J. B., *Cancer Etiology: Ionizing Radiation* Lea and Febiger, Malvern, PA, (1991).
4.  Nishizuka, Y. *J. Natl Cancer Inst.* 76: 363 (1986).
5.  Kikkawa, U., Nishizuka, Y. *Ann. Rev. Cell. Biol.* 2: 149 (1986).
6.  Hokin, L. E. *Annu. Rev. Biochem.* 54: 205 (1985).

7.   Horiguchi, J., Spriggs, D., Immamura, K., *et al. Mol. Cell. Biol.* 9: 252 (1989).

8.   Rozengurt, E., Rodriguez-Pena, A., Coombs, M., *et al. Proc. Natl. Acad. Sci. USA.* 81: 5748 (1984).

9.   Hallahan, D. E., Sukhatme, V. P., Sherman, M. L., *et al. Proc. Nat'l Acad. Sci.* 88: 2152 (1991).

10.  Lin, C. S., Goldthwaite, D. A., Samuels, D. *Proc. Natl. Acad. Sci. USA.* 87: 36 (1990).

11.  Yasuda, I., Kishimoto, A., Tanaka, S.-I., *et al. Biochem. and Biophys Res Comm.* 166: 1220 (1990).

12.  Kishimoto, A., Takai, Y., Mori, T., *et al. J. Biol. Chem.* 255: 2273 (1980).

13.  Hallahan, D., Virudachalam, S., Sherman, M., *et al.* Submitted: (1991).

14.  Stumpo, D. J., Graff, J. M., Albert, K. A., *et al. Proc. Natl. Acad. Sci USA.* 86: 4012 (1989).

15.  Stein, B., Rahmsdorf, H. J., Steffen, A., *et al. Mol. Cell Biol.* 9: 5169 (1989).

16.  O'Brian, C. A., Ward, N. E., Weinstein, B., *et al. Biochem. and Biophys Res Comm.* 155: 1374 (1988).

17.  Strassle, M., Stark, G., Wilhelm, M. *Int. J. Radiat. Biol.* 51: 265 (1987).

18.  Blakeborough, M. H., Owen, R. W., Bilton, R. F. *Free Rad. Res. Comms.* 6: 359 (1989).

19.  Larsson, R., Cerutti, P. *Cancer Research.* 49: 5627 (1989).

20.  Singh, S. P., Lavin, M. F. *Molec Cell Biol.* 10: 5279 (1990).

21.  Ghosh, S., Baltimore, D. *Nature.* 344: 678 (1990).

22.  Morrison, D. K., Kaplan, D. R., Rapp, U., *et al. Proc. Natl Acad Sci.* 85: 8855 (1988).

23.  Kolch, W., Heidecker, G., Lloyd, P., *et al. Nature.* 349: 426 (1991).

24.  Al-Bagdadi, F., Singh, B., Arlinghaus, R. B. *Oncogene.* 5: 1251 (1990).

25.  Borner, C., Weinstein, I. B. *Cell Growth Diff.* 1: 653 (1990).

26.  Woloschak, G., Chang-Liu, C., Shearin-Jones, P. *Cancer Research.* 50: 3963 (1990).

27.  Hsiao, W. L., Housey, G. M., Johnson, M. D., *et al. Molec Cell. Biol.* 9: 2641 (1989).

28.  Sherman, M. L., Datta, R., Hallahan, D. E., *et al. Proc. Natl. Acad. Sci.* 87: 5663 (1990).

29.  Rodriguez-Pena, A., Rozengurt, E. *Biochem. Biophys. Res. Comm.* 120: 1053 (1984).

30.  Hidaka, H., Inagaki, M., Kawamoto, S., *et al. Biochemistry.* 23: 5036 (1984).

31.  Asano, T., Hidaka, H. *Pharm. Exper. Therap.* 231: 141 (1984).

32. Ryseck, R.-P., Harai, S. I., Yaniv, M., *et al. Nature (London)*. 334: 535 (1988).
33. Bohmann, D., Bos, T. J., Admon, A., *et al. Science.* 238: 1386 (1987).
34. Lamph, W. W., Wamsley, P., Sassone-Corsi, P., *et al. Nature (London)*. 334: 629 (1988).
35. Angel, P., Allegretto, E. A., Okino, S. T., *et al. Nature.* 332: 166 (1988).
36. Sakai, M., Okuda, A., Hatayama, I., *et al. Cancer Research.* 49: 5633 (1989).
37. Bernstein, L. R., Colburn, N. H. *Science.* 244: 566 (1989).
38. Angel, P., Hattori, K., Smeal, T., *et al. Cell.* 55: 875 (1988).
39. Borek, C., Ong, A., Stevens, V., *et al. Proc Natl Acad Sci, USA.* 88: 1953 (1991).
40. Toda, T., Shimanuki, M., Yanagida, M. *Genes Devel.* 5: 60 (1991).
41. Abe, K., Yoshida, M., Usui, T., *et al. Exp. Cell. Res.* 192: 122 (1991).
42. Matsumoto, H., Sasaki, Y. *Biochem. Biophys. Res. Commun.* 158: 105 (1989).
43. Sukhatme, V. P. *J. Am. Soc. Nephrol.* 1: 859 (1990).
44. Sloan, S. R., Newcomb, E. W., Pellicer, A. *Mol. Cell. Biol.* 10: 405 (1990).
45. Hallahan, D. E., Spriggs, D. R., Beckett, M. A., *et al. Proc Natl Acad Sci U S A.* 86: 10104 (1989).
46. Sherman, M. L., Datta, R., Hallahan, D., *et al. J. Clin. Invest.* In press: (1991).
47. Witte, L., Fuks, Z., Haimovits-Friedman, A., *et al. Cancer Res.* 49: 5066 (1989).

# DETECTION OF TRANSFORMING GENES FROM RADIATION TRANSFORMED HUMAN EPIDERMAL KERATINOCYTES BY A TUMORIGENICITY ASSAY


P. Thraves, S. Reynolds, Z. Salehi, W. K. Kim,
J. H. Yang, J. S. Rhim, and A. Dritschilo
Georgetown University School of Medicine,
Washington, D.C. 20007; NIEHS, Research Triangle
Park, NC 27709; Laboratory of Cellular & Molecular
Biology, NCI, Bethesda, MD 20892


Carcinogenic action of ionizing radiation in humans has been well recognized from epidemiological data. There have been, however, very few studies on radiation-induced neoplastic transformation of human cells, particularly, those of epithelial origin, in culture. Recently, we have developed an *in vitro* human keratinocyte multistep model suitable for the study of human epithelial cell carcino-genesis (1). This was developed following an infection of primary human epidermal keratinocytes with Ad12-SV40 virus leading to the acquisition of an indefinite lifespan in culture, but not the development of malignant phenotype. These immortalized human keratinocytes (RHEK-1) when treated subsequently with either Kirsten murine sarcoma virus (Ki-MSV) (1) or chemical carcinogens, (2) led to the induction of morphological alterations and the development of a malignancy. The availability of this human keratinocyte system led us to determine the potential of X-rays as a carcinogenic agent in human epithelial cells and to characterize the molecular events involved in the development of a radiation-induced malignancy.

We have recently shown that nontumorigenic RHEK-1 cells can be transformed by exposure to x-ray irradiation (3). Such transformants showed morphological alterations, formation of colonies in soft agar, and induced carcinoma when transplanted into nude mice, whereas primary human epidermal keratinocytes exposed to radiation in this manner failed to shown any evidence of transformation. These findings demonstrate the malignant transformation of

human primary epithelial cells in culture by the combined
action of a DNA tumor virus and radiation, indicating a
multistep process for radiation-induced neoplastic
conversion (3).

### *Ras oncogenes were not activated in the radiation-transformed RHEK-1 cell lines.*

Since RHEK-1 cells could be transformed by Ki-MSV
infection and become tumorigenic (1), we analyzed the *ras*
oncogene products in the radiation-transformed as well as
KiMSV-transformed RHEK-1 cells using antibody to p21
protein and SDS-PAGE. In comparison to the KIMSV
transformed RHEK-1 cells, the radiation transformed
keratinocytes showed neither altered mobility or increased
expression of the p21 protein (3). This observation
indicated that the activation of a *ras* gene was not
involved in the radiation-induced transformation of
immortalized human epidermal keratinocytes.

While the activation of cellular *ras* oncogenes has
been demonstrated in rodent tumors induced by ionizing
radiation (4, 5), the activation of unique non-*ras*
oncogenes has been shown in malignant radiogenic
transformed rodent cells (6). The reproducible neoplastic
transformation of the RHEK-1 human epithelial cell line by
x-ray irradiation suggests that cellular oncogenes may be
activated as part of the process. Our evidence further
indicates that *ras* oncogenes, which have been commonly
implicated in radiation-induced animal tumors (4-5) and
spontaneous human tumors (7), were not activated in the
transformation. Thus, this system may be useful in
efforts to detect and characterize other cellular genes
that can contribute to the neoplastic phenotype of human
epithelial cells.

### *Isolation of dominant human sequences from radiation transformed RHEK-1 cells by a tumorigenicity assay.*

As we described (3), we have been unsuccessful in
isolating human sequences using the NIH/3T3-focus
formation assay. Since the majority of tumor DNAs fail to
induce transformed foci in the NIH/3T3 focus formation
assay (8, 9, 10), probably due to this system having a
bias for *ras* genes containing structural mutations, an
alternative assay was required. We have used as an
alternative the NIH 3T3 DNA transfection-nude mouse

tumorigenicity assay as previously described by Fasano *et al.* (11). This approach has been shown to be more sensitive than the NIH/3T3 focus assay for detecting transforming genes (12, 13, 14).

This system is a modification of the one described by Blair *et al.* (13). It relies on the ability of transformed NIH/3T3 cells to form tumors in nude mice, but also incorporates the use of a co-transfection with a selectable marker to increase the sensitivity (15). More recently, Yuasa *et al.*, using this tumorigenicity assay, have been able to isolate transforming genes from the cells of patients with familial adenomatous polyposis (16).

*Primary transfection.* The DNA from the RHEK-1 unirradiated-nontumorigenic cells gave rise to a single small tumor after 11 weeks which proved not to contain human Alu sequences when analyzed by restriction enzyme digestion and Southern-blot analysis. The DNA from the isolated clonal transformants (RHEK-1/200R C1.5 and RHEK/400R C1.10) each gave rise to two slow growing large tumors, 9 and 11 weeks, respectively.

These four tumors were then re-established as cell lines, DNA was isolated from them and then analyzed for the presence of human Alu-sequences. One of the RHEK-1/200R C1.5 derived primary tumors and both RHEK-1/400R C1.10 primary tumors proved positive for human Alu sequences. These DNAs isolated from these primary mouse tumors were then used to transform the recipient cells again, to demonstrate that the transforming potential could be transmitted serially.

*Secondary transfection.* Both Alu positive primary nude mouse tumor DNAs derived from RHEK-1/400R C1. 10 retransmitted the transforming potential with a much higher frequency and shorter latency period. The single Alu-positive primary nude mouse tumor DNA derived from RHEK-1/200R C1.5 retransmitted its tumorigenic potential with a moderate frequency and latency period (Table 1). We have subsequently established NIH/3T3 cell lines from these nude mouse tumors as a source of DNA for the molecular analysis of the transforming genes.

## Table 1. Secondary Transfection

| Donor DNA | Tumor/<br>Injection Sites | Tumor Latency |
|---|---|---|
| NIH/3T3<br>(- control) | 2/8<br>(very small tumors) | 10 weeks |
| Human T24<br>(+ control) | 8/8<br>(large tumors) | 3 weeks |
| PNMT -3<br>(RHEK 200R C1.5) | 3/8<br>(large to intermediate<br>tumors) | 7 weeks |
| PNMT -2<br>(RHEK 400R C1.10) | 8/8<br>(very large tumors) | 5 weeks |
| PNMT-7<br>(RHEK 400R C1.10) | 6/8<br>(very large tumors) | 5 weeks |

PNMT = primary nude mouse tumor


### *Preliminary molecular characterization of transforming human sequences.*

The fact that human sequences can be serially transmitted in the NIH/3T3-nude mouse assay demonstrates that there are dominant transforming human sequences in the tumorigenic clones derived from the radiation treated RHEK-1 cells. The next phase of the study was to characterize the human sequences in order to answer the following questions.

What are the sizes and frequency of these sequences? Are these transforming sequences related to any known proto-oncogene?

Following the successful testing for tumorigenicity (Table 1), two of the secondary mouse tumors from each group, PNMT-2 and PNMT-7, and three from group PNMT-3 were re-established as mouse fibroblasts lines in culture. The two cell lines derived from the PNMT-2 group tumors were designated 49-7A and 49-7G, while the two cell lines from group PNMT-7 were designated 49-7B and 49-7D. The three cell lines from group PNMT-3 were designated 49-8C, 49-8E, and 49-8F. The seven cell lines were then grown and their genomic DNA was isolated. The DNAs from these cell lines were subsequently analyzed for the presence of Alu positive sequences (Fig. 1). The subsequent autoradiographic analysis revealed that the secondary nude mouse tumors 49-7A and 49-7G (Lanes 4 and 5) and their respective cell lines **49-7A** and **49-7G** (Lanes 11 and 12) contain strongly Alu-positive bands. The other tumors and cell lines gave weakly positive Alu bands which could only be visualized by prolonged exposure of the autoradiogram.

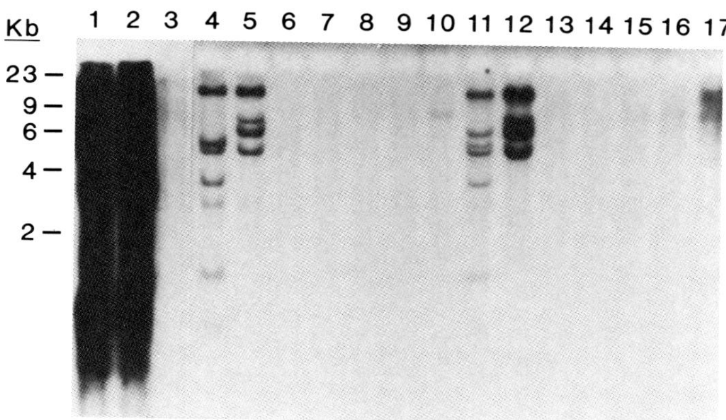

FIGURE 1: Twenty micrograms of genomic DNA were digested with restriction endonuclease EcoRI (5/µg DNA) and the digestion products electrophoresis on a 1% agarose gel. Following Southern blotting onto nylon, the blots were probe with $^{32}$P-labeled BLUR-8 probe. Lane 1, RHEK-1/200R, soft agar clones #5; Lane 2, RHEK-1/400/soft agar clone #10; Lane 3, NIH/3T3 mouse fibroblast DNA; Lanes 4-10, Secondary nude mouse tumor DNAs, 49-7A, 49-7G, 49-8C, 49-8E, 49-8F, 49-9B, 49-9D, respectively. Lanes 11-17, mouse fibroblast cell line established from 49-7A, 49-7G, 49-8C, 49-8E, 49-8F, 49-9B, and 49-9D, respectively.

A subsequent study, in which these two cell lines, 49-7A and 49-7G, were digested with either EcoRI or BamHI restriction endonuclease, provided more information of the molecular sizes of these human sequences. In particular, a restriction enzyme analysis of nude mouse tumor DNA, 49-7G, with EcoRI yielded four strongly Alu positive bands with approximate molecular weights of 20, 8, 6, and 5Kb, Lane 3 (Fig. 2). This same analysis demonstrated that there were two common bands in both the EcoRI and BamHI digests of the 49-7G DNA. These two common bands had

molecular weights of about 20 and 8Kb, respectively, Lanes
3 and 4.

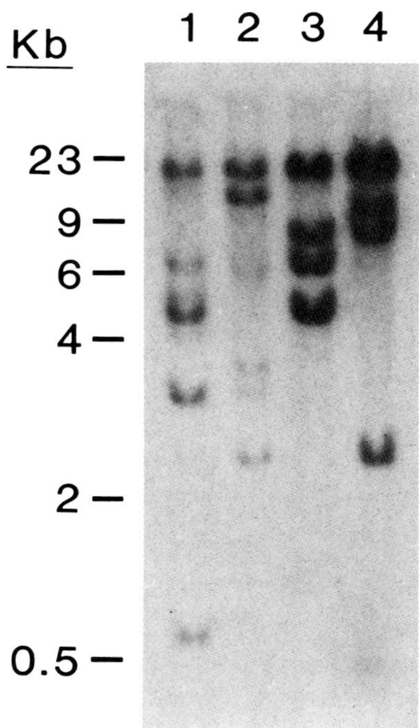


FIGURE 2: Twenty micrograms of genomic DNA from secondary
nude mouse tumor DNAs, 49-7A and 49-7G, were digested with
restriction endonucleases EcoRI and BamHI both at 5
units/μg DNA; Lanes 1 and 2, 49-7A, digested with EcoRI
and BamHI, respectively; Lanes 3 and 4, 49-7G digested
with EcoRI and BamHI, respectively. Following digestion,
the products were electrophoresed on a 1% agarose gel,
blotted onto nylon, and probed with 32-labeled BLUR-8
probe.


We have attempted to identify the transforming
sequences we have isolated to determine if they have any
homology with any of the known proto-oncogenes associated
with epithelial cell transformation or radiation-induced
transformation *in vitro* or *in vivo*.

Our approach has involved the digestion of the genomic DNA from the secondary mouse tumor (49-7G), which contains the human sequences, with the restriction enzymes BamHI and EcoRI. Following electrophorasis on agarose gels and blotting, the blots were then hybridized with radiolabelled probes homologous with known proto-oncogenes. Similar restriction enzyme digestions were performed on the genomic DNAs from the original unirradiated RHEK-1 cells, the isolated radiation transformed clone, RHEK-1/400R/SAC-10 and the rodent recipient cell line, NIH/3T3 cells. This type of analysis will verify the existence of human sequences in addition to the endogenous mouse sequences in the secondary nude mouse transformed cell line.

Two proto-oncogenes we have studied are the *ras* and *myc* genes. Since these genes have been shown to be involved in radiation-induced tumorigenesis *in vivo* (4, 5, 17, 18, 19). Sawey *et al.* (17) have found an activated K-*ras* oncogene as well as amplification of c-*myc* oncogene in irradiated rat tumors. Pellicer and his associates (4, 18, 19) have demonstrated the 12th codon-mutated Ki-*ras* oncogene activation in radiation-induced thymic lymphomas in mice. In addition, they found that some radiation-induced thymic lymphomas did not contain any activated *ras* gene (19). Subsequently the activation of distinct non-*ras* oncogenes has repeatly been shown in malignant x-ray transformed rodent cells as well as in rodent tumors induced by x-ray irradiation (6, 20, 21).

The initial results of our proto-oncogene characterization of the DNA from these secondary nude mouse tumors containing the isolated transforming human sequences have demonstrated that there is no homology with any of the genes of the *ras* family. None of the bands positive for human DNA had homology with N-, Ki-, or H-*ras*. Subsequent analysis has also eliminated the myc family of genes (c-*myc*, N-*myc*, and L-*myc*). To this point, we have so far found no homology between these human sequences and the proto-oncogenes v-*raf*, v-*src*, v-*mos*, v-erbA, v-erbB, v-*fos*, v-*sis*, and c-*met*. Further characterization and subsequent cloning of these transforming sequences is in progress.

## SUMMARY

Immortalized human epidermal keratinocytes have been morphologically transformed and made tumorigenic with ionizing radiation. DNA from a highly tumorigenic soft

agar clone-derived line (8 Gy clone 10) induced Alu
positive tumors in nude mice by a tumorigenicity assay.
These tumor DNA's were also Alu positive in second round
analysis of the tumorigenicity assay.  Restriction enzyme
analysis of these secondary nude mouse tumor DNAs with
EcoRI yielded four strongly Alu-positive bands with
approximate molecular weights of 20, 8, 6, and 5Kb.  The
DNA from these Alu positive secondary nude mouse tumors
were also screened for homology with probes for the *ras*
and *myc* gene families.  None of the Alu positive bands
were found to have homology with N-, K-, or H-*ras*.  No
homology was observed with probes for the myc family of
genes (c-*myc*, N-*myc*, or L-*myc*).  Subsequent analysis has
also eliminated the c-raf gene.  Further characterization
and cloning of these transforming sequences is in
progress.

These studies were supported by Grant Number CA52945
the National Cancer Institute, National Institutes of
Health, USPHS and by the funding from the Department of
Radiation Medicine, Georgetown University School of
Medicine.

## LITERATURE CITED


1.   Rhim, J.S., Jay, G., *et al.*, <u>Science</u> 227:1250 (1985).
2.   Rhim, J.S., Fujita, G., *et al.*, <u>Science</u> 232:385
     (1986).
3.   Thraves, P., Salehi, Z., *et al.*, <u>Proc Natl Acad Sci
     USA</u> 87:1174 (1990).
4.   Guerrero, I., Villasanta, A., *et al.*, <u>Science</u> 225:1159
     (1984).
5.   Guerrero, I., Calzada, P., *et al.*, <u>Proc Natl Acad Sci
     USA</u> 81:202 (1984).
6.   Borek, C., Ong, A., *et al.*, <u>Proc Natl Acad Sci USA</u>
     84:794 (1984).
7.   Weinberg, R.A., <u>Adv Cancer Res</u> 36:49 (1982).
8.   Krontiris, T.G., Cooper, G.M., <u>Proc Natl Acad Sci USA</u>
     78:1181 (1981).
9.   Perucho, M., Goldfarb, M., *et al.*, <u>Cell</u> 27:467 (1981).
10.  Pulciani, S., Santos, *et al.*, <u>Proc Natl Acad Sci USA</u>
     79:2845 (1982).
11.  Fasano, O., Birnbaum, D., *et al.*, <u>Mol Cell Biol</u> 4:1695
     (1984).
12.  Ananthaswamy, H.N., Price, J.E., *et al.*, <u>J Cell
     Biochem</u> 36:137 (1988).
13.  Blair, D.G., Cooper, C.S., *et al.*, <u>Science</u> 281:1122
     (1982).

14. Tainsky, M.A., Cooper, C.S., *et al.*, <u>Science</u> (Wash., D.C.) 225:643 (1984).
15. Wigler, M.R., Sweet, R., *et al.*, <u>Cell</u> 16:777 (1979).
16. Yuasa, Y., Kamiyama, T., *et al.*, <u>Oncogene</u> 5:589 (1990).
17. Sawey, M.J., Hood, A.T., *et al*, <u>Mol Cell Biol</u> 7:932 (1987).
18. Diamond, L.E., Guerrero, I., *et al.*, <u>Mol Cell Biol</u> 8:2233 (1988).
19. Newcomb, E.W., Steinberg, J.J., *et al.*, <u>Cancer Res</u> 49:5514 (1988).
20. Jaffe, D.R.. Bowden, G.T., <u>Carcinogenesis</u> 10:2243 (1989).
21. Krolewski, B., Little, J.B., <u>Mol Carcinogenesis</u> 2:27 (1989).



From: *Neoplastic Transformation in Human Cell Culture,*
Eds.: J. S. Rhim and A. Dritschilo ©1991 The Humana Press Inc., Totowa, NJ

# NEOPLASTIC TRANSFORMATION OF HUMAN EPITHELIAL CELLS BY IONIZING RADIATION


T. C. Yang[1], M. R. Stampfer[2], and J. S. Rhim[3]

[1]NASA JSC, Houston, TX 77058, USA, [2]Lawrence Berkeley Laboratory, Berkeley, CA 98720, USA, [3]National Cancer Institute, Bethesda, MD 20892, USA


## ABSTRACT


Ionizing radiation can induce cancers in humans and animals and can cause _in vitro_ neoplastic transformation of various rodent cell systems. There has been, however, very litter studies on radiogenic transformation of human epithelial cells, especially with high-LET radiation. Using energetic heavy ions, we have been able to transform human epidermal keratinocytes and mammary epithelial cells to various stages of transformation. Both cell lines are immortal, anchorage dependent for growth, and non-tumorigenic in athymic nude mice. Experimental results indicated that radiogenic transformation of these cells is a multistep process and that a single exposure of ionizing radiation can cause only one step of transformation. Multihits may be required for transforming human epithelial cells to fully tumorigenic. Simple chromosome analysis with cells cloned at various stages of transformation showed no consistant large termianl deletion in the transformed cells. Some changes of total number of chromosomes, however, were found in the radiation-transformed epidermal keratinocytes.

## INTRODUCTION

Ionizing radiation can cause cancers in humans, can induce tumors in various tissues and organs in animals, and can transform mammalian cells in culture. There has been, however, very little studies on radiogenic transformation of human epithelial cells, especially with high-LET (Linear Energy Transfer) radiations. Neoplastic transformation of immortalized human epidermal keratinocytes by X-ray irradiation has recently been reported (1). For a better assessment of radiation risk, an understanding of the responses of human cells, especially the epithelial cells, to low- and high-LET radiation is essential. At Lawrence Berkeley Laboratory, the accelerator facilities provide a wide range of particle radiations, which can be highly effective in transforming cells in culture (2,3,4) and in producing tumors in animals (5,6). Using these energetic heavy ion beams, we have been able to transform immortalized human epidermal keratinocytes and mammary epithelial cells to various stages of transformation with repeated irradiation. The growth properties and the karyotype of selected transformants were examined, and the experimental results are reported here.

## METHODOLOGY

Human mammary epithelial cells (H185B5) used for present studies were from primary cells treated with benzo(a)pyrene. They are immortal and nontumorigenic and require medium enriched with growth factors to grow (7). The human epidermal keratinocytes (RHEK) were immortalized by a transfection of pSV3-neo (8). These RHEK cells have a flat epithelial morphology, form monolayer with density inhibition, show no anchorage independent growth, and are nontumorigenic in athymic nude mice.

For neoplastic transformation studies, the irradiation was done with a 250 kVp Philips X-ray machine and heavy ions accelerated at BEVALAC in Lawrence Berkeley Laboratory. The dosimetry and exposure condition for X rays and heavy ions have been reported in detail (9). Confluent or log-phase cells were irradiaed at room temperature with X rays or monoener-getic heavy ion beams. The dose rates and beam uniformity for both X rays and heavy ions were 100-300 cGy/min and ±5-10% respectively.

To study the morphological transformation of human epidermal keratinocytes, we used the focus assay, similar to that for C3H10T1/2 cells. The anchorage independent growth was determined by plating cells into 0.33% agar medium, and colonies containing more than 50 cells were counted as transformants. The tumorigenic test was done by injecting $10^6$-$10^7$ cells in 0.2 ml serum free media subcutaneously on the back of athymic nude mice. A result was considered positive only when a nodule was formed at the site of injection and continued to grow into a size greater than 0.5 cm in diameter.

For transformation studies with human mammary epithelial cells in vitro, log-phase cells were irradiated and plated into dishes with enriched media (MCDB-170). At weekly interval, cells were subcultured and part of the cell population was seeded into MEM containing 10% new born calf serum to select for growth variants. The tests for anchorage independent growth and for the tumorigenic capacity of cells were the same as that used for human epidernal keratinocytes.

## RESULTS

We have successfully transformed human mammary epithelial cells from the stage of immortalization to the stage of anchorage independent growth. Immortalized cells (H184B5) were irradiated by 2.2 Gy of iron particles (600 MeV/u; LET=200 keV/um) and selected for growth variants in MEM supplemented with 10% serum. Growth variants were found at frequency about $10^{-4}$ to $10^{-3}$ per survivor, and were cloned. A growth rate comparison between H184B5 and a growth variant (H184B5-F5) is shown in Figures 1 and 2. Both cell lines grew well in medium MCDB 170. The growth variants actually appeared to grow somewhat better than H184B5. In the MEM, H184B5 did not grow and slowly died

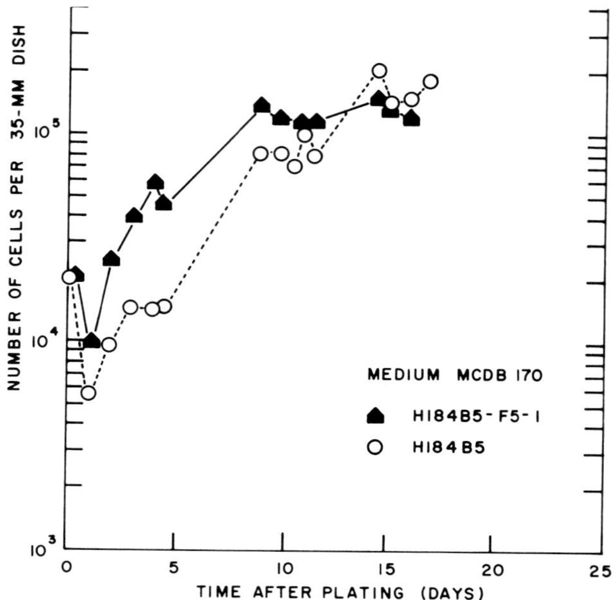


Figure 1. A comparison of growth in enriched media (MCDB-170) between human mammary epithelial cells (H184B5) and a growth variant (H184B5-F5).

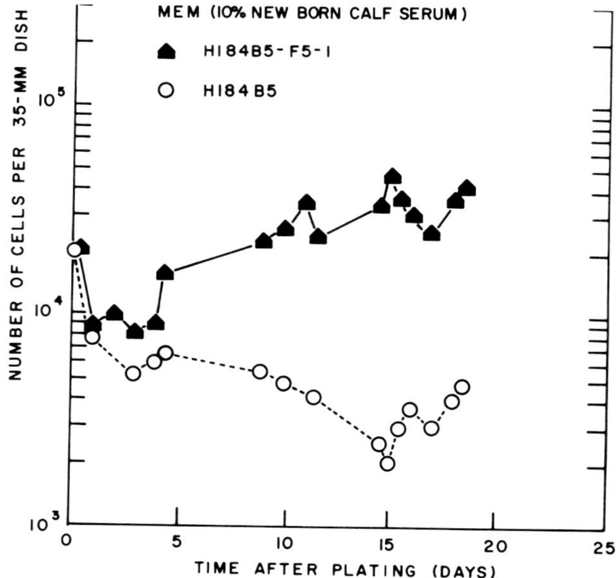


Figure 2. A comparison of growth in MEM between H184B5 and a growth variant (H184B5-F5) induced by iron particles.

off, while the growth variants proliferated steadily. Although the growth variants can grow well in the medium with less growth factors, they cannot grow in soft agar media. A second exposure of radiation was found to be necessary to transform these growth variants into the next stage of transformation, i.e., anchorage independent growth. The sequence of transformation stages appears to be definite. In spite of much effort, we have not been able to transform H184B5 cells, with a single exposure of radiation, into the stage of anchorage independent growth. Recently we have obtained transformants, which can grow in soft agar media, by irradiating the growth variants with 2.2 Gy iron beam (600 MeV/u). Figure 3 shows a colony of transformant found in soft agar media. These anchorage independent growth variants did not form tumor when they were injected into athymic nude mice. Additional irradiation may be needed to change these variants into tumorigenic.

Human epidermal keratinocytes immortalized by pSB3-neo can grow in regular MEM supplemented with serum and 2 ug/ml hydrocortisone and form monolayer in dish (Figure 4). Ionizing radiation can cause morphological transformation of these cells. In general, after 5-6 weeks incu-bation, foci can be found in the dishes of irradiated cells. There is an extensive piling up of cells in the focus, as shown in Figure 5. These transformed cells can grow in soft agar media, but do not form a tumor in athymic nude mice. When these transformed cells were given another exposure of radiation, they became tumorigenic in athymic nude mice, as shown in Figure 6.

Human epidermal keratinocytes transformed by radiation to various stages of progression were obtained and analyzed for chromosome changes. The model number of chromosomes of RHEK cells was about 50 with a range from 49-50. Similar analysis was done for cells transformed by X rays and/or heavy ions, and in general less number of chromosomes and a broader range of chromosome number was observed, as compared with nontransformed ones. There was no large terminal deletion of chromosomes in transformed cells when the karyotype of these cells was examined.

                                    

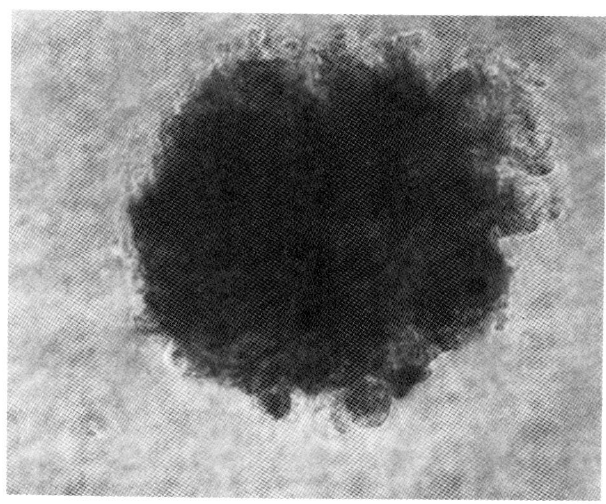

Figure 3.  A colony of H184B5-F5 cells,  transformed by iron particles, found in soft agar medium.

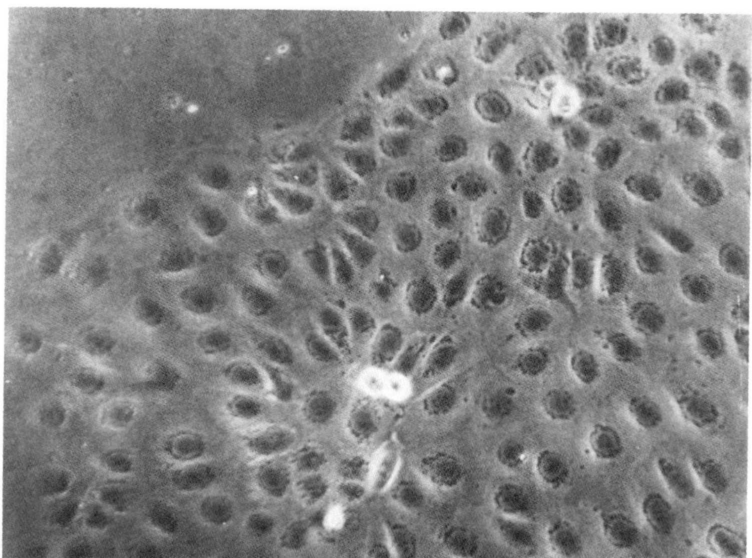

Figure 4.  Monolayer of human epidermal keratinocytes (RHEK), showing density inhibition of growth.  These cells were cultured in a tissue culture dish for one week.

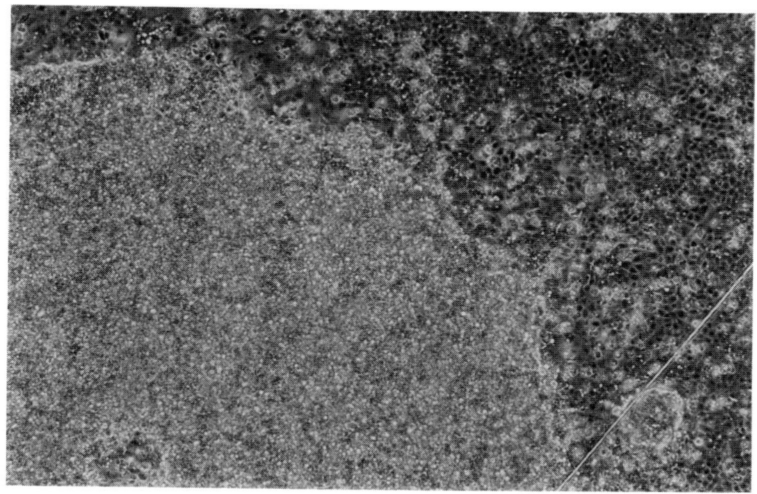

Figure 5. A close-up picture of a transformed focus of human epidermal keratinocytes. There is extensive pilling up of cells in the focus.

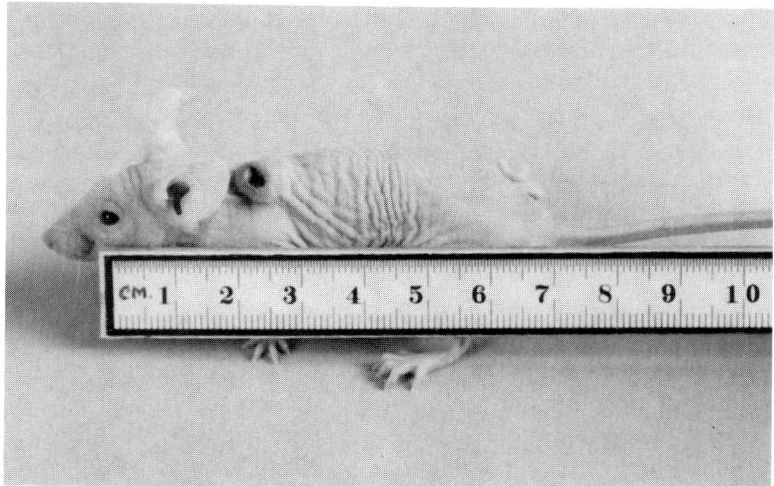

Figure 6. A tumor found in an athymic nude mouse at the site of injection of transformed human epidermal keratinocytes which first received 5 Gy X rays and then 2 Gy iron ions (600 MeV/u).

## DISCUSSION

Most studies with rodent cell systems showed that a single radiation dose could transform cells to tumorigenic stage. Our present results suggest that human epithelial cells can only be transformed one step after each exposure to ionizing radiation. There appears to be a definite sequence of steps in the multistage process of transformation. The sequence of these steps are growth variant, anchorage independent growth, and tumorigenic. Neoplastic transformation of human epithelial cells by ionizing radiation, thus, requires multi hits, as shown recently by Thraves et al (1) and by present work. This finding has an important implication for radiation risk assessment. It suggests that a single exposure to radiation is unlikely to cause a normal human cell tumorigenic and that protracted irradiation can be much more hazardous than acute exposure. This finding also suggest that several genes may have to be altered by radiation before a human epithelial cell become tumorigenic.

Shortly after the discovery of X rays, the carcinogenic effect of radiation was noticed. Since then, the question how radiation causes cancer in man has been a major interest in radiobiology. With the success of transforming human epithelial cells in vitro, we now have an unprecedented opportunity to search for the answer at cell and molecular level. In our laboratory, we have just begun to study systematically the genetic changes in transformed human epithelial cells. It has been shown that ionizing radiation, especially high-LET heavy ions, can cause large deletions in DNA. For this very reason, we did simple chromosome preparations and expected to find some large terminal deletions. Contrary to our expectation, preliminary results showed no consistent large terminal deletions in transformed cells. A decrease of total chromosome number, however, was observed in some transformants. The significance of the changes of total chromosome number is unclear at present and requires further investigation.

## ACKNOWLEDGMENTS

We would like to thank Laurie M. Craise and John C. Prioleau for their excellent technical help, the BEVALAC crew for providing the heavy ion beams needed for these studies. The dosimetry and operation help from Dr. B. Ludewigt and other BioMed operators are highly appreciated. We also thank Marco Durante for his valuable help in chromosome preparation. These studies were supported by NASA (Contract #1391M).

## REFERENCES

1. P. Thraves, Z. Salehi, A. Dritschilo, and J. S. Rhim. <u>Proc. Natl. Acad. Sci. USA</u>. 87, 1174 (1990)
2. T. C. H. Yang and C. A. Tobias. <u>Adv. in Biol. and Med. Phys</u>. 17, 417-461 (1980)
3. T. C. Yang and C. A. Tobias. <u>Adv. Space Res</u>. 4, #10, 207-218 (1984)
4. M. Suzuki, M. Watanabe, K. Suzuki, K. Nakano, and I. Kaneko. <u>Radiat. Res.</u> 120, 468-476 (1989)
5. R. J. M. Fry, P. Powers-Risius, E. L. Alpen, and E. J. Ainsworth. <u>Radiat. Res</u>. 104, S188 (1985)
6. F. J. Burns, S. Hosselet, and S. Garte. In: <u>Low Dose Radiation Biological Bases of Risk Assessment</u>. Taylor and Francis, London (1989)
7. M. S. Stampfer and J. C. Bartley. <u>Proc. Natl. Acad. Sci. USA</u> 82, 2394-2398 (1985)
8. R. Gantt, K. K. Sanford, R. Parshad, F. M. Price, W. D. Peterson, Jr., and J. S. Rhim. <u>Cancer Res</u>. 47, 1390-1397 (1987)
9. T. C. Yang, L. M. Craise, M. Mei, and C. A. Tobias. <u>Radiat. Res</u>. 104, S-177-S-187 (1985)

From: *Neoplastic Transformation in Human Cell Culture,*
Eds.: J. S. Rhim and A. Dritschilo ©1991 The Humana Press Inc., Totowa, NJ

# EFFECTS OF IONIZING RADIATION ON HUMAN PAPILLOMAVIRUS IMMORTALIZED HUMAN BRONCHIAL EPITHELIAL CELLS

James C. Willey, Jim Greene, Alberec Bressoud, Peter Cerutti, Tom Hei, Nancy Wang, David Maillie, Chris Cox, and Ellen Miles

University of Rochester School of Medicine and Dentistry, Environmental Health Sciences Center and Departments of Biophysics, Pediatrics and Biostatistics, Rochester, N.Y., 14642, Columbia University, Center for Radiobiological Research, New York, N.Y. 10032, Department of Carcinogenesis, Swiss Institute for Experimental Cancer Research, CH-1066 Epalinges S./Lausanne, Switzerland

The carcinogenic action of ionizing radiation in humans has been well recognized from epidemiologic data. Despite this fact there has been only one report on the radiogenic transformation of human epithelial cells (1). We have established immortalized, non-tumorigenic human bronchial epithelial cell lines following transfection with human papillomaviruses (HPV) 16 or 18 (2) and are employing them in experiments designed to identify genetic mechanisms involved in neoplastic transformation of human bronchial epithelial cells by ionizing radiation. The specific investigations are 1) analysis for specific genetic alterations in transformants (cells that have altered morphology, growth in soft agar or tumorigenicity in immunosuppressed mouse); and 2) identification of mechanisms involved in differentiation of human bronchial epithelial cells by evaluation of the differentiation-specific transcription of the E6/E7 transforming genes in radiated cells.

## Effects of Radiation on the Immortalized Cell Lines BEP2D and BEP3D

We are comparing the effects of low linear energy transfer (LET) radiation from a $^{137}$Cs source to that of high LET radiation (150 KeV/μM) from a Van de Graaf accelerator on colony forming efficiency (CFE), morphology, karyotype, and growth in soft agar for the human papillomavirus (HPV) 16 or 18 immortalized human bronchial epithelial

"

cell lines BEP2D and BEP3D respectively.  We used conditions similar to those previously described (1).  We have determined that  high LET radiation is more cytotoxic than low LET radiation for these cells. While the $D_0$ for low LET radiation is about 2 Gy the $D_0$ for high LET radiation is 0.4 Gy.  After two irradiations with 8 or 10 Gy from the $^{137}$Cs source, colonies with an altered morphology developed in the BEP2D line, and in the BEP3D cells after three irradiations with 8 Gy. The alteration in morphology included smaller size and piling up. BEP2D cells twice irradiated with 2, 4, 6, 8, or 10 Gy from the $^{137}$Cs source were evaluated for ability to grow in soft agar.  Colonies developed in the 8 and 10 Gy irradiated samples but not in the control. While both the control and the twice  irradiated cells had karyotypes similar to previous evaluations of BEP2D (2), including a 12:13 translocation, twice 10 Gy irradiated cells possessing the morphological transformation had new consistent alterations, including a numerical aberration of chromosome 9 and a structural aberration of chromosome 11p15.  These data are preliminary but suggest that there is a step-wise process in malignant transformation caused by radiation, as recently described  (1).  The significance of the chromosomal alterations described here is unclear and will await evaluation of additional independently induced radiation-transformants.


**Genetic Alterations in Transformants**

Based on epidemiologic (3) and experimental (4) data, we believe that many different genes are involved in malignant transformation of human bronchial epithelial cells.  It is widely believed that at least seven or eight different genes must be mutated in the same human bronchial epithelial cell for that cell to become malignant (3).  In addition,  there is the possibility that these seven or eight genes may come from an even larger pool of genes, that if altered in the correct combination, will lead to loss of growth control.  Due to rapid advances in understanding of the interactions between components involved in controlling cell proliferation and differentiation (5), there are many genes now known that logically may act as tumor suppressor genes.

Application of molecular genetic techniques to epidemiology studies have allowed recent identification of specific genes involved in human bronchogenic carcinogenesis, including K-*ras* oncogene (6) and the p53 and retinoblastoma (Rb) tumor suppressor genes (7,8).

In order to augment molecular epidemiology studies we propose to use immortalized, non-tumorigenic human bronchial epithelial cells in carcinogenicity studies.  The advantages of this approach are the following.  First, the problems resulting from stroma and from lack of heterozygosity are avoided.  One may test restriction fragment length (RFLP) probes for heterozygosity on the parent cell line; any tumorigenic cell lines that result from treatment with carcinogens will be derived from the informative parent line and will thereby also be informative. Second, it is possible to compare the ability of different carcinogens to induce malignant transformation, and associate neoplastic transformation with alterations in particular genes known from molecular epidemiology studies to be involved in human bronchogenic carcinogenesis. Third, it may be possible to identify genetic mechanisms for a multistep process in malignant transformation.

The BEP2D cell line is being used primarily in these studies because it has a near diploid karyotype with one stable marker chromosome (2). Consequently, any changes occurring as a result of radiation exposure will more readily be detected.

Two stages of immortalization by HPV virus detectable by morphological changes have been observed (2,9). Presumably, alterations in cellular genes are responsible for the additional changes in confluence density and soft agar growth described above as well. As has been described recently for colon carcinoma, a clear step-wise progression involving particular genes may be identified.

## Differentiation-Specific Effects on E6/E7 Transcription

By use of reverse transcriptase technology, it is possible to evaluate the level of transcription of the E6/E7 transforming genes in these immortalized cell lines. Transcription of both E6 and E7 are regulated by the same promoter. HPV virus replication is sensitive to the state of cellular differentiation (10), perhaps in part due to interactions between differentiation-specific cellular enhancer proteins and the HPV upstream regulatory region. Theoretically, another mechanism by which HPV viral gene expression may be regulated in a differentiation-specific manner is through alternative splicing; for example, it is known that troponin RNA may be spliced in a differentiation-specific manner in muscle cells (11). It is known that the E6/E7 transcript may undergo alternative splicing in the strains of HPV that are associated with malignant transformation in vivo. We are evaluating HPV16 or 18 immortalized cells for potential to differentiate in a squamous metaplastic pathway at different passages. In conjunction with these studies, we are evaluating the level of production of the full-length E6/E7 message versus the spliced message. In a human bronchial epithelial cell line established from normal cells following transfection with HPV16 both the full-length and shortened transcript were present at passage 8 (fig.). By treating these cells with agents that induce differentiation in normal human bronchial epithelial cells such as tetradecanoyl-12-phorbol-13-acetate (TPA) (12) we may determine whether induction of differentiation causes a change in the splicing pattern.

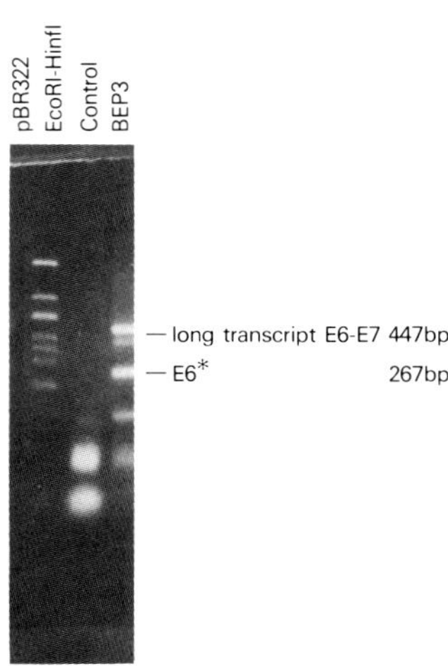


Reverse transcriptase-polymerase chain reaction amplification analysis of E6/E7 RNA messages of a clonal isolate of a HPV16 transfected bronchial epithelial cell line. Lane 1: marker, EcoRI-HinfI digest of pBR322; Lane 2: control with no template DNA: Lane 3; BEP3 DNA amplified with primers for E6/E7 region of HPV16. The amplification of the full-length E6/E7 transcript results in a 447 bp long product, while amplification of the spliced E6* transcript results in a 267 bp transcript. The bands in the control lane are primers and primer dimers. The authenticity of the indicated bands were confirmed by diagnostic restriction enzyme cuts.

## REFERENCES


1.  Thraves, P., Salehi, Z. et al. <u>Proc. Natl. Acad. Sci. U.S.A.</u> 87, 1174 (1990).
2.  Willey, J.C., Bressoud, A. et al, <u>Cancer Research</u>, in press, 1991..
3.  Cook, P.J., Doll, R., Fellingham, S.A. <u>International Journal of Cancer</u> 4, 93 (1969).
4.  Willey, J. and Harris, C.C. <u>CRC Critical reviews in Oncology/Hematology</u> 10, 18 (1990).
5.  Hunter, T. <u>Cell</u> 64, 249 (1991).
6.  Bos, J.L. <u>Mutation Research</u> 195, 255 (1988)

7.  Hollstein, M.M., et al., <u>Science</u> 253, 49 (1991).
8.  Harbour, J.W., Lai, S.-L., et al. <u>Science</u> 353, 241 (1988).
9.  Barbosa, M.S. and Schlegel, R.  <u>Oncogene</u> 4, 1529 (1989).
10. Stoler, M.H., Wolinsky, S.M., et al. <u>Virology</u> 172, 331 (1989).
11. Breitbart, R.E., Nguyen, H.T., et al. <u>Cell</u> 41, 67 (1985).
12. Willey, et al. <u>Carcinogenesis</u> 5, 209 (1984).

From: *Neoplastic Transformation in Human Cell Culture,*
Eds.: J. S. Rhim and A. Dritschilo ©1991 The Humana Press Inc., Totowa, NJ

# BIOCHEMICAL PURIFICATION OF A CSF-1 LIKE MOLECULE RELEASED DURING MALIGNANT TRANSFORMATION OF IL-3 DEPENDENT HEMATOPOIETIC PROGENITOR CELL LINES COCULTIVATED WITH GAMMA IRRADIATED CLONAL MARROW STROMAL CELL LINES

J.S. Greenberger, J. Lief, P. Anklesaria, M.A. Sakakeeny, D. English, D. Crawford, and T.J. FitzGerald

Department Of Radiation Oncology, University Of Massachusetts Medical Center, Worcester, MA 01655

Cocultivation of IL-3 dependent hematopoietic progenitor cell line FDC-P1JL26 with 5000 cGy irradiated clonal bone marrow stromal cell line D2XRII has been demonstrated to stimulate selection of factor independent hematopoietic cell lines that produce tumors _in vivo_ (1,2). Hematopoietic stem cell specific and stromal cell specific variables in this experiment have been described (3). The precise molecular mechanism of the malignant transformation of hematopoietic cells and the growth factor or cell membrane contact which is responsible for the transformation have not yet been elucidated. Biochemical purification of several liters of conditioned medium from D2XRII cells revealed a 75,000 molecular weight protein that was neutralized by a polyclonal antiserum to M-CSF. This growth factor stimulated formation of macrophage colonies in fresh mouse bone marrow cells _in vitro_. A biochemical purification scheme utilizing a Pellicon cassette system concentration, followed by lentil lectin chromatography, ion exchange high pressure liquid chromatography, gel filtration high pressure liquid chromatography, and reverse phase HPLC yield biological activity using tritiated thymidine incorporation into microwell cultures of FDC-P1JL26 cells (4). Active fractions were run out on NaDodSO$_4$/PAGE gel electrophoresis and revealed a band consistent in size with 75,000 molecular weight.

Since several bands of activity were detected using this biochemical scheme, an alternative biochemical purification scheme was chosen to confirm that the activity of differing molecular weights (other than 75,000) might represent other growth factor species or, alternatively, varying degrees of glycosylation of M-CSF, (CSF-1).

In an attempt to determine if another humoral factor distinct from M-CSF was released from irradiated D2XRII stromal cells, a second purification method was initiated. Partially purified D2XRII stromal cell conditioned medium at the DEAE step, was applied to a 10-20% nondenaturing polyacrylamide gradient gel. After running two hours at 140 volts and initially, 25 milliamps, duplicate lanes were cut out into four equal pieces each extending to the dye front. Proteins from each fragment were then electroeluted for 90 minutes at 200 volts, 20 milliamps using an Amicon microelectroeluter into Centricon-10's (Amicon; 10,000 molecular weight cutoff). This volume (1.7 ml) was then spun, concentrated to approximately 150 ul and directly tested for mitogenic activity using tritiated thymidine incorporation with FDC-P1 cells that had been adapted for growth in D2XRII conditioned medium (termed FDC-P1-LSF for leukemogenic stromal factor adapted cells). All activity was located in the first quadrant. Coomassie Blue staining of an identical adjacent lane revealed a major band of Rf 0.25. To address the possibility of glycosylation, the DEAE fraction was pretreated with glycosidase, then run out on a polyacrylamide gel, and the locations of mitogenic activity again tested using the FDC-P1 LSF adapted cells. DEAE preparations were tested with multiple glycosidases using sequential N-glycanase, neuraminidase, and O-glycanase. The extensively glycosylated protein fetuin was included as a control in these studies. The results showed a decrease in relative mitogenic activity of the 0.2 - 0.25 Rf gel fragment for FDC-P1-LSF cells. A broad band of activity was detected at Rf 0.05 - 0.20. The positive control molecule fetuin also exhibited a similarly altered mobility on the SDS gel following the sequential glycosidase treatment. We next treated D2XRII cells in culture with the glycosylation inhibitor tunicamycin to both eliminate the contaminating effect of multiple glycosidase treatments on the preparation and to search for a more effective resolution of mitogenic activity on SDS gels. The results indicated a different peak distribution of the broad band of activity (Rf 0.05 - 0.10 and 0.15 - 0.25) as compared with both multiple glycosidase treatment of material obtained from nontunicamycin treated D2XRII cells (peak 0.05 - 0.20) and nontreated, fully glycosylated LSF.

Neither procedure described above resolved the activity to a single band. Tunicamycin pretreatment was chosen as an initial purification step, then SDS-gel electrophoresis was tested as a second step to recover protein after denaturation but in the absence of DTT reduction. DEAE fractions from nontunicamycin treated D2XRII conditioned medium were run on a 9.0% SDS gel using Laemmli buffers. Eight equal gel sections (down to the dye front) were cut and the proteins electroeluted and concentrated. Electroeluted gel segments 1-7 from the above tunicamycin study, were also run out and sliver-stained to determine how these proteins distributed across the gel. In addition, activity in each of these seven samples was tested for its neutralization by polyclonal M-CSF antiserum at 1:18 dilution in the preincubation (45 minutes, room temperature), and 1:360 in the final assay. The results indicated that mitogenic activity for FDC-P1-LSF was recoverable from SDS gels and most of the applied DEAE activity localized to the second gel segment. Molecular weight standards indicated that this segment contained proteins of molecular weight 60-100,000 daltons. In contrast, tunicamycin fractions 1-7, were distributed widely across the SDS gel lanes. All activity was strongly neutralized by polyclonal anti-M-CSF antiserum.

A different two-step gel purification of LSF was next carried out using a sequential 10-20% nondenaturing gradient and 9% SDS denaturing polyacrylamide gel electrophoresis. Conditioned medium from tunicamycin-treated D2XRII cells was used as a source of LSF. Six lanes each containing 432 ugs of LSF from the tunicamycin-treated cell preparation were run on the 10-20% gradient gel. The area corresponding to known mitogenic activity from previous studies (approximate Rf 0.12 - 0.22) was excised from five of the lanes and electroeluted. The rest of the gel was then stained with Coomassie Blue. The electroelute was then put on 9% SDS gel (75 ugs and 9,200,000 CPM) in triplicate lanes. After the run, one lane was cut into 8 equal sections down to the dye front, electroeluted and concentrated. Activity was localized to the second and third segments corresponding to 40-110,000 molecular weight. The remaining gel was then stained with 0.2% Coomassie Blue in 50% methanol and 5% acetic acid and destained in 50% methanol. Nine bands were visible between molecular weights 40,000 and 105,000 and these were excised and electroeluted, the last two (42,000 and 41,000) together. A ninth area of the gel where no stained band was present was excised as a background control. The results revealed that LSF activity could not be resolved to a single band but rather extend it over at least three protein species ranging in molecular weights from 60-81,000 with a peak at 75,000.

These and other results (4) indicated that LSF was similar, of not identical, to M-CSF.

Other studies have demonstrated that FDC-P1JL26, or LSF adapted cells grown in suspension culture in LSF, generated factor independent subclones at higher frequency than if the cells were cultured in a source of IL-3 (4). Furthermore, when single cell structures of FDC-P1-LSF were cocultivated in microwell plates (96 well dish) with a monolayer of 5,000 cGy irradiated D2XRII cells, the frequency of evolution of factor independent cell lines was 40-80-fold increased. This data suggested that the effect of LSF/M-CSF was to provide for selection of a variant of FDC-P1 cells with factor independence.

Other data indicate that one factor independent subclonal cell line derived by cocultivation with irradiated D2XRII cells produces mRNA for M-CSF and c-fms (M-CSF receptor), suggesting an autocrine mechanism of factor independence (4). However, concentrated conditioned medium from this factor independent cell line, which produces tumors in vivo at high frequency, did not contain detectable growth factor, for parent cells FDC-P1JL26, or for fresh mouse bone marrow. Thus, if an autocrine mechanism of factor independence is, in fact selected by cocultivation, there is no detectable secretion of the growth factor into concentrated conditioned medium from the factor independent cell line.

Prior studies have demonstrated that nonirradiated D2XRII, or other mouse bone marrow stromal cell lines compared with 5000 cGy irradiated stromal cells of the same clones, have a decreased efficiency at inducing factor independent subclones from FDC-P1JL26 (3). The mechanism by which gamma irradiation alters bone marrow stromal cell interaction with hematopoietic stem cells clearly involve hematopoietic cell binding . to the stroma by a mechanism that is separable from M-CSF (since the interaction was not inhibited by antiserum to M-CSF or monoclonal antibody to murine c-fms) (4).

Elucidation of the molecular biologic mechanism of factor independent cell line evolution in this model of indirect gamma irradiation leukemogenesis through the marrow stroma may prove very relevant to understanding the late effects of ionizing irradiation on the bone marrow.

## REFERENCES:

1. E. Naparstek, J.H. Pierce, D. Metcalf, et al. **Blood, 67:139 (1986).**

2. E. Naparstek, T.J. FitzGerald, M.A. Sakakeeny, et al. **Cancer Res, 6:4677 (1986).**

3 J.S. Greenberger, E. Wright, S. Henault, et al. **Exp Hematol, 18:48 (1990).**

4. J.S. Greenberger, J. Leif, D. Crawford, et al. **Exp Hematol, (Submitted).**

From: *Neoplastic Transformation in Human Cell Culture,*
Eds.: J. S. Rhim and A. Dritschilo ©1991 The Humana Press Inc., Totowa, NJ

AN INHERITED P53 POINT MUTATION IN A CANCER PRONE FAMILY

WITH LI-FRAUMENI SYNDROME

S. Srivastava[1 & 2], Z. Zou[1], K. Pirollo[1], D. Tong[1],
V. Sykes[1], K. Devadas[1], J. Miao[1], Y. Chen[1], W.
Blattner[3], and E.H. Chang[1 & 2].
Departments of Pathology[1] and Surgery[2], USUHS,
Environmental Epidemiology Branch[3], NCI,
Bethesda, MD 20814.

## ABSTRACT

Somatic cells derived from members of a cancer-
prone family representing three generations were used to
assess mutations in selected regions of p53. Fibroblast
DNAs from four family members--the proband, his brother,
their father and a paternal aunt, yielded an identical
point mutation in codon 245 in only one allele of the
p53 gene. This mutation, involving G to A transition
(GGC -> GAC) leads to substitution of aspartic acid for
glycine at that codon in p53 protein and is not present
in NSF DNAs of the proband's mother or his paternal
grandfather, neither of whom are in the cancer-prone
lineage. Despite the observed mutation, the level of
p53 protein detected in these fibroblasts is comparable
to low levels observed in normal control fibroblasts.
This is in contrast to the high levels of mutant p53
usually found in tumor cell lines. Thus the mutant p53
in these fibroblasts appears to behave differently as
compared to the mutant p53 previously detected in
transformed cells. Given the inherited nature of this
p53 mutation, the demonstrated role of p53 in
tumorigenesis and the location of mutation in a region
of the gene known to be critical for its function, it
appears that we have identified a primary genetic
alteration in this Li-Fraumeni family, a defect which
may predispose them to increased susceptibility to
cancer.

     Familial cancer syndromes provide opportunities to
examine the mechanisms of inherited susceptibility to
cancer as well as more general processes involved in the
development of malignancy.  Tumor suppressor genes have
been implicated in many inherited as well as in sporadic
form of malignancies (for reviews see ref. 1-3).  A
large body of experimental evidence supports the concept
of tumor formation by loss-of-function mutations in
suppressor genes as predicted by the two-hit model of
Knudson (4) and DeMars (5) involving inactivation of
both alleles for manifestation of the tumorigenic
phenotype.  The tumor suppressor gene, p53, has been
shown to have sustained numerous genetic alterations in
diverse neoplasm, usually exhibiting loss of one allele
and point mutation in the other.  We have been studying
predisposing genetic factors in a specific cancer-prone
family diagnosed as having Li-Fraumeni syndrome, which
is characterized by the early onset of diverse
neoplasms, as well as occurrence of multiple primaries
in single individuals (6,7).  Although p53 mutations in
other studies are reported to be tumor specific (for
reviews see refs. 8 and 9), we reasoned that if a defect
in the p53 gene was central to the tumorigenesis in this
cancer-prone family, the alterations in p53 gene may be
detected in at least one allele in noncancerous somatic
cells.  Normal skin fibroblast (NSFs) derived from
members of this family, representing three generations,
were analyzed for alterations in the mutational hot
spots of the p53 gene by polymerase chain reaction (PCR)
amplification and direct sequencing of the PCR product.
Recently we (10) and others (11) have described germ-
line p53 mutations in Li-Fraumeni cancer-prone families.
Here, we briefly summarize our findings on the inherited
codon 245 mutation in the p53 gene of fibroblasts
derived from members of a specific cancer-prone family.
**GERM-LINE P53 MUTATION IN MEMBERS OF A CANCER-PRONE
FAMILY:**
     NSF cell lines derived from members of three
generations of a cancer-prone family (Fig. 1) were
utilized to assess the status of p53 gene.  Utilizing
p53 cDNA as a probe, we did not detect any major
alteration in the p53 gene by Southern or Northern blot
analyses (data not shown).
     We, therefore, analyzed the family NSFs for subtle

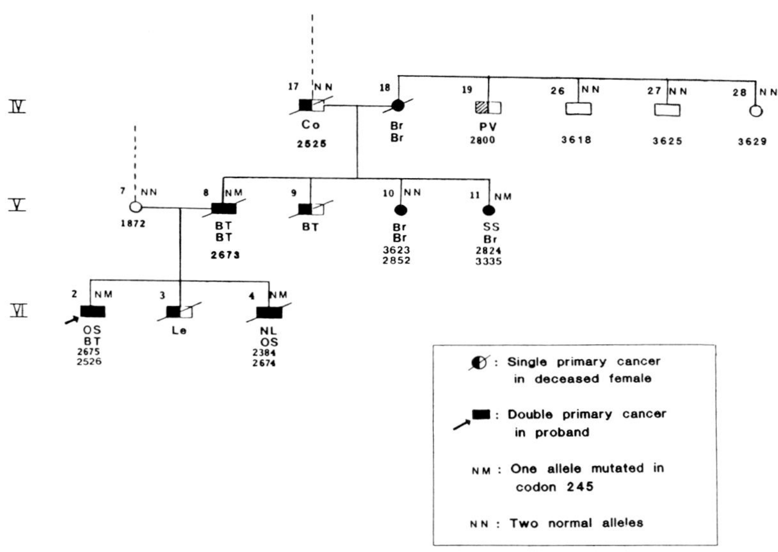



FIGURE 1. PARTIAL PEDIGREE OF A CANCER-PRONE FAMILY:
Shown here is a branch of a much larger pedigree in
which cancer can be traced through six generations in
three separate lineages from a woman who died with
breast cancer in 1865 (refs. 7,10) Normal skin
fibroblast (NSF) cell line designations are given for
each individual, where available. NM, individuals in
whom the G -> A transition in codon 245 of one p53
allele was found; NN, presence of two normal alleles;
▬ or ◖ , double primary cancer in deceased male or
female. Abbreviations: OS, osteogenic sarcoma; SS,
soft-tissue sarcoma; BT, brain tumour; Br, breast
cancer; PV, polycythemia vera; Le, leukaemia; Co, colon
cancer; NL, neurilemmoma.

alterations of p53 gene namely, point mutations, which
have been frequently identified in a wide variety of
neoplasms (12) in one of the four conserved regions of
p53 (region A, encompassing codons 132-143; B, codons
174-179; C, codons 236-248; D, codons 272-281).  The
family NSF DNA samples were amplified by PCR to yield a
2.9 kbp fragment encompassing all the four of the
mutational hot spots (12).  This fragment was then
reamplified by asymmetric PCR utilizing one set of
primers encompassing region A and B and a second set of
primers encompassing regions C and D.

  The nucleotide sequences of these regions were then
determined, leading to the identification of a single
base substitution, a G -> A transition, in codon 245 of
p53 (Fig. 2).  This mutation, which results in the
substitution of an aspartic acid for glycine in the p53
protein, was found in DNA from four different NSF cell
lines of the family: 2675, 2674, 2673 and 3335.  These
cell lines were obtained from the proband (VI-2), his
brother (VI-4), their father (V-8) and a paternal aunt
(V-11), respectively.  These individuals were
heterozygous for this mutation, with one allele
retaining the normal GGC sequence.  It is important to
note that all four of these individuals had suffered
from cancer (Fig. 1).  Moreover, a separate isolate of
NSF cells from the proband, his brother and their aunt
possessed the same mutation as that detected in the
original cell lines, confirming that the mutation was
genetically inherited rather than an artefact of cell
culture or PCR amplification.  This mutation was not
observed in the NSF DNAs from a second paternal aunt
(2852, V-10) with breast cancer or from a genetically
unrelated normal control.  More importantly, the
mutation was not found in NSF DNAs derived from the
mother (1872, V-7), or the paternal grandfather (2525,
IV-17) of the proband, both of whom married into the
cancer-prone lineage.  Unfortunately, neither NSF cell
lines nor lymphocytes from the deceased paternal
grandmother of the proband in the cancer-prone lineage,
who died from bilateral breast cancer, were available
for analysis.  DNAs from NSFs cell lines of two paternal
great uncles and a great aunt (Fig. 1), all unaffected,
did not reveal a mutation in codon 245.    The finding
that the mother (V-7) and paternal grandfather (IV-17)
of the proband did not possess the mutation lends

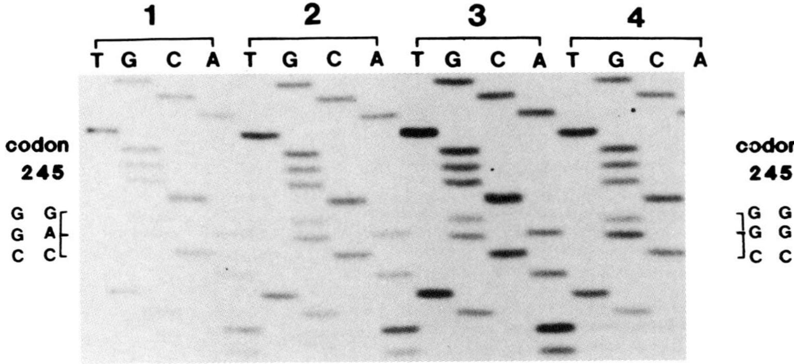



FIGURE 2. IDENTIFICATION OF A POINT MUTATION IN THE P53 GENE OF NSF CELL LINES FROM MEMBERS OF A CANCER-PRONE FAMILY: Shown is a representative sample of the sequence data obtained from seven different NSF cell lines representing four individuals in the cancer-prone family, as described in the text. The sequence data shown is for the area surrounding and including codon 245 where the point mutation was observed and is identical for all seven cell lines (10) representing proband 2675(1), his brother, 2674(2), their father 2673(3) and a genetically unrelated normal control, 196(4).

credence to the conclusion that the proband and his
brother acquired this mutation genetically from their
father.  In addition, the father and his sister (aunt
V-11) most probably inherited the mutation from their
mother (IV-18) who is directly in the lineage of the
cancer-prone family.  Two independent NSF cell lines
from one of the paternal aunts with breast cancer, V-10
did not have the p53 mutation in codon 245.  With
mendelian inheritance of a specific genetic trait, one
would not expect it to be carried by every individual in
a generation.  Although bilateral breast cancer has been
considered to be one of the primary characteristics of
the Li-Fraumeni Syndrome, the previously identified
elevated c-myc expression in the NSFs of this family
(13), as well as the contribution of additional genetic
influences inherited from her father's (IV-17) branch of
the family, might contribute to her susceptibility to
bilateral breast cancer.  In fact, other incidences of
cancer have been reported in the pedigree of IV-17 (ref.
7).  The finding of a heritable mutation in the p53 gene
in family NSFs is analogous to similar mutations in
somatic cells of individuals with a defective Rb gene
and predisposition to retinoblastoma (for a review, see
ref. 1-3), suggesting that a heritable defect in the p53
gene in the family that we studied results in a
heightened risk of cancer.

## ANALYSIS OF P53 PROTEIN IN FAMILY NSFS:

In order to understand the functional significance of
the inherited p53 mutation detected in the NSF DNA
derived from members of this Li-Fraumeni cancer syndrome
family (10), we have analyzed the expression of p53
protein in family NSFs.  The high level of mutant p53
protein observed in transformed cell lines is believed
to exert its effect by complexing with the endogenous
wild type p53 and inactivating the function of the
latter (8,9). Therefore, it is all the more important to
assess how the expression of mutant p53 is regulated in
the Li-Fraumeni family NSFs.  Utilizing anti p53
monoclonal antibody, p53 Ab2, we have detected low
levels of p53 protein in family NSFs (Fig. 3). These
levels are similar to the levels of p53 in family
fibroblasts harboring only wild type p53 or unrelated
fibroblasts controls.  Although NSF cell lines in our
study carry different mutation in codon 245 of p53 gene,
these observations are in agreement with the **report**

credence to the conclusion that the proband and his
brother acquired this mutation genetically from their
father.  In addition, the father and his sister (aunt
V-11) most probably inherited the mutation from their
mother (IV-18) who is directly in the lineage of the
cancer-prone family.  Two independent NSF cell lines
from one of the paternal aunts with breast cancer, V-10
did not have the p53 mutation in codon 245.  With
mendelian inheritance of a specific genetic trait, one
would not expect it to be carried by every individual in
a generation.  Although bilateral breast cancer has been
considered to be one of the primary characteristics of
the Li-Fraumeni Syndrome, the previously identified
elevated c-myc expression in the NSFs of this family
(13), as well as the contribution of additional genetic
influences inherited from her father's (IV-17) branch of
the family, might contribute to her susceptibility to
bilateral breast cancer.  In fact, other incidences of
cancer have been reported in the pedigree of IV-17 (ref.
7).  The finding of a heritable mutation in the p53 gene
in family NSFs is analogous to similar mutations in
somatic cells of individuals with a defective Rb gene
and predisposition to retinoblastoma (for a review, see
ref. 1-3), suggesting that a heritable defect in the p53
gene in the family that we studied results in a
heightened risk of cancer.

**ANALYSIS OF P53 PROTEIN IN FAMILY NSFS:**

In order to understand the functional significance of
the inherited p53 mutation detected in the NSF DNA
derived from members of this Li-Fraumeni cancer syndrome
family (10), we have analyzed the expression of p53
protein in family NSFs.  The high level of mutant p53
protein observed in transformed cell lines is believed
to exert its effect by complexing with the endogenous
wild type p53 and inactivating the function of the
latter (8,9). Therefore, it is all the more important to
assess how the expression of mutant p53 is regulated in
the Li-Fraumeni family NSFs.  Utilizing anti p53
monoclonal antibody, p53 Ab2, we have detected low
levels of p53 protein in family NSFs (Fig. 3). These
levels are similar to the levels of p53 in family
fibroblasts harboring only wild type p53 or unrelated
fibroblasts controls.  Although NSF cell lines in our
study carry different mutation in codon 245 of p53 gene,
these observations are in agreement with the report

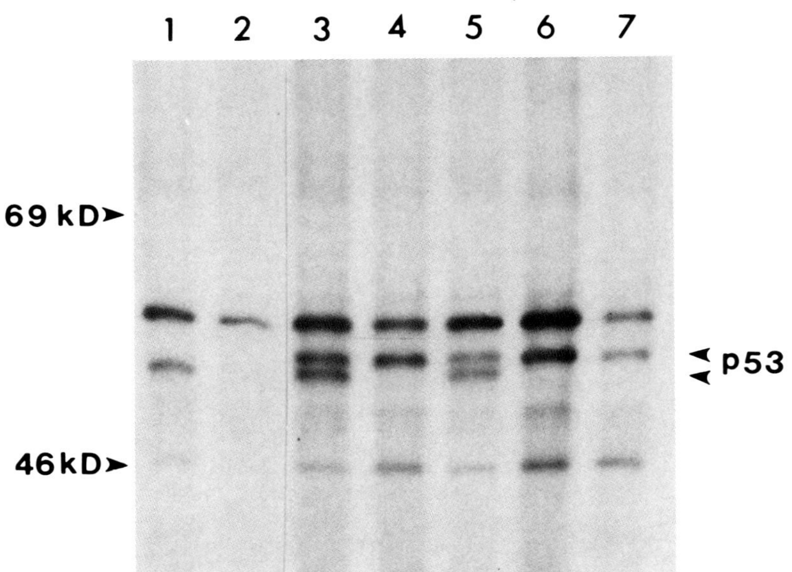



**FIGURE 3.**

P53 PROTEIN IN NSF CELLS OF THE CANCER-PRONE FAMILY:
NSF cell lines derived from proband, 2675 (lane 6), his
brother, 2674 (lane 5) and his father, 2673 (lane 4) and
unrelated normal skin fibroblast, GM0038A (lane 7), 308
(lane 3) and 196 (lane 1) were labelled with $^{35}$S-
methionine and cleared lysates equivalent to 5 X 10$^6$ TCA
precipitable counts were immunoprecipitated with anti
p53 monoclonal antibody Ab2 (Oncogene Science Inc.).  As
a control, lysate from cell line, 196 (lane 2) was
processed without antibody under similar conditions.
The immunoprecipitates were analyzed by SDS/8% PAGE and
autoradiography.

describing the low levels of p53 in other Li-Fraumeni
family NSFs carrying germ line mutations in codons 248,
252, 258, and 245 (11). However, in both instances, it
was not clear whether the mutant p53 is expressed in
family NSFs.  Our recent analysis of family NSF RNA by
PCR sequencing has clearly revealed that both the mutant
and normal p53 alleles are expressed in roughly equal
proportion in these family fibroblasts (to be published
elsewhere).  A recent study (14) describing the non-
tumorigenic phenotype of transfected cells carrying one
copy each of the mutant and normal p53 alleles supports
our observation that the skin fibroblasts under study
exhibit a non-tumorigenic phenotype and that the wild
type p53 function may be dominant when the mutant p53 is
not overexpressed.  Therefore, some sort of competition
may exist between the wild type and the mutant p53 for
the putative target(s) and the quantity of wild type p53
may affect the function of mutant p53 and vice versa.
However, it is also possible that the mutant p53
observed in germ-line configuration exhibit a biological
property, which is different from previously analyzed
mutant p53 proteins in murine system (9).  This low
level expression of mutant p53 observed in family NSFs
may manifest its phenotypic effect only upon loss of the
normal p53 allele or upon quantitative increase of
mutant allele encoded protein in transformed cells.
Moreover, this hypothesis is confirmed by our recent
analysis (to be published elsewhere) of tumor DNAs from
the family members showing the loss of the wild type p53
allele.
 Therefore, it appears that we have identified an
inherited defect in the tumor suppressor gene, p53 in
this Li-Fraumeni family.  In view of the fact that the
location of this defect is in a region known to be
important for the function of p53 gene and its
correlation to the development of cancer in these
individuals, it is likely that we have identified the
primary genetic defect which predisposes them to cancer.

## ACKNOWLEDGEMENTS

We thank Dr. R.F. Friedman for the helpful discussion
during the course of this work.  We also thank Shawna
Taylor for typing this manuscript.

## REFERENCES


1. Scrable H.J., Supienza, C., and Cavanee, W. <u>Adv. in Cancer Res</u>. 54, 25 (1990).
2. Ponder, B.A.J. <u>Trends in Genetics</u> 6, 213 (1990).
3. Marshall, C.J. <u>Cell</u> 64, 313 (1991).
4. Knudson, A.G. <u>Proc. Natl. Acad. Sci.</u> 68, 820 (1971).
5. DeMars, R. in 23rd <u>A. Symp. Fund Cancer Res.</u> 105-106 (1969) William and Wikings, Baltimore.
6. Li, F.P. and Fraumeni, J.F. Jr. <u>Ann. Intern Med.</u> 71, 747 (1969).
7. Blattner, W.A. <u>et al</u>. <u>J. Am. Med. Ass.</u> 241, 259 (1979).
8. Vogelstein, B. <u>Nature</u> 348, 681 (1990).
9. Levine, A.J. <u>Virology</u> 177, 419 (1990).
10. Srivastava, S., Zou, Z., Pirollo, K., Blattner, W. and Chang, E.H. <u>Nature</u> 348, 747 (1990).
11. Malkin D. <u>et al</u>. <u>Science</u> 250, 1233 (1990).
12. Nigro, J. M <u>et al</u>. <u>Nature</u> 342, 705 (1989).
13. Chang, E.H. <u>et al</u>. <u>Science</u> 237, 1036 (1987).
14. Chen, P.L. Chen, Y., Bookstein, R., and Lee, W.H. <u>Science</u> 250, 1576 (1990).



From: *Neoplastic Transformation in Human Cell Culture,*
Eds.: J. S. Rhim and A. Dritschilo ©1991 The Humana Press Inc., Totowa, NJ

# p53 A DIRECT TARGET OF MUTATIONAL ACTIVATION BY CHEMICAL CARCINOGENS?


M. Nagarajan, M. Bowman, L. Rigby, J. S. Rhim and S. Sukumar

MBBC Laboratory, The Salk Institute, N. Torrey Pines Rd, La Jolla, CA 92037 USA and National Cancer Institute, Bethesda, MD 20892 USA


Tumor suppressor genes are emerging as major participants in the development and progression of a variety of human neoplasms. Loss of normal function of tumor suppressor genes as negative regulators of cell growth is believed to lead to tumor development. Loss of function of these genes may occur in the germ line, their absence predisposing the individual to cancer. More frequently, progressive loss of function in tumor suppressor genes occurs through an accumulation of somatic mutations.

The tumor suppressor gene, p53, encodes a 53-kDa nuclear phosphoprotein. Mutated p53 genes have been found in a large percentage of most common types of human cancer, such as colon, lung, liver, and B-cell leukemias. Unlike dominant tumor suppressor genes typified by the retinoblastoma gene, RB, p53 is unique in the potential of the mutant protein to act as a dominant oncogene. This is supported by its ability to co-operate with *ras* oncogenes to mediate transformation *in vitro*, despite the presence of two or more normal copies of the p53 gene in the cell (reviewed in 1).

Since the p53 protein is associated with malignant transformation, Masuda *et al.* surveyed 134 human malignancies that included carcinomas, sarcomas, leukemias and lymphomas for gene rearrangements in the p53 locus (2). p53 gene rearrangements were found in half (3/6) of the osteogenic sarcomas. Two of these sarcomas with

rearranged p53 also expressed high levels of the protein.
Along the same lines, Mulligan *et al.* screened 241 tumors
for aberrations in the p53 locus (3). Again, p53 changes
were confined to sarcomas. The changes that the p53 locus
had undergone in rhabdomyosarcomas included deletion of
both p53 alleles, deletion of one allele with or without
point mutation of the remaining allele, and absence of
detectable RNA. Similarly homozygous deletions and lack
of p53 mRNA or aberrant expression of the p53 protein were
seen in the osteosarcomas. These results indicate that in
tumors, gross gene rearrangements in p53 are not common.
On the other hand, loss of one allele, with mutation in
the remaining allele, appears to be the most common
mechanism of inactivation of the tumor suppressor function
of p53 gene in human tumors.

The fact that altered p53 has been implicated in
such a wide spectrum of tumors implies that inactivation
of this gene is a fundamental step in cellular transformation. If, as *in vitro*, the presence of mutated p53
genes bestows the property of immortality to primary cells
in culture, primary events in the initiation of malignancy
could be those involving p53 gene alterations. Some clue
that this may be the case is provided by recent data on
hepatocellular carcinomas from two geographically distant
regions, where the majority of p53 mutations were confined
to the specific codon 249 (4,5). The nature of the base
changes implicates specific mutagenesis by aflatoxin, long
suspected to be an etiological agent in this type of
cancer. On the other hand, somatic mutations in the p53
gene could be late events, as seen in human colon cancers,
pushing the tumor into the more aggressive phenotypes,
characteristic of progression.

The origin of somatic mutations in DNA are often
traceable to exposure to radiation or environmental,
chemical or physiological carcinogens, infection by
viruses, or faulty DNA repair. In the case of proto-
oncogenes, these alterations activate the gene and result
in malignancy. This has been frequently found in
carcinogen-induced animal tumors as well as in some types
of human tumors (6). The carcinogen-induced animal tumor
models offer some of the most dramatic examples of
involvement of *ras* oncogenes in carcinogenesis and the
reflection of the mutagenic specificities of the chemicals
used for initiation (6). In addition, such models provide
the opportunity to study genetic events involved in the
initiation, promotion and progression of cancer. Similar
model systems are provided by carcinogen-treated human
cells in culture.

The HOS cell line, derived originally from an aneuploid, human osteosarcoma, grows densely, forms small colonies in agar and is non-tumorigenic in nude mice. When treated with N-methyl-N'-nitro'N-nitrosoguanidine (MNNG), a potent carcinogen, (7), the cells acquired an altered phenotype, growing as aggregates, formed large colonies in agar and were tumorigenic in nude mice. In addition to MNNG, cell lines derived by treatment with 3-methylcholanthrene (MCA), 7, 12,-dimethyl benzo(a)-anthracene (DMBA) and benzo(a)pyrene [B(a)P] (8) as well as by infection with Kirsten sarcoma virus (Ki-SV) had similar properties (9). The conversion of the nontumorigenic parental HOS line to differing degrees of tumorigenicity following treatment with potent carcino-genic agents provides an *in vitro* model for studying additional genetic alterations involved in tumor progression. In fact, MCA-HOS cells contain activated H-*ras* oncogenes (10), and MNNG-HOS cells contain activated *met* oncogenes (11). To further elucidate the molecular mechanisms underlying multistep tumorigenesis, we examined the role of the p53 gene in the initiation and progression of the HOS cell lines. Secondly, since the chemical specificity of each of these carcinogens is well known, we considered the potential of this system to determine if the p53 gene, like *ras* oncogenes, is a direct target for mutational effects of carcinogens.

We examined the p53 gene and its expression in the parental cell line HOS, and its derivatives, MNNG-HOS, MCA-HOS, DMBA-HOS, B(a)P-HOS and K-HOS. Immunoprecip-itation of p53 using a polyclonal antibody, pAB122 showed that elevated levels (2-5 fold) of p53 protein were present in each of the carcinogen treated cell lines in comparison to the levels expressed by the parental cell line HOS (Table 1), whereas the level of p53 in K-HOS was in the same range as the parental HOS cells. In our experience and those of others, elevated levels of p53 protein are often indicative of the presence of point mutations in the conserved regions of the gene. We therefore sequenced the codons 30 to 300 (encompassing exons 4-8) to determine whether introduction of single base changes in p53 DNA was a consequence of treatment with the carcinogens. The results of these experiments are summarized in Table 1.

**TABLE 1.**

| Cell Line | Mutation at | Codon | Amino Acid Substitution | Expression levels of p53 |
|---|---|---|---|---|
| HOS | CGC->CCC | 156 | Arg->Pro | + |
| K-HOS | CGC->CCC | 156 | Arg->Pro | + |
| MNNG-HOS | CGC->CCC | 156 | Arg->Pro | |
| | TTT->CTT | 270 | PhA->Leu | +++ |
| MCA-HOS | CGC->CCC | 156 | Arg->Pro | |
| | GCC->GTC | 82 | Pro->Leu | +++ |
| DMBA-HOS | CGC->CCC | 156 | Arg->Pro | +++ |
| | ATG->ACG | 243 | Met->Thr | |
| BP-HOS | CGC->CCC | 156 | Arg->Pro | |
| | TAC->CAC | 163 | Tyr->His | +++ |

The p53 gene in the parental HOS cell line contained
a missense mutation in codon 156.  Each of the carcinogen-
treated cell lines had acquired a second point mutation in
the p53 gene.  These results suggest that the codon 156
mutation in HOS cell line was not sufficient for full
expression of the malignant phenotype.  These properties
could be attributed to the second point mutation that the
cell lines acquired in response to exposure to the
carcinogens.  Whether this is the case could be
determined, in future, by transfecting HOS cells with p53
genes carrying the second mutation.

Next, we took a more direct approach to study the
ability of carcinogens to introduce cancer-causing
mutations in DNA.  The wild type p53 cDNA in plasmid pSLVH
p53c-62 (12), was treated with two different doses of
MNNG, NMU, DMBA, BP, ethylmethane sulfonate (EMS),
hydroxylamine, and UV.  After carcinogen inactivation, the
plasmid DNA was transfected with mutated *ras* oncogene and
pSV2neo into primary and secondary cultures of rat cells.
Transformed foci were scored between 14-21 days.  Foci
appeared in plates that received carcinogen-treated
pSLVH.p53 plasmids.  The first cycle rat transformants
contain multiple copies of the p53 gene.  Further cycles

of transfection are being done to isolate p53 genes that
are responsible for the transformed phenotype. Examination of the presence of mutations in p53 by SSCP
analysis, followed by sequencing of the PCR products will
reveal the nature of mutations that endowed transforming
properties to the p53 transgene. These studies will
provide answers to whether there are any hot spots of
mutation in p53 genes and more importantly, whether there
is specificity in the type of mutation in p53 caused by a
particular carcinogen, implying a direct interaction
between the two.

## REFERENCES

1.    A.J. Levine, and J. Momand.  __Biochem Biophys Acta__
      1032, 119 (1990).
2.    H. Masuda, C. Miller, *et al*.  __Proc. Natl.__
      __Acad. Sci. USA__ 84, 7716 (1987).
3.    L. Mulligan, G.J. Matlashewski, *et al*.  __Proc.__
      __Natl. Acad. Sci. USA__ 87, 5863 (1990).
4.    B. Bressac, M. Kew, *et al*.  __Nature__ 35, 429
      (1991).
5.    I.C. Hsu, R.A. Metcalf, *et al*.  __Nature__ 350, 427
      (1991).
6.    S. Sukumar.  __Cancer Cells__ 2, 199 (1990).
7.    J.S. Rhim, D.P. Park, *et al*.  __Nature__ 256, 751
      (1975).
8.    H.Y. Cho, J.S. Rhim, *et al*.  __Int. J. Cancer__ 21, 22
      (1978).
9.    J.S. Rhim, H.Y. Cho, *et al*.  __Int. J. Cancer__ 15, 23
      (1975).
10.   J.S. Rhim, J. Fujita, *et al*.  __Carcinogenesis__ 8, 1165
      (1987).
11.   C.S. Cooper, D.G. Blair, *et al*.  __Cancer Res.__ 44, 1
      (1984).
12.   R. Zakut-Houri, B. Bienz, D. Givol, M. Oren.  __EMBO__
      4, 1251 (1985).

From: *Neoplastic Transformation in Human Cell Culture,*
Eds.: J. S. Rhim and A. Dritschilo ©1991 The Humana Press Inc., Totowa, NJ

# III. Viral Transformation
## and Oncogenes

# THE HIV *tat* GENE INDUCES EPIDERMAL HYPERPLASIA *IN VIVO* AND TRANSFORMS KERATINOCYTES *IN VITRO*

Jonathan A. Rhim, Jonathan Vogel, Chang-Min Kim, Johng S. Rhim* and Gilbert Jay

Laboratory of Virology, Jerome H. Holland Laboratory, American Red Cross, Rockville, MD, *Laboratory of Cellular and Molecular Biology, National Cancer Institute, Bethesda, MD

Many dermatologic disorders are associated with the acquired immune deficiency syndrome (AIDS). Kaposi's sarcoma, psoriasis, seborrheic dermatitis, squamous cell carcinoma, basal cell carcinoma, and melanoma are all increased in frequency in the AIDS population (1,2). Multiple pathologic processes are likely to be at work in inducing the complex manifestations of AIDS, including the direct effects of infection with the human immunodeficiency virus (HIV), the indirect effects of profound immune dysfunction, and the involvement of multiple other infectious agents (3,4).

We chose to study the *tat* gene of HIV to better understand the contributions of viral gene expression in the pathogenesis of AIDS. We believe that the product of the *tat* gene is important in HIV pathology for the following reasons: [1] it is essential for viral replication, and [2] it is a transactivator gene, capable of upregulating viral gene expression (5,6). In the course of *tat* gene expression and HIV replication, *tat* not only influences the expression of other viral genes but also of cellular genes. The resulting perturbation of normal cellular functions and differentiation is likely to induce cell proliferation.

Previous study of the *tat* gene in transgenic mice under the control of the HIV regulatory sequences demonstrated cutaneous disorders, namely, epidermal hyperplasia and dermal lesions resembling Kaposi's sarcoma (7,8). *Tat* expression was confined to the epidermis in these mice, suggesting that a target cell was present within the epidermis that could interact with the *tat* gene product and result in epidermal hyperplasia (9). The epidermal changes are multifocal and can be extensive (Fig. 1).

There are multiple cell types present within the mouse epidermis, including keratinocytes, Langerhans' cells, and Thy1-positive cells (10,11). Although the CD4-positive Langerhans' cells are hypothesized to be the major reservoir of HIV (12,13), keratinocytes have also been suggested to be infected (14). The abundant proliferation of keratinocytes in our transgenic mice suggested that these cells could be targets for *tat* gene expression, and prompted us to study this interaction in cultured human cells.

To examine the effect of the Tat protein on human keratinocytes, we transfected RHEK-1 cells with the *tat* gene under the control of the HIV long terminal repeat (7). The RHEK-1 cell line is a keratinocyte cell line established from human foreskin (15). The cells were immortalized by transfection with an Ad12-SV40 hybrid virus. RHEK-1 cells grow as a flat monolayer in culture, do not grow in soft agar, express appropriate human keratinocyte differentiation markers, and are not tumorigenic in nude mice.

Initially, the transfected cells gave no detectable transformed foci but acquired a transformed morphology only after multiple passages. This observation suggested that small numbers of transfected cells expressing the *tat* gene were being obscured by the large number of nontransformed cells in the culture, and required many passages to manifest their growth properties. We sought to enrich for these transformed cells by cotransfection with a plasmid containing the neomycin-resistant gene, followed by selection with neomycin (Geneticin). Of 7 neomycin-resistant clones that were found to contain the transfected gene, 5 expressed *tat* mRNA (16). These clones showed a transformed phenotype characterized by foci of piled cells (Fig. 2). Southern blot hybridization analysis confirmed that each represented an independently-derived clone.

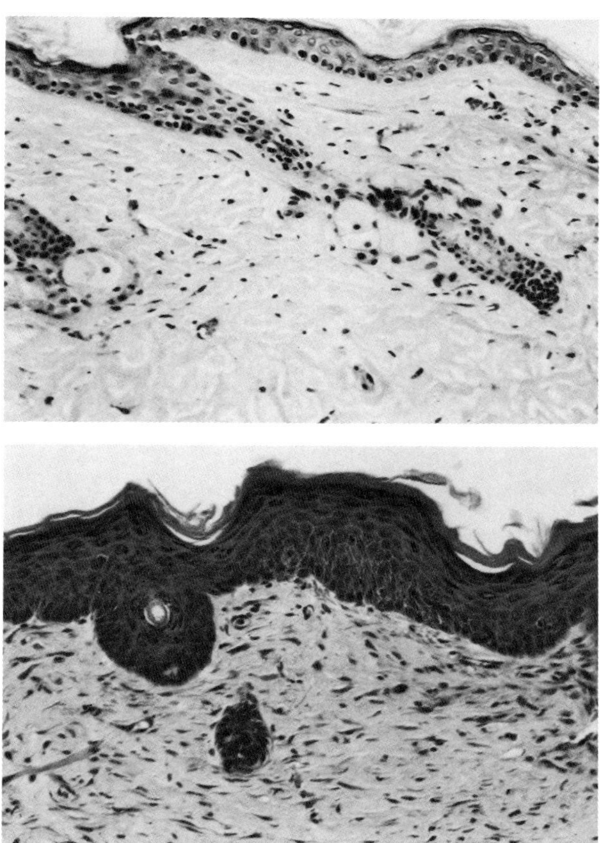

**Figure 1.** Microscopic examination of the skin from mice carrying the HIV *tat* gene. Skin biopsies from a control mouse (A) and a transgenic mouse (B) were placed in 10% buffered formalin for 24 hours, embedded in paraffin, sectioned and stained with hematoxylin-and-eosin.

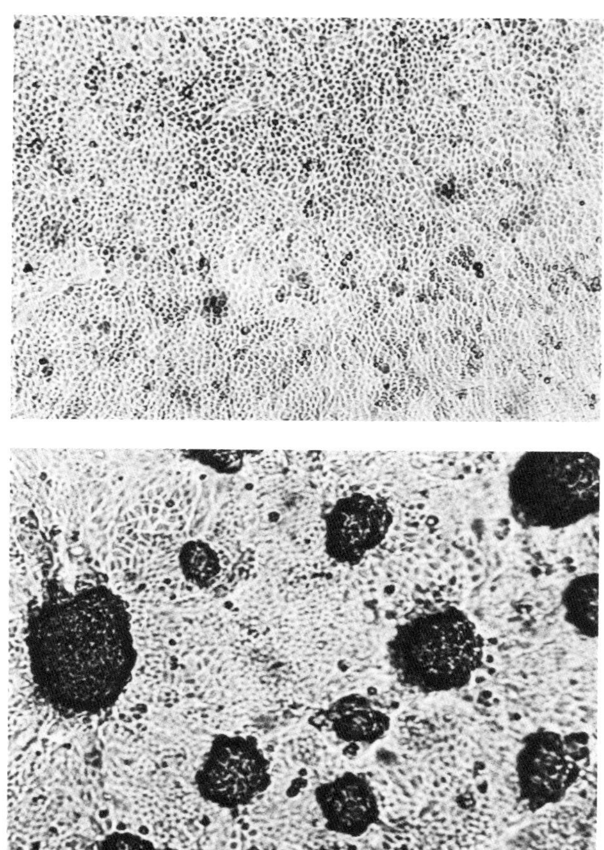

**Figure 2.** Growth characteristic of human keratinocytes transfected by the HIV *tat* gene. Growth morphology in monolayer cultures of the nontransfected RHEK-1 cells (A) and a neomycin-resistant and *tat*-expressing clone (B). Cells were placed on plastic dishes in Dulbecco's modified essential medium containing 10% fetal bovine serum.

No piled-up morphology was detected in nontransfected or neomycin-transfected controls. Tat expressing cells grew to an increased density, displayed a faster doubling time, and were able to grow in soft agar; features which correlated with the level of *tat* mRNA expression. Most significantly, subcutaneous injections of $10^7$ cells in nude mice resulted in tumors within 3-4 weeks. Nontransfected RHEK-1 cells showed no tumor formation. Cell lines established from the tumors continued to express Tat.

To summarize, transfection of the HIV *tat* gene into human epidermal keratinocytes resulted in neoplastic transformation as demonstrated by piling up of cells in culture, anchorage-independent growth in soft agar, and tumorigenicity in nude mice. Transfected cells expressed the *tat* gene, indicating that subcellular targets exist within keratinocytes capable of interacting with this critical gene product of HIV, and suggesting that keratinocytes may be a target cell for HIV infection and pathogenicity.

The interaction of HIV and keratinocytes may contribute to the dermatologic disorders seen in individuals with AIDS. Psoriasis has been associated with HIV infection (17,18). Psoriatic lesions have appeared at all stages of HIV infection, not only in profoundly immunosuppressed AIDS patients but also in asymptomatic, AIDS-related complex (ARC) patients (6). Most have not had a previous family history of psoriasis. In general, psoriasis in the HIV-infected population is more severe, occurs in unusual areas, and over a larger area of the body. It is less amenable to therapy.

Psoriasis is one of the papulosquamous disorders of the skin and is characterized clinically by hyperkeratotic plaques and scales. Histologically, the lesions show thickening of the epidermis, elongation of dermal papillae, hyperkeratosis, parakeratosis, prominence of dermal papillary vessels, and an inflammatory cell infiltrate (19,20). Exacerbations of psoriasis include stress, sunlight, infection, and trauma. The development of psoriatic lesions after trauma in previously normal-appearing skin of patients with psoriasis is well established. This phenomenon suggests that the fine controls governing keratinocyte proliferation in even normal appearing skin in patients with psoriasis are altered. The process of wound healing might add stress to these controls on epidermal growth, and bring out the clinical lesions. Immunologic dysfunction has also been suggested in the pathogenesis of psoriasis (20). Moreover, the disease responds to immunosuppressive medications, such as cyclosporine (21). Arthritis of presumed immune etiology is associated with psoriasis (22).

Keratinocytes are able to express a variety of growth factors and immunoregulatory molecules in both normal as well as pathologic states. HIV infection and expression of *tat* in keratinocytes could result in abnormally high levels of endogenous keratinocyte growth factors or inappropriate expression of genes promoting keratinocyte growth. Transforming growth factor alpha (TGF-α) is an attractive candidate in the pathogenesis of psoriasis. It is mitogenic for a variety of cancer cells and normal cells in culture. Keratinocytes produce TGF-α in culture and are stimulated by it to divide (23). TGF-α has sequence homology to epidermal growth factor (EGF), binds the EGF receptor, and is able to mediate similar physiologic properties as EGF, including supporting the growth of keratinocytes in culture. TGF-α has been implicated in skin homeostasis *in vivo,* where it is detected immunohistochemically in the normal epidermis. Application of TGF-α promotes wound healing in experimental animals, perhaps by stimulation of keratinocyte proliferation (24,25). Recently, TGF-α expression has been shown to be increased in psoriatic lesions (26).

In general, HIV expression in infected individuals is very low. Even in CD4-positive T-cells, a cell type that is profoundly affected in HIV infection, viral sequences can be detected in only approximately 1:1000 circulating cells (27). In order to account for such global dysfunction of this population of cells in the absence of widespread viral infection, soluble factors produced by infected cells may be considered. Indeed TGF-α is a secreted molecule capable of stimulating keratinocyte proliferation in both a paracrine and autocrine manner (23). A few infected keratinocytes expressing *tat* may result in release of factors affecting many. In addition, paracrine action of TGF-α may influence other cell types in the vicinity as well. Endothelial cells are stimulated to divide in response to TGF-α exposure (24). Endothelial cell proliferation and vascular prominence, seen in psoriatic plaques, may be a consequence of keratinocyte overproduction and release of TGF-α.

Inappropriate expression of immunoregulatory molecules in *tat*-expressing keratinocytes may contribute to immune-mediated keratinocyte proliferation. Disrupted immune function has been implicated in the pathogenesis of psoriasis (28). Psoriatic keratinocytes express HLA antigens, while keratinocytes in normal skin do not (29). Increased numbers of activated T-cells are present in psoriatic skin (30). The most convincing evidence for the involvement of the immune system in the pathogenesis of psoriasis is the response of the disease to cyclosporin A (21), an immunosuppressive agent with many effects on T-cell functions and antigen presentation.

Keratinocytes are a rich source of immunoregulatory molecules (11). Many of these inflammatory mediators may also cause keratinocyte proliferation. Interleukin-1 (IL-1) is a potential mediator of the inflammatory processes at work in psoriasis (31). Implicated in a wide variety of inflammatory processes, IL-1 is expressed in and is a mitogen for keratinocytes. Two major species of IL-1 are expressed by normal keratinocytes, IL-1$\alpha$ and IL-1$\beta$. The altered expression and activities of the two species of IL-1 in psoriasis may uniquely reflect the complex immunologic abnormalities of the keratinocytes in this disorder.

Although many cytokines with the potential to stimulate keratinocyte proliferation are expressed in normal skin, two appear to be increased in psoriatic skin. Interleukin-6 (IL-6), a mitogen for keratinocytes, is usually not detected in normal skin. Its expression and activity are increased in psoriatic skin (32). Interferon-$\gamma$ induced protein IP-10 is found in keratinocytes of psoriatic skin but not in normal skin (33). The consequences of this molecule for keratinocyte proliferation is unknown at present.

Tat expression in keratinocytes may result in different patterns of keratinocyte proliferation in different patients. Seborrheic dermatitis has recently been recognized as a common manifestation of AIDS, occurring in up to 80% of patients (18). Histologically the lesions show epidermal hyperplasia and a dermal infiltrate of lymphocytes. Although the epidermal hyperplasia is distinct histologically, seborrheic dermatitis may have a psoriasiform appearance clinically, perhaps due to the hyperplasia.

Neoplastic transformation has been shown fundamentally to involve successive genetic events in its development and progression. Often one of these events involves a growth-promoting change, which then increases the probability of secondary genetic events leading to a malignant change. HIV integration and *tat* gene expression may represent an early growth-promoting step in keratinocyte progression to malignancy in AIDS patients. Subsequent genetic events may then lead to squamous cell carcinoma or basal cell carcinoma, invasive cancers whose incidence is increased in the AIDS population. Certainly the contribution of decreased immune surveillance and UV irradiation may also be of importance in the development of these tumors. UV irradiation, causing direct damage to DNA, may lead to oncogene activation and tumor development. On the other hand, UV-mediated damage to keratinocytes and activation of genes that promote *tat* expression may also lead to inappropriate keratinocyte proliferation. The relationship between UV irradiation, immune activation, wound healing, other dermal infectious agents and *tat* expression in keratinocytes deserve further investigation.

In conclusion, we have demonstrated that transfection of the *tat* gene into human epidermal keratinocytes results in uncontrolled proliferation, implicating keratinocytes as a potential target cell for HIV infection. Altered keratinocytes, through the elaboration of cytokines may account for some of the cutaneous manifestations of AIDS, including psoriasis, and may provide an early step towards neoplastic transformation. *Tat* gene expression in HIV-infected keratinocytes may provide a common pathway for the many triggers of psoriasis. The identification of a particular gene product of HIV with pathogenic potential provides a potential target against which future AIDS therapies can be directed.

# REFERENCES


1. Harawi, S. J. In *Pathology and Pathophysiology of AIDS and HIV-related Disease*, (eds. Harawi, S. J. and O'Hara, C. J.). Pp. 47-56 (C. V. Mosby Company, St. Louis, 1989).

2. Sadick, N. S., McNutt, N. S., and Kaplan, M. H. 1990. *J. Am. Acad. Dermatol.* 22:1270-1277.

3. Gallo, R. C., and Montagnier, L. 1988. *Sci. Am.* 259:40-48.

4. Rosenberg, Z. F., and Fauci, A. S. 1991. In *The Human Retroviruses* (eds. Gallo, R. C. and Jay, G.). Pp. 140-160 (Academic Press, San Diego).

5. Dayton, A. I., Sodroski, J. G., Rosen, C. A., Goh, W. C., and Haseltine, W. A. 1986. *Cell* 44:941-947.

6. Varmus, H. 1988. *Genes Develop.* 2:1055-1062.

7. Vogel, J., Hinrichs, S. H., Reynolds, R. K., Luciw, P. A., and Jay, G. 1988. *Nature* 335:606-611.

8. Vogel, J., Rhim., J. A., Jay, D. B., and Jay, G. 1991. In *The Human Retroviruses* (eds. Gallo, R. C. and Jay, G.). Pp. 277-295. (Academic Press, San Diego).

9. Vogel, J., Cepeda, M., Tschachler, E., Napolitano, L., and Jay, G. Submitted for publication.

10. Shimada, S., and Katz, S. 1988. *Arch. Pathol. Lab. Med.* 112:231-234.

11. Saunder, D. N. 1990. *J. Invest. Dermatol.* 95:27S-28S.

12. Tschachler, E., Groh, V., Popovic, M., Mann, D. L., Konrad, K., Sasai, B., Eron, L, diMarzo Veronese, F., Wolff, K., and Stingl, G. 1987. *J. Invest. Dermatol.* 88:233-237.

13. Stingl, G., Rappersberger, K., Tschachler, E., Gartner, S., Groh, V., and Mann, D. L. 1990. *J. Am. Acad. Dermatol.* 22:1210-1217.

14. Chesebro, B., Bullar, R., Portis, J., and Wehrly, K. 1990. *J. Virol.* 64:215-221.

15. Rhim, J. S., Jay, G., Arnstein, P., Price, F. M., Sanford, K. K., and Aaronson, S. A. 1985. *Science* 227:1250-1252.

16. Kim, C.-M., Vogel, J., Jay, G., and Rhim, J. S. Submitted for publication.

17. Lazar, A. P., and Roenigk, H. H. 1987. *Cutis* 39:347-351.

18. Mathes, B. M., and Douglass, M. C. 1985. *J. Am. Acad.*

*Dermatol.* 13:947-951.

19.  Krueger, J. G., Krane, J. F., Carter, D. M., and Gottlieb, A. B. 1990. *J. Invest. Dermatol.* 94:1355-1405.
20.  Gottlieb, A. B. 1990. *J. Invest. Dermatol.* 95:185-195.
21.  Ellis, C. N., Gorsulowsky, D. C., Hamilton, T. A., Billings, J. K., Brown, M. D., Headington, J. T., Cooper, K. D., Baadsgaard, O., Duell, E. A., Annesley, T. M., Turcotte, J. G., and Voorhees, J. J. 1986. *J. Am. Med. Assoc.* 256:3110-3116.
22.  Gladman, D. D. 1985. In *Psoriatic Arthritis.* Gerber, L. H. and Espinoza, L. R. (eds.). Grune and Stratton, Orlando.
23.  Nickoloff, B. J., Mitra, R. S., Elder, J. T., Fisher, G. J., and Voorhees, J. J. 1989. *Br. J. Dermatol.* 121:161-174.
24.  Schreiber, A. B., Winkler, M. E., and Derynck, R. 1986. *Science* 232:1250-1253.
25.  Schultz, G. S., White, M., Mitchell, R., Brown, G., Lynch J., Twardzik, D. R., and Podaro, G. 1987. *Science* 235:350-352.
26.  Elder, J. T., Fisher, G. J., Lindquist, P. B., Bennett, G. L., Pittelkow, M. R., Coffey, R. J., Ellingsworth, L., Derynck, R., and Voorhees, J. J. 1989. *Science* 243:811-814.
27.  Ho, D. D., Moudgil, T., and Alam, M. 1989. *New Engl. J. Med.* 321:1621-1625.
28.  Gottlieb, A. B. 1990. *J. Invest. Dermatol.* 95:18S-19S.
29.  Gottlieb, A. B., Lifshitz, B., Fu, S. M., Staiano-Coico, L., Wang, C. Y., and Carter, D. M. 1986. *J. Exp. Med.* 164:1013-1028.
30.  Baker, B. S., Swain, A. F., Fry, L., and Valdimarsson, H. 1984. *Br. J. Dermatol.* 11:555-564.
31.  Cooper, K. D., Hammerberg, C., Baadsgaard, O., Elder, J. T., Chan, L. S., Taylor, R. S., Voorhees, J. J., and Fisher, G. 1990. *J. Invest. Dermatol.* 95:245-265.
32.  Grossman, R. M., Kruegar, J., Yourish, D., Granelli-Piperno, A., Murphy, D. P., May, L. T., Kupper, T. S., Sehgal, P., and Gottlieb, A. B. 1989. *Proc. Natl. Acad. Sci. USA* 86:6367-7371.
33.  Gottlieb, A. B., Luster, A. D., Posnett, D. N., and Carter, D. M. 1988. *J. Exp. Med.* 168:941-948.

IMMORTALIZATION AND TUMORIGENIC TRANSFORMATION OF
NORMAL HUMAN CERVICAL EPITHELIAL CELLS TRANSFECTED
WITH HUMAN PAPILLOMAVIRUS DNAs

Craig D. Woodworth

Laboratory of Biology, National Cancer
Institute, Bethesda, Maryland, 20892

## ABSTRACT

An _in vitro_ - _in vivo_ model useful for
investigating etiologic factors involved in
cervical cancer is described. Cultures of normal
human epithelial cells derived from foreskin or
cervix were transfected with recombinant human
papillomavirus (HPV) DNAs and a series of immortal
cell lines were established. These cell lines
contained integrated and transcriptionally active
HPV DNAs, they were not tumorigenic in nude mice,
and they retained the ability to undergo terminal
squamous differentiation when tested at early
passages. With continued propagation in culture
the cells progressively became dysplastic and lost
responsiveness to normal regulatory factors such
as transforming growth factors beta 1 and 2 (TGF$\beta$1
and 2). Transfection of immortal lines at early
passage with activated v-Ha-_ras_ or herpes simplex
virus type 2 DNAs, which are often present in
cervical cancer, led to malignant progression and
formation of squamous carcinomas when cells were
innoculated in nude mice. Thus, HPV-immortalized
cervical cells are an appropriate model for
studying the importance of specific environmental
or host factors in cervical malignancy.

## INTRODUCTION

Cervical cancer is a major public health problem and ranks second worldwide as a cause of cancer deaths in women (1). Clinical and epidemiologic data support an etiologic role for specific human papilloma virus (HPV) types in cervical cancer (1-3). HPV DNAs have been detected in the majority (>90%) of cervical intraepithelial neoplasias and invasive cervical cancers (4-6). This association is specific as certain HPV types (in particular HPV16 and 18) occur consistently in advanced cervical intraepithelial neoplasia and in cervical carcinomas whereas others such as HPV6 and 11 are frequently found in benign lesions, suggesting a difference in oncogenic potential. Progression of HPV infection to invasive cervical cancer is often associated with integration of the HPV genome into the host cell DNA. The tumors are often monoclonal with respect to the virus integration pattern suggesting that integration represents an early and important event in tumor development (6). Furthermore, the HPV E6 and E7 genes are characteristically retained and actively expressed in tumors or tumor-derived cell lines (7-8), implying a role for these proteins in oncogenesis.

Although HPVs have been implicated as important agents in the development of cervical cancer, the presence of the virus alone appears insufficient to cause malignant disease. Thus, additional alterations or insults are required. The nature of these agents is poorly understood, however clinical and epidemiologic work suggests the importance of other viruses (9), cigarette smoking (10), and alterations in cellular protooncogenes such as _myc_ and _ras_ (11-12).

_In vitro_ and _in vivo_ models have been developed to study the interaction between HPVs and cervical cells. Normal human epithelial cells have been cultured from the cervical transformation zone in which most cervical cancers originate, or from foreskin epithelium which serves as a reservoir for HPV infection _in vivo_.

Transfection of these cultures with recombinant HPV DNAs associated with cervical cancer has led to immortalization and establishment of a series of cervical and foreskin cell lines. This review summarizes experiments in our laboratory that have utilized this *in vitro/in vivo* system to examine the role of HPVs in altering cell growth, differentiation, and contributing to malignant disease.

## RESULTS AND DISCUSSION

Tissue samples obtained from foreskin or cervical epithelium were placed in MCDB153-LB medium (13) containing 0.25% collagenase and allowed to digest for 18 - 24 hours (14). The mucosa was gently scrapped to dislodge clumps of epithelial cells and these were transferred to 100 mm collagen-coated culture dishes and maintained overnight to allow cell attachment. Cultures were composed mainly of small round cells with a few larger cells that had undergone squamous differentiation. Secondary cultures were transfected with recombinant plasmids containing HPV types frequently associated with cervical malignancy (HPV16, 18, 31, or 33), or types with low or no association (HPV1, 6b, and 11). Cells were selected for resistance to G418 due to the presence of a cotransfected neomycin resistance gene. Within 7 - 10 days resistant colonies arose; these grew rapidly, could be subcultured repeatedly, and closely resembled normal cells in morphology (14).

Recombinant HPVs could be classified into two groups on the basis of their ability to immortalize (15). Cells transfected with HPV16, 18, 31, or 33 DNAs formed rapidly growing colonies in a reproducible manner when tested on cells derived from different individuals. In contrast, recombinant HPV1, 6b, and 11 DNAs induced G418-resistant colonies that grew transiently, but quickly senesced. Thus, the ability of specific HPV DNAs to immortalize cultured epithelial cells is related to their association with cervical

carcinoma        (15),        suggesting        that        the
immortalization   function   is   important   in   the
pathogenesis of cervical cancer (15-17).

A series of immortal cell lines derived from
cervical or foreskin epithelium were established
(14,15).  These lines all contained integrated and
rearranged HPV genomes when examined by Southern
analysis.  Most cell lines also retained one or
more intact HPV genomes.  Further analyses showed
that these lines expressed several HPV RNAs and
that   these   hybridized   strongly   to   probes
containing the HPV E6 and E7 genes (15).  These
cell lines represent an appropriate model for
studying factors that regulate HPV gene expression
in cervical epithelial cells and examining the
influence   of   cocarcinogens   on   neoplastic
progression.

HPV DNAs are detected in the majority of
cervical intraepithelial neoplasias, suggesting
that    HPVs    directly    stimulate    dysplastic
differentiation.  To test this hypothesis, normal
cervical and foreskin epithelial cells and HPV-
immortalized cell lines were transplanted beneath
a   skin-   muscle   flap   in   nude   mice   (18,19).
Xenografts containing normal cells formed well
differentiated stratified squamous epithelia but
cells immortalized by HPV16, 18, 31 or 33 DNAs
exhibited dysplastic morphology (19). Dysplastic
changes   were   particularly   striking   when   the
immortalized     cell     lines     were     maintained
continuously in culture (more than 180 population
doublings)   prior   to   transplantation.   These
changes consisted of altered mitoses, an increased
nuclear to cytoplasmic ratio, and often a total
absence of cell flattening in superficial layers
of  epithelium.   Grafts  containing  normal  or
immortalized   cells   were   also   examined   for
expression of involucrin, a structural protein
that is a marker for squamous differentiation in
normal  cervical  epithelium  (20).   Involucrin
expression was confined to the suprabasal layers
in grafts of normal cervical or foreskin cells and
thus resembled the pattern seen <u>in situ</u>.  In

contrast, involucrin localization in grafts containing dysplastic cells was often altered. Specifically, the protein was either not detectable or was present in a diffuse disorganized pattern (21).

Replicate cultures of normal or immortal cells were examined by Northern analysis to determine whether immortality resulted in alterations in expression of genes involved in squamous differentiation. Steady state levels of keratin 1 and involucrin RNAs were decreased in several immortal lines. Most cells with decreased expression of these two RNAs *in vitro* also formed severely dysplastic epithelia in xenografts, suggesting a correlation between *in vitro* and *in vivo* gene expression (19). These results show that specific HPV DNAs commonly detected in most anogenital intraepithelial neoplasias and carcinomas stimulate dysplasia *in vivo* in normal human epithelial cells derived from genital tract epithelium. Because dysplasias have the potential to undergo malignant progression, our results imply that HPVs might contribute to the multistage carcinogenesis process by virtue of their ability to alter normal differentiation.

Both experimental and epidemiologic studies indicate that HPVs are necessary, but not sufficient factors for the development of cervical cancer. Recent studies have demonstrated that some invasive cervical carcinomas have an activated c-Ha-*ras* gene (11) and amplification and/or over expression of the c-*myc* gene (12). Because activation of these two protoncogenes was found in conjunction with HPV16 DNA, the possibility exists that activation of *ras* or *myc* is sufficient to convert the HPV-containing cervical cells into a tumor-producing cell line. To test this possibility an HPV-immortalized cervical line was cotransfected with either the v-Ha-*ras* or c-*myc* genes in combination with a gene encoding multi-drug resistance (MDR). Colonies expressing resistance to colchicine were isolated, pooled, and cells containing either MDR/c-*myc*, MDR/v-Ha-*ras* or MDR alone were established. The tumorigenicity of these lines was assessed after innoculation of 1x10$^7$ cells subcutaneously into nude mice. Only cells transfected with MDR/<u>ras</u> formed tumors (22). These tumors were well differentiated cystic squamous cell carcinomas that exhibited both squamous and glandular elements. Tumor cell lines were derived by disaggregation of these carcinomas and subsequent selection by growth in medium containing colchine. These tumor-derived cell lines produced carcinomas when tested in nude mice (22).

Molecular studies indicated that the transfected v-Ha-<u>ras</u> gene was expressed in the tumorigenic cells, and that the HPV E6 and E7 proteins were also produced at a level comparable to the parent immortalized cells (22). Thus, addition of <u>ras</u> did not alter quantitatively the expression of HPV transforming genes. The development of tumorigenicity after addition of <u>ras</u> is significant because addition of <u>ras</u> alone is not effective in normal human keratinocytes (23) or cervical cells (22). These observations are relevant to the <u>in vivo</u> situation because Ha-<u>ras</u> may be amplified, overexpressed or mutated in some cervical cancers (11).

The regulation of HPV gene expression and papilloma formation is influenced by a variety of host factors. Normal genital epithelial cells possess an intracellular control mechanism directed against HPV gene transcription (6,24). Cellular functions down-regulating HPV expression are absent in genital carcinoma cells (24) suggesting that this loss represents an important step in the development of cancer. The beta transforming growth factors (TGFβs) are members of a family of polypeptides that modulate cell proliferation and gene expression in diverse cells (25). Normal genital epithelial cells secrete and respond to TGFβ1 suggesting that it might act as an autocrine regulator of growth and gene expression in normal epithelium. In addition, alterations in expression or responsiveness to TGFβs often occur in malignancy (26).

A series of immortal and tumorigenically transformed cervical cell lines was used to characterize the effect of TGF$\beta$s on cell growth, differentiation, and HPV gene expression (27). TGF$\beta$1 and 2 reversibly inhibited expression of the HPV16 E6 and E7 oncoproteins in several different immortal cell lines. The loss of E6 and E7 protein expression followed a dramatic time- and dose- dependent decrease in E6 and E7 RNA levels and was accompanied by cessation of cell proliferation. Nuclear run on transcriptional analyses showed that regulation of HPV gene expression occurred at the level of transcription. Interestingly, TGF$\beta$1 concommitantly induced a 5-6 fold increase in expression of its own RNA, thereby providing a means of amplifying and sustaining its inhibitory effects on HPV gene expression. These results suggest that TGF$\beta$1 may have an autocrine function in down-regulating HPV gene expression in infected anogenital epithelium.

The biological significance of TGF$\beta$1 in the multistage carcinogenesis process was investigated by comparing the effects of the cytokine on normal cervical cells, cells that had been immortalized, cells that exhibited aberrant differentiation (induced by continuous passage in culture), or cells that had been malignantly transformed <u>in vitro</u> (22,28). Although TGF$\beta$1 dramatically down-regulated growth and virus gene expression in immortal cells, the inhibition was often less pronounced in similar cells maintained extensively in culture. HPV16 RNA was decreased only minimally in two cervical carcinoma cell lines QGU and SiHa, however, virus gene expression was down-regulated significantly in another line, QGH. Furthermore, HPV RNA expression decreased only slightly after TGF$\beta$1 treatment of immortal lines that had been malignantly transformed <u>in vitro</u> with either the v-Ha-<u>ras</u> gene or the herpes simplex virus type 2 <u>Bgl</u> II N fragment (28). These results indicate that loss of responsiveness to TGF$\beta$1 often precedes or accompanies malignant development in cultured genital epithelial cells. Different tumorigenic lines also varied significantly in their response to TGF$\beta$1, and one line (QGH) was partially sensitive.  Therefore, while acquisition of resistance to TGF$\beta$1 might contribute to the carcinogenesis process, this study as well as others (25) indicates that resistance to TGF$\beta$1 is not a prerequisite.

Work from our laboratory has focused on understanding the multistage progression of cervical cancer.  The *in vitro/in vivo* model discussed is unique because it involves relevant etiologic agents in combination with the actual target cells from which cervical carcinomas arise *in vivo*.  Future work in our laboratory will focus on several important questions.  HPVs influence normal cell growth and differentiation. Therefore, what are the molecular mechanisms by which specific HPV proteins alter cell regulation? What are the roles of host defense mechanisms such as the immune response in combating HPV infection or in reversing preneoplastic lesions?  Most importantly, are there additional cofactors that contribute to the development of cervical cancer and what are the molecular mechanisms underlying their cocarcinogenic effects?

## REFERENCES


1.    J. Waterhouse, C., et al (eds.).  Cancer Incidence in Five Continents.  Vol 4, IARC, Lyon France, 1982.
2.    D. J. McCance. <u>Biochim Biophys. Acta.</u> 823, 195 (1986).
3.    W. C. Reeves, W. E. Rawls, <u>et al</u>. <u>Rev. Inf. Dis.</u> 11, 426 (1989).
4.    M. Boshart, L. Gissmann, <u>et al</u>. <u>EMBO J.</u> 3, 1151, (1984).
5.    M. Durst, L. Gissmann, <u>et al</u>. <u>Proc. Natl. Acad. Sci. (USA)</u> 80, 3812 (1983).
6.    H. zur Hausen. <u>Cancer Res.</u> 49, 4677 (1989).
7.    A. Schneider - Gadicke, and E. Schwarz. <u>EMBO J.</u> 5, 2285 (1986).
8.    D. Smotkin, and F. O. Wettstein. <u>Proc. Natl Acad. Sci. (USA)</u> 83, 4680 (1986).
9.    V. Vonka, J. Kanka, <u>et al</u>. <u>Adv. Cancer Res.</u> 48, 149 (1987).

10. L. Brinton, C. Schairer, *et al.*JAMA 255, 3265 (1986).
11. G. Riou, M. Barrois, *et al.* Oncogene 3, 329 (1988).
12. H. Shirasawa, Y. Tomita, *et al.* J. Gen Virol. 68, 583 (1987).
13. L. Pirisi, S. Yasumoto, *et al.* J. Virol 61, 1061 (1987).
14. C. D. Woodworth, P. Bowden, *et al.* Cancer Res. 48, 4620 (1988).
15. C. D. Woodworth, J.Doniger, *et al.* J. Virol. 63, 159 (1989).
16. R. Schlegel, W.C. Phelps, *et al.* EMBO J. 7, 3181. (1988).
17. G. Pecoraro, D. Morgan, *et al.* Proc. Natl. Acad. Sci (USA) 86, 563 (1989).
18. Y. Barrandon, V. Li, and H. J. Green. J. Invest. Dermatol. 91, 315 (1988).
19. C. D. Woodworth, S. Waggoner, *et al.* Cancer Res. 50, 3709 (1990).
20. M. J. Warhol, G. S. Pinkus, *et al.* Int. J. Gynecol, Pathol. 3, 71 (1984).
21. C. D. Woodworth, S. Waggoner, *et al.* In, P. Howley and T. Broker (eds.), Papillomaviruses, UCLA Symposium on Molecular and Cellular Biology, pp. 231–238, Wiley-Liss, NY.
22. J. A. DiPaolo, C.D. Woodworth, *et al.* Oncogene 4, 395 (1989).
23. M. Durst, D. Gallahan, *et al.* Virology 173, 767 (1989).
24. F. Rosl, M. Durst, and H. zur Hausen. EMBO J. 7, 1321 (1988).
25. A. B. Roberts, and M. B. Sporn. Handb. Exp. Pharmacol. 45, 419 (1990).
26. L. Braun, M. Durst, *et al.* Cancer Res. 50, 7324 (1990).
27. C. D. Woodworth, V. Notario, and J. A. DiPaolo. J. Virol. 64, 4767 (1990).
28. J. A. DiPaolo, C. D. Woodworth, *et al.* Virology 177, 777 (1990).

# USING THE PAPILLOMAVIRUS E6/E7 GENES TO GENERATE WELL-DIFFERENTIATED EPITHELIAL CELL LINES.


M. Conrad[1], J. Yankaskas[2], R. Boucher[2], and R. Schlegel[1]

[1]Department of Pathology, Georgetown University, Washington, D.C. 20007 and

[2]Department of Medicine, University of North Carolina, Chapel Hill, N.C.


## INTRODUCTION

The study of normal cell growth and differentiation would be greatly augmented by the development of an efficient method for obtaining human immortalized cell lines which would retain their ability to differentiate and respond to external regulatory signals. One critical research area which would greatly benefit from such an approach would be the study of cystic fibrosis (CF). Not only would CF cell lines permit the analysis of the altered ion permeability properties of these cells and their alteration by pharmacologic agents, but they would also serve as a substrate for future gene therapy experiments. In an attempt to generate such cell lines, the SV40 large T antigen has been used to immortalize CF cells. Unfortunately, the derived cell lines lose many of their differentiated properties and are inadequate for biochemical, physiological, and molecular analysis. Recently the E6/E7 genes of the human papillomaviruses (HPV's) have been shown capable of immortalizing human epithelial cells [1]. Interestingly, these E6/E7 immortalized cell lines remain non-tumorigenic in nude mice and often display normal responses to negative regulators of cell growth (e.g. TGF-beta) [2]. When injected subcutaneously into nude mice, these cells form well-differentiated epithelial cysts which mimic normal epithelial cells [3]. To determine whether the HPV E6/E7 genes would be useful for generating well-differentiated cell lines from CF patients, these genes were transfected into primary cultures of tracheal epithelial cells from a patient with cystic fibrosis.

## METHODS AND RESULTS

<u>Primary culture.</u>  Donor tissue was obtained postmortem from a 24 year old man with cystic fibrosis who was homozygous for the phenylalanine 508 deletion in the Cystic Fibrosis Transmembrane Conductance Regulator (CFTR) gene.  The trachea was cut into 2 x 2 cm pieces and washed with Joklik's modified essential medium (MEM) containing antibiotics, dithiothreitol (0.5 mg/ml), and DNAse (10μg/ml) at 4 degrees C for 3 hours.  The tissues were then incubated in fresh supplemented MEM plus protease ( Sigma Type XIV, 0.1 μg/ml) at 4 degrees for 18 hours. The epithelial cells were dislodged by gentle agitation and plated in  in hormone-supplemented F12 medium (F12 + 7x; supplements: insulin 5 μg/ml, endothelial cell growth supplement 3.7 μg/ml, epidermal growth factor 25 ng/ml, triiodothyronine 3 x 10-8 M, hydrocortisone 1 x 10-6 M, transferrin 5 μg/ml, and cholera toxin 10 ng/ml, plus ceftazidime, tobramycin, and amphotericin B).

<u>Transfection with HPV-18 E6 and E7 genes.</u>  A  pUC19-based plasmid containing the HPV-18 nucleotides 6273-2440 encoding the intact E6 and E7 open reading frames, a partial E1 open reading frame, and the upstream regulatory region [4] was transfected by lipofection as described [5]. After a 2 hr incubation at 37, 12 ml of fresh F12 + 7x medium was added.  On the following day the cells were fed with fresh medium.

<u>Culture and Clonal selection.</u>   At 14-18 days post-seeding, clusters of 30-200 dividing cells of apparent clonal origin developed and were isolated using cloning cylinders.   Between passages 1-4, most subclones were co-cultured with lethally irradiated NIH3T3 fibroblasts, which were removed by differential trypsinization at passage 4.   Eleven clones were isolated and developed a polygonal morphology typical of airway epithelial cells in primary culture.

<u>Presence and expression of HPV genes in immortalized cell lines.</u> The presence of the HPV-18 genome in selected clones was assayed using  polymerase  chain  reaction  (PCR)  technology  with oligonucleotide primers specific for the HPV-18 E6-E7 region.  The 5' primer corresponds to HPV-18 nucleotides 105-124 and the 3' primer to nucleotides 888-907 of the HPV-18 DNA sequence. Extracts of 6 x $10^3$ cells of selected clones were analyzed by PCR for 30 cycles with the following conditions: 94 C for 1 min, 50 C for 2 min, and  72  C  for  3  min.   An  HPV-18  transformed  human keratinocyte cell line (18Nco) and an SV40-transformed keratinocyte

cell line were used as positive and negative controls. Agarose gel electrophoresis of PCR products demonstrated the 802 bp E6-E7 amplified product in the positive control and in all CF clones examined (data not shown).

<u>Expression of the HPV-18 E7 protein</u> . Ten cm dishes of selected clones were metabolically labelled with $^{35}$S-cysteine for 4 hours following a 2 hr starvation in cysteine-free media. Total protein was extracted following labelling and immunoprecipitated with 20 µl of a rabbit polyclonal antibody specific for the HPV-18 E7 protein. The immunoprecipitated proteins were separated electrophoretically on a 14% acrylamide-SDS gel. Autoradiography of the gel showed the presence of the 17 kD E7 protein in both of the CF clones examined (CF1 and 2) as well as the 18-Nco positive control and absent from the SV40 negative control (Fig.1). A combined immunoprecipitation/immunoblotting procedure was also used to detect the E7 protein. Cell extracts were immunoprecipitated as above (without label) and electrophoretically separated. The gel was then blotted onto nitrocellulose and the E7 protein was detected by Western blotting using a Protoblot (Promega) kit using a 1:100 dilution of the rabbit polyclonal antibody as primary antibody. The 17 kD E7 protein was detected in all clones examined (data not shown).

<u>Ion Transport Properties</u>. To screen for the development of functional tight junctions, clones were passaged onto a collagen matrix support. Beginning on day 2 following passage, transepithelial resistance (Rt) and spontaneous transepithelial potential difference (Vt) were measured daily using a WPI electrometer connected to the apical and basolateral media with calomel half-cells. Measurements were taken daily until the Vt declined or the cells senesced. Resistance was calculated from the voltage deflections induced by +/- 7 µamp current pulses passed through silver- silver chloride electrodes placed in the mucosal and submucosal bathing solutions. The results for all clones are shown in **Table 1**. Transepithelial resistance (Rt) for the CF lines (CFT1) is similar to that observed in primary cultures of human airway epithelial cells, indicating the presence of tight junctions, while $R_t$ for SV40-transformed cells (CF/T43) is markedly decreased. Additionally, the transepithelial potential difference ($V_t$) in CF lines is -13.3 which is approximately 5-fold higher than $V_t$ in SV40-transformed airway epithelial cells.

## DISCUSSION

Immortalization of human airway epithelial cells with HPV E6/E7 genes produces cell lines which retain the differentiated phenotype of

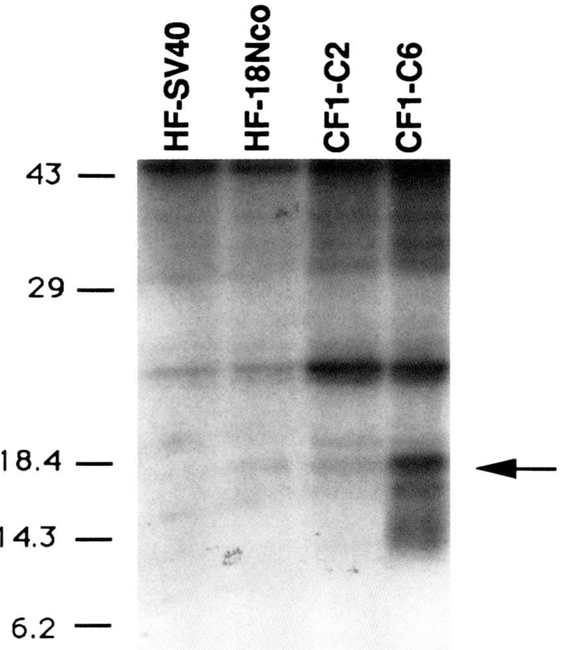



**Figure 1.  Immunoprecipitation of the HPV-18 E7 protein in two CF1 lines.** Cells from CF1-C2 and CF1-C6 were labeled with $^{35}$S cysteine and extracts were immunoprecipitated with rabbit polyclonal antibody to the HPV-18 E7 protein. Human foreskin keratinocytes transformed by the HPV-18 genome (18Nco) and SV40 were used as positive and negative controls.  The 17 kD E7 protein is present in both CF lines along with the 18Nco positive control.

primary airway epithelial cultures.  This differentiated phenotype is evidenced by the development of transepithelial resistances, indicating the formation of functional tight junctions  similar to those in primary cultures.  The transepithelial potential differences in these CF lines is approximately fivefold higher than that of SV40-transformed cells. The HPV E6 and E7 genes play well-recognized roles in the process of cell immortalization.  The E6 and E7 proteins have been shown to bind to the gene products of the tumor suppressor genes, p53 and Rb, respectively [6,7].  Although the SV40 large T viral oncoprotein has also been shown capable of binding p53 and Rb gene products [8,9], cell lines immortalized by SV40 undergo a loss of differentiation. This undifferentiated phenotype may be due to additional functions of the large T antigen, such as its role in DNA replication.

Interestingly, it is also possible to immortalize human keratinocytes using only the HPV E7 gene, although this occurs with markedly decreased efficiency. It will be important to determine whether E7-immortalized cells display an even more differentiated phenotype than those immortalized by both E6 and E7.

|                        | $V_t$ (mV)   | $R_t$ ($\Omega$-cm2) |
|------------------------|--------------|----------------------|
| CFT1 (n=10)            | -13.3 ±1.8   | 440 ±60              |
| CF/T43 (n=18)          | -2.3 ±0.3    | 125 ±12              |
| Primary Cultures (n=28)| -29.2 ±4.4   | 435 ±42              |

**Table 1.** Transepithelial potential difference ($V_t$) and transepithelial resistance ($R_t$) measurements for CF cell lines immortalized by HPV E6/E7 (CFT1), SV40-immortalized CF cell lines (CF/T43), and primary cultures of human airway epithelial cells.

## REFERENCES


1. Pirisi, L., et. al. J Virol. 1987, 61:1061-1066.
2. Braun, L., et. al.  Cancer Research 1990, 50:7324-7332.
3. Dürst, M., et. al. J Virol. 1991, 65:796-804.
4. Barbosa, M., and R. Schlegel. Oncogene 1989, 4:1529-1532.
5. Felgner, P., et. al. PNAS USA 1987, 84:7413-7417.
6. Werness, B., et. al. Science 1990, 248:76-79.
7. Dyson, N., et. al. Science 1989, 243:934-937.
8. Schmieg, F.I., and D.T.Simmons. Virology 1988, 164:132-140.
9. DeCaprio, J., et. al. Cell 1988, 54:275-283.

# TUMOR PROGRESSION IN BREAST CANCER

Vimla Band and Ruth Sager

Dana Farber Cancer Institute

44 Binney Street, Boston, MA  02115

Breast cancer is one of the leading cause of cancer-related deaths of women in North America and Europe. Progress in understanding the cellular and molecular biology of mammary tumorigenesis has been impeded by lack of suitable _in vitro_ models. The availability of normal tissue from reduction mammoplasty, and pathological tissue samples from biopsies and mastectomies provides a unique opportunity for studying human cancer. The importance of growing normal and tumor-derived cells for comparative studies of gene expression, drug resistance, surface antigens, mechanism of cell cycle control and prognostic markers can hardly be overstated. While some information can be obtained from fixed and frozen tissues, they are not useful for indepth studies involving biochemical and molecular analyses. There are no _in vivo_ or _in vitro_ models of tumor progression in human breast cancer. In fact, cells from mammary carcinomas have been among the most difficult human tumor-derived cells to grow in culture (1,2) and have poorly grown as xenografts in the nude mouse model (3). Very few primary mammary tumor cell lines are available (4-6).

## DEVELOPMENT OF A MEDIUM TO GROW NORMAL
## AND TUMOR MAMMARY EPITHELIAL CELLS

When we began working with breast cancer system about 5 years back no single medium was available to grow normal, primary tumor and metastatic tumors from mammary gland.  Conventionally, mammary tumor cell lines have been isolated from metastases or pleural effusions and grown in medium containing standard salts e.g. Eagle's minimum essential medium with 10 % fetal calf serum (7), whereas normal mammary epithelial cells have been grown in MCDB-170, a serum-free medium containing bovine pituitary extract (8).  Hence, the first challenge we faced was to develop a medium that should allow the establishment and long term growth of normal and tumor mammary

TABLE 1.

COMPOSITION OF DFCI-1 MEDIUM

<u>Salts:</u>   α- MEM / Ham's F12 (1:1)
<u>Supplements:</u>

| | |
|---|---|
| Insulin | 1.0 μg/ml |
| Hydrocortisone | 2.8 μM |
| Epidermal Growth Factor | 12.5 ng/ml |
| Transferrin | 10.0 μg/ml |
| Ethanolamine | 0.1 mM |
| Phosphoethanolamine | 0.1 mM |
| Bovine Pituitary Extract | 35.0 μg/ml |
| Estradiol | 2.0 nM |
| Triiodothyronine | 10.0 nM |
| Cholera Toxin | 1.0 ng/ml |
| L-Glutamine | 2.0 mM |
| Ascorbic Acid ( freshly made ) | 50.0 μM |
| Sodium Selenite | 15.0 nM |
| HEPES | 10.0 mM |
| Fetal Calf Serum | 1% |
| Penicillin | 100 units/ml |
| Streptomycin | 100 μg/ml |

$CO_2 = 6.5\%$
pH  = 7.4

epithelial cells under identical conditions. We developed a medium called
DFCI-1 (Table 1) which allowed us to establish normal epithelial cells from
reduction mammoplasty specimens, and supported long-term growth of
normal mammary epithelial cells and established metastases-derived cell lines
(9).


## MARKERS TO DISTINGUISH NORMAL
## AND TUMOR MAMMARY EPITHELIAL CELLS

One major problem in establishing normal and tumor mammary
epithelial cells from a mixture of tumor tissue was the unavailability of markers
to distinguish these cells in <u>in vitro</u> cell culture. We have shown two criteria that
distinguish normal from tumor mammary epithelial cells. i)  Rhodamine-123 (R-
123) retention.  R-123 is a mitochondrial specific fluorescent dye that is
preferentially taken up and retained longer by the mitochondria of tumor cells
as compared to normal cells (10, 11).  We found this was true for normal and
tumor mammary epithelial cells grown <u>in vitro</u> under identical conditions.  R-
123 retention changes if cells are grown in different media (9). ii)  HMFG-2
epitope expression : second criterion which differentiates normal and tumor
mammary epithelial cells grown <u>in vitro</u> is the expression of human milk fat

globule-2 antigen epitope on tumor cells. HMFG-2 antibody is known to recognize epitopes expressed on tumor cells but not on normal cells in tissue sections (12, 13). We found that all mammary tumor cell lines but not normal cells tested to date express HMFG-2 antigen epitope (9).

## PRIMARY AND METASTATIC TUMOR CELL LINES
## FROM PATIENT # 21

We developed a series of cell lines from a patient # 21 diagnosed of infiltrating and intraductal carcinoma of the breast. 21PT and 21NT cell lines were derived from the primary tumor and 21MT was derived from the pleural effusion (Fig.1). Two morphologically distinct cell lines were derived from 21MT cell line based on differential trypsin sensitivity and these are designated as 21MT-1 and 21MT-2 (Fig.1). These four tumor cell lines have distinct phenotypic and genotypic characteristics (14). We have shown by DNA finger print analysis that all of these cell lines are derived from a single patient (14). The similarities and differences of these four tumor cell lines are shown in Table 2. Morphologically 21NT, 21PT and 21MT-2 cells are very similar whereas 21MT-1 cells are clearly different (Fig.1 and Table 2). 21PT is nontumorigenic whereas 21NT and 21MT make tumors in nude mice system. All of these cell lines exhibit abnormal karyotypes and have many marker chromosomes. All the four cell lines express HMFG-2 epitope and retain R-123 longer than normal cells (9, 14). Three of these cell lines, 21PT, 21NT and 21MT-2 can be grown in completely defined medium , called D3 (DFCI-1 minus bovine pituitary extract, fetal calf serum, epidermal growth factor (EGF), insulin, triiodothyronine, cholera toxin, and hydrocortisone (HC) ) supplemented with EGF, HC, and  linsulin. However, 21MT-1 cells do not grow in this defined medium,and require serum for growth. In this respect 21MT-1 cells resemble

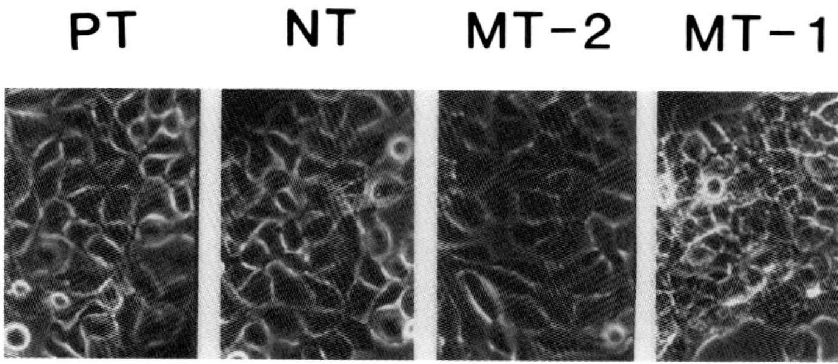


Fig. 1.   Morphology of primary (21PT, 21NT), and metastatic (21MT-2, 21MT-1) tumor-derived cell lines grown in DFCI-1 medium (phase-contrast optics X230).

TABLE 2

CHARACTERISTICS OF 21T SERIES AND NORMAL CELLS

| | Normal | 21PT | 21NT | 21MT-2 | 21MT-1 |
|---|---|---|---|---|---|
| Morphology | Homogenous flat-spindle | Homogenous flat-polygonal | Homogenous flat-polygonal | Homogenous flat-polygonal | Heterogenous 3D clusters |
| Tumor | - | - | + | + | + |
| Karyotype | Normal | 54-55 Chromo 20% near diploid 6-24 mar | 54-55 Chromo - 6-24 mar | 55-60 Chromo - >34 mar | 55-60 Chromo - >34 mar |
| HMFG-2 expression | - | + | + | + | + |
| R-123 retention | Low | High | High | High | High |
| Growth factors | Undefined | Defined | Defined | Defined | Undefined |
| RB protein | Normal | Normal | Normal | Normal | Normal |
| ErbB2 expression | - | + | + | + | ++ |
| ErbB2 amplification | - | + | + | + | +++ |
| EGF receptor mRNA | 5-6x | 2x | 2x | 2x | 1x |
| TGF alpha mRNA | 10x | 10x | 10x | 10x | 1-2x |
| Estrogen receptor | - | - | - | - | - |

other pleural effusion- and ascites-derived metastatic mammary tumor cell lines reported in the literature, all of which require serum for optimal growth.

We also investigated the expression of certain genes which are suspected to be involved in mammary tumorigenesis. These are EGF receptor, erbB2, myc, retinoblastoma, and 52 kD cathepsin D. Compared to normal cells EGFR mRNA expression is 2-3 fold lower in 21PT, 21NT, and 21MT-2 cell lines, and about 5 fold lower in 21MT-1 cells. Since TGF$\alpha$ is a ligand for the EGFR we examined expression of its RNA. Levels of TGF$\alpha$ mRNA were equal to normal cells in 21PT, 21NT and 21MT-2 cells whereas 21MT-1 had 5-10 fold less TGF$\alpha$ (14). The basis of lower levels of EGFR and TGF$\alpha$ mRNA expression in 21MT-1 cells is not known.

ErbB2 is known to be overexpressed in more than 25 % of breast cancers (15). We examined the expression of erbB2 at mRNA and protein levels, and assessed the amplification of erbB2 gene. 21T series cell lines overexpress erbB2 mRNA and protein compared to normal cells. 21MT-1 showed higher expression and DNA amplification as compared to other three cell lines (14). No significant differences were observed between normal and 21T series cell lines in the levels of mRNA expression for c-myc, Rb and 52kD cathepsin D. We propose that 21T series cell lines represent a tumor progression model in this patient. We rank them in the following order:

21PT-------> 21NT-------> 21MT-2-------> 21MT-1

## IN VITRO CELL TRANSFORMATION

As tumorigenesis is a multistep process, the tumor-derived cells that we have examined are likely to have already undergone several steps in this process. It is important to define and characterize the very early stages in tumor progression. One way to do so experimentally is to start with normal cells and immortalize them, since immortalization is a crucial event in oncogenesis. Human cells are extremely difficult to immortalize in culture (16, 17), although two immortalized mammary epithelial cell lines were recovered after long-term exposure to benzo[a] pyrene (18). This was an extremely rare event and it is difficult to determine the molecular basis of carcinogen-induced genetic changes. Availability and success of human papilloma virus DNA to immortalize human keratinocytes prompted us to use this in mammary cells. HPV is known to be involved in cervical carcinomas (19) and keratinocytes are squamous epithelial cells which are known targets of HPV. At present there is no evidence of the involvement of HPV in mammary carcinomas. Surprisingly, HPV16 and HPV18 DNA reproducibly and efficiently immortalized human mammary epithelial cells (20). DFCI-1 medium allowed us to select for immortal cells easily as normal cells plated at low density do not form colonies in this medium, whereas immortal cells make colonies. Further, immortalized cells show reduced growth factor requirements such that they could be grown in a completely defined medium containing only one growth factor i.e EGF, whereas normal cells require all the growth factors present in DFCI-1 medium.

These immortal cells also show chromosomal rearrangements (20 and K. Swisshelm et al unpublished).

## HPVE6 ALONE IS SUFFICIENT FOR NORMAL MAMMARY EPITHELIAL CELL IMMORTALIZATION

Two transforming genes of HPV, E6 and E7, are essential for immortalization of keratinocytes (21). Recently, using retroviral infection, E7 gene alone was shown to immortalize keratinocytes, although the frequency of immortalization was quite low and increased considerably when E6 and E7 were used together (22).

We have transfected HPV constructs with mutations in open reading frames (ORFs) of various early genes (obtained from Dr. Peter Howley) (21) into normal mammary epithelial cells. Disruption of ORFs of E1, E2, E4 and E7 did not affect the immortalizing capacity of HPV16 genome, whereas mutation in E6 completely abolished its transforming ability. Further, transfection of E6 alone under control of the actin promoter was sufficient and as efficient as E6+E7 to immortalize mammary epithelial cells. Further, HPVE6-immortalized cells have the same reduced growth factors requirement as do whole genome transfectants. These results demonstrate that E6 alone is sufficient for immortalization and change in growth factor requirements of normal mammary epithelial cells (manuscript submitted).

## IMMORTALIZATION OF NORMAL EPITHELIAL AND MESOTHELIAL CELLS FROM PATIENT # 21

Since HPV-induced immortalization of mammary epithelial cells is quite efficient, we used this method to immortalize normal cells from patient # 21. These cells grow only for 5 to7 passages before they senesce. Availability of immortalized normal cells would provide an early stage of tumor progression model from this patient  to complement the cell series that we established from the  primary and metastatic tumors. Due to limited quantities of available normal cells from patient #21, cells in two 100 mm dishes at passage 4 were transfected with HPV16E6+E7 construct using actin promoter (no selectable marker ). These cells were subcultured every other week for two months without any drug selection. Immortal cells (H16N-2 and H16N-3) were obtained from the progeny of both original culture dishes and are in culture for > 6 months. These cells are morphologically different from parent cells (Fig. 2), and express  HPV genes as assessed by Northern analysis (Fig. 3). Similar to other HPV-immortalized cells H16N-2 and H16N-3 cells lack the expression of HMFG-2 epitope while all the tumor-derived 21T series cell lines express this marker. In contrast to high erbB2 expression in the 21T series tumor cell lines, H16N-2 and H16N-3 lack erbB2 mRNA (Fig. 3) thus resembling other normal and HPV-immortalized mammary epithelial cells.

## 21N  H16N-2 21MTF1 H16F1

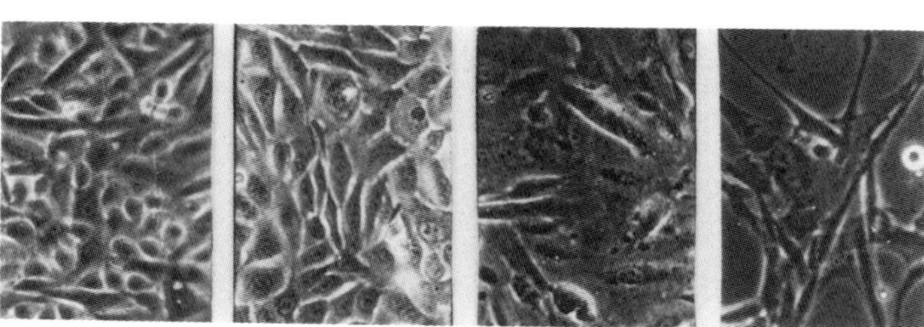

Fig. 2.  Morphology of normal (21N) and immortalized (H16N-2) epithelial, and normal (21MTF1) and immortalized (H16F1) mesothelial cells grown in DFCI-1 medium (phase-contrast optics X230).

To serve as non-mammary/non-epithelial controls for genetic and biochemical experiments, we have also obtained mesothelial cells (21MTF1) derived from pleural effusion of the patient # 21 (23).  These cells usually grow for about 16 passages in culture.  We transfected these cells with HPV16E6+E7 DNA construct under actin promoter and have obtained an immortal cell line, H16F1 (Fig 2) that is in culture for > 6 months.

### p53 AND RB IN HPV-IMMORTALIZED CELLS

It has been shown in *in vitro* reticulocytes system that HPV E6 and E7 gene products  bind to two well known tumor suppressor gene products p53 and RB respectively (24, 25, 26).  This binding has been speculated to account for the transforming activity of these two HPV genes. Therefore, we examined RB and p53 protein in E6 and E6+E7 transfectants.  RB  protein is normal in these transfectants as judged by its phosphorylation pattern and binding to SV40 large T antigen.  On the contrary these transfectants have markedly reduced levels of immunoprecipitable p53 as compared to the parent line ( manuscript submitted ).  These results suggest that  alteration of p53 but not RB protein may be important in HPV-induced immortalization of normal mammary epithelial cells.

The immortalized mammary cells are not tumorigenic but have undergone significant preneoplastic changes.  Thus, they represent valuable starting material for experimental induction of further events in mammary cell

                                                          *Band and Sager*

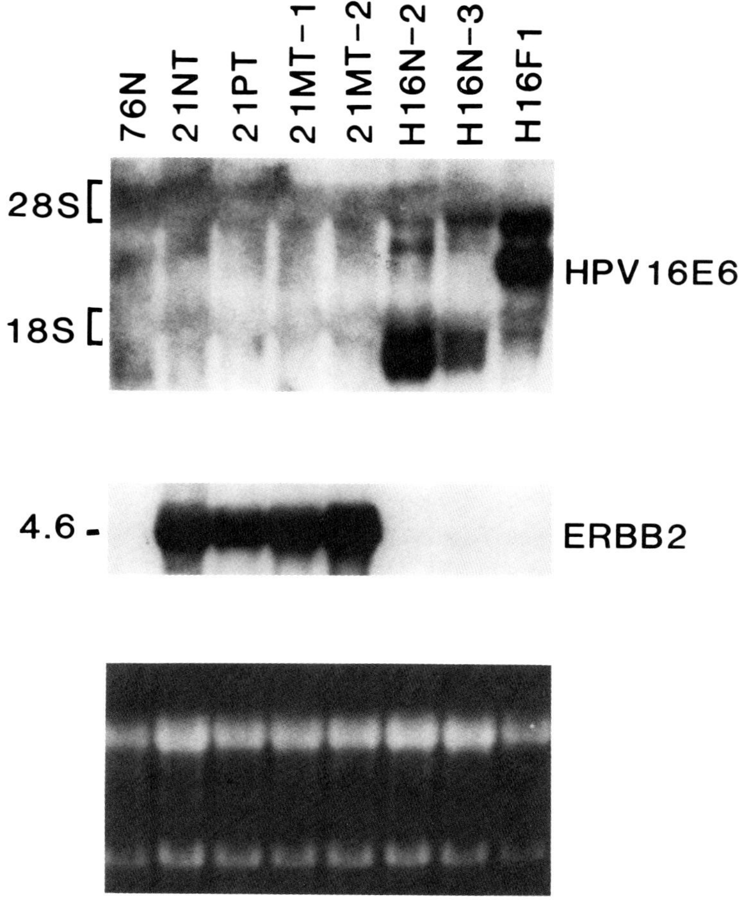


Fig. 3.  Upper panel : HPV 16E6 mRNA expression in mammoplasty-derived normal cells (76N), and tumor cell lines (21PT, 21NT, 21MT-2 and 21MT-1), immortalized normal epithelial (H16N-2, H16N-3) and immortalized mesothelial (H16F1) cells from patient # 21.  Middle panel: ErbB2 mRNA expression in normal, tumor and immortalized cells.  Lower panel: equivalent loading and integrity of RNA were verified by ethidium bromide staining of rRNA bands.

oncogenesis. Further, this method may be generally applicable to other epithelial and mesothelial cell systems.

In conclusion, we have established two models, one patient derived and second in vitro immortalization model, which are available to study various cellular, biochemical and molecular changes at various steps of mammary tumorigenesis.

## ACKNOWLEDGEMENT

We thank Drs. D. Zajchowski, K. Swisshelm, J. A. De Caprio for helping in certain experiments, V. Kulesa and L. Delmolino for technical help, and S. Budd for preparing the manuscript.

## REFERENCES

1.    J. Taylor-Papadimitriou, M. Shearer, and M. G. P. Stoker. Int. J. Cancer 20, 903 (1977).
2.    H. S. Smith, S. Lan, R. Ceriani, A. J. Hackett, and M. R. Stampfer. Cancer Res. 41, 4637 (1981).
3.    H. S. Smith, S. R. Wolman, and A. J. Hackett. Biochim. Biophys. Acta. 738, 103 (1984).
4.    E. Y. Lasfargues, W. G. Coutinho, and E. S. Redfield. J. Natl. Cancer Inst. 61, 967 (1978).
5.    S. Minafra, V. Morello, et al. Br. J. Cancer 60, 185 (1989).
6.    O. W. Petersen, B. van Deurs, et al. Cancer Res. 50, 1257 (1990 ).
7.    H. S. Smith, S. R. Wolman, et al. J. Natl. Cancer Inst. 78, 611 (1987).
8.    S. L. Hammond, R. G. Ham, and M. R. Stampfer. Proc. Natl. Acad. Sci. USA 81, 5435 (1984).
9.    V. Band, and R. Sager.  Proc. Natl. Acad. Sci. USA 86, 1249 (1989).
10.    L. V. Johnson, M. L. Walsh, and L. B. Chen.Proc. Natl. Acad. Sci. USA 77, 990 (1980).
11.    I. C. Summerhayes, I. C. Lampidis, et al. Proc. Natl. Acad. Sci. USA 79, 5292 (1982).
12.    J. Burchell, H. Durbin, and J. Taylor-Papadimitriou. J. Immunol. 131, 508 ( 1983).
13.    J. Taylor-Papadimitriou, L. B. Lane, and S. E. Chang. In: M. Rich, J. C. Hager and P. Furmanski (eds.),  Understanding Breast Cancer: Clinical and Laboratory Concepts, 215-246, Marcel Dekker Inc, New York, 1983.
14.    V. Band, D. Zajchowski, et al. Cancer Res. 50, 7351 (1990).
15.    R. Seshadri, C. Matthews et al. Int. J. Cancer 43, 270 (1989).
16.    R. Sager. Cancer Cells 2, 487 (1984).
17.    J. A. DiPaolo. J. Natl. Cancer Inst. 70, 3 (1983).
18.    M. R. Stampfer, and J. C. Bartley. Proc. Natl. Acad. Sci. USA 82, 2394 (1985).
19.    H. Z. Hausen, Adv. Viral Oncol. 8 , 1 (1989).

20.  V. Band, D. Zajchowski, V. Kulesa, and R. Sager. Proc. Natl. Acad. Sci. USA 87, 463 (1990).
21.  K. Munger, W. C. Phelps, et al. J. Virol. 63, 4417 (1989).
22.  C. L. Halbert, G. W. Demers, and D. A. Galloway. J. Virol. 65, 473 (1991).
23.  V. Band, D. Zajchowski, et al. Genes Chromo. Cancer. 1, 48 (1989).
24.  B. A. Werness, A. J. Levine, and P. M. Howley. Science 248, 76 (1990).
25.  M. Scheffner, B. A. Werness, et al. Cell 63, 1129 (1990).
26.  K. Munger, B. A. Werness, et al. EMBO J. 8, 4099 (1989).



From: *Neoplastic Transformation in Human Cell Culture,*
Eds.: J. S. Rhim and A. Dritschilo ©1991 The Humana Press Inc., Totowa, NJ

# Growth Regulation of HPV-Positive Keratinocytes by TGF-$\beta$1


L. Braun,[1] M. Dürst,[2] R. Mikumo,[1] A. Blaschke,[1] A. Crowley,[1] K. Rowader[1]

[1]Department of Pathology and Laboratory Medicine, Brown University, Providence RI 02912, USA, [2]Institute fur Virusforschung, Deutsches Krebsforschungszentrum, Heidelberg, Germany


## INTRODUCTION

Human papillomaviruses (HPV) are epitheliotropic DNA viruses, some of which have been implicated in the development of cervical cancer (1). Despite intensive research, little is known about the molecular and cellular events in cervical carcinogenesis, in large part because of the lack of *in vitro* models for HPV infection. Although it is still not possible to propagate human papillomaviruses in tissue culture, immortalized cell lines which constitutively express the E6 and E7 transforming proteins of two 'high risk' HPVs, HPV 16 and HPV 18, have recently been established in several laboratories by transfection of HPV DNA into foreskin and cervical keratinocytes (2). Such cell lines contain transcriptionally active HPV sequences, display variable patterns of keratinocyte differentiation in monolayer culture, and produce epithelium morphologically indistinguishable from cervical intraepithelial neoplasia when grown on three-dimensional collagen/fibroblast rafts (3). Thus, the availability of HPV-positive cell lines with many phenotypic similarities to HPV-induced lesions *in vivo* represents a significant advance for mechanistic studies of the transformation events triggered by HPV infection.

Using HPV-immortalized cell lines, it has been shown that the transforming proteins of HPVs form protein/protein complexes with the products of cellular tumor suppressor

genes, E6 with p53 (4) and E7 with the retinoblastoma
protein pRB (5). Although it is thought that binding of
viral oncoproteins genes leads to functional inactivation
of these two cellular genes, the significance of complex
formation in terms of cell growth has yet to be demonstrated. These studies have, however, provided insight into
potential mechanisms by which HPVs transform keratinocytes.
Furthermore, the demonstration that phosphorylation of pRB
is regulated by transforming growth factor (TGF)-$\beta$1 has
revealed a possible link between intracellular proteins
involved in transcriptional regulation and extracellular
regulators of cell proliferation (6).

The family of proteins termed TGF-$\beta$ are prototypical
examples of molecules which have functionally diverse
effects on cells, depending on the cellular microenvironment. TGF-$\beta$1, the first isoform of TGF-$\beta$ to be purified
and cloned, is inhibitory to many epithelial cells in
culture, including human keratinocytes. However, some
tumor-derived cell lines are refractory to TGF-$\beta$-mediated
growth inhibition. Since TGF-$\beta$1 is produced by multiple
cell types in the skin, it has been suggested that this
molecule may be a negative autocrine regulator of keratinocyte  growth.

To understand the sequential steps in HPV-associated
transformation, we are studying the response of several
different HPV-positive cell lines at various stages of
transformation to growth factors. In this report, we have
used these cell lines to investigate whether human papillomavirus infection of squamous epithelial cells is associated with an altered sensitivity to the growth inhibitor TGF-
$\beta$1 and whether sensitivity is modulated by the cellular
microenvironment.

**METHODS**

*Growth of cells on collagen/fibroblast gels.*

HPV 16-immortalized HPKIA cells were maintained as
described (7). Collagen rafts were prepared using VITROGEN
100 collagen (Collagen Corp, Palo Alto, CA) according to
manufacturer's instructions and established protocols (3).
Briefly, NIH 3T3 fibroblasts were suspended in liquid
collagen and incubated for two days. HPKIA cells

were seeded on top of the gels and allowed to proliferate
in DMEM:F12 with growth factor supplements as described (7)
until semi-confluent (approximately 2 days).  TGF-β1 was
then added to the cultures at a concentration of 10 ng/ml
for 48 h and [$^3$H]-thymidine was added for the last 24 h, at
which point the cultures were fixed and processed for
autoradiography.  Dishes were stained with Giemsa and
labeled nuclei/cm$^2$ were counted.

**RESULTS**

*Effects of TGF-β1 on HPV 16-immortalized keratinocyte
growth and gene expresion.*

We have previously reported that TGF-β1 has differential effects on the proliferation of immortalized, nontumorigenic HPV-positive keratinocytes and tumor-derived
cervical carcinoma cell lines (8-10).  As summarized in
Table 1, the differential effects on growth are reflected
at the level of gene expression. In normal and immortalized
keratinocytes, exposure of cells to TGF-β1 leads to a rapid
induction of c-*jun* and c-*fos* mRNA transcripts and a decrease in the steady-state levels of c-*myc* mRNAs.  On the
other hand, c-*myc* is unaffected by TGF-β1 in four cervical
carcinoma cell lines which are also resistant to the growth
inhibitory effects of TGF-β1.  C-*jun* transcripts are induced in all keratinocyte lines, regardless of tumorigenicity, indicating that TGF-β1 sensitive and resistant cells
express functional cell surface receptors for TGF-β1.
These results suggest that altered sensitivity to TGF-β1
produced by cells in squamous epithelium may be one mechanism for escape from growth control which occurs as cervical cells undergo malignant transformation.

*Growth  of HPKIA cells in modified 'organotypic'  cultures.*

Previous studies by Rollins *et al.* (11) have shown
that co-culture of mouse 3T3 fibroblasts with normal human
kerotinocytes can reduce the sensitivity of keratinocytes
to TGF-β1.  In this experimental system, it appears that
fibroblasts scavenge TGF-β1, degrading the protein within
two days.  We have also found that normal and HPV-
immortalized keratinocytes are less inhibited by TGF-β1
when grown on an irradiated  3T3 feeder layer with serum
(10).  To determine if the response of HPV 16-immortalized
keratinocytes might differ when epithelial cells were grown

**Table 1:  Summary of TGF-β1 effects on HPV-positive cell lines**

| Cells | Source | HPV Type | TGF-β1[a] Sensitivity | mRNA expression[b] | | | |
|---|---|---|---|---|---|---|---|
| | | | | c-*jun* | c-*fos* | c-*myc* | HPV |
| keratinocytes | normal foreskin | – | sensitive | ↑ | ↑ | ↓ | – |
| keratinocytes | normal cervix | – | sensitive | ↑ | ↑ | ↓ | – |
| HPK1A[c] | transfection | 16 | sensitive | ↑ | ↑ | ↓ | ↓ |
| HPKII[c] | transfection | 16 | sensitive | ND | ND | ↓ | ↓ |
| HPKIII[c] | transfection | 16 | sensitive | ND | ND | ↓ | ↓ |
| Siha[d] | tumor-derived | 16 | resistant | ↑ | 0 | 0 | 0 |
| Caski[d] | tumor-derived | 16 | resistant | ND | ND | 0 | 0 |
| ME-180[d] | tumor-derived | ? | resistant | ND | ND | ND | ND |
| C4-I[d] | tumor-derived | 18 | resistant | ND | ND | 0 | 0 |

[a]Measured by [3H]-thymidine incorporation, followed by autoradiography (10); [b]Measured by Northern blot analysis of cells exposed to TGF-β1 (10 ng/ml) for 1-3 h (10); [c]These cell lines are immortalized but not tumorigenic; [d]Cell lines obtained from American Type Culture Collection; ↑-induced, ↓-suppressed, 0-no effect, ND-not done

on a three-dimensional reconstituted equivalent of dermal
tissue, we examined the effects of TGF-β1 on the proliferation of HPKIA cells plated on a collagen lattice in which
3T3 fibroblasts have been embedded.  Rather than raising
the cells to the air-liquid interface, these studies were
performed on submerged cultures to obtain adequate labeling
of cells.  This set of conditions is referred to as modified 'organotypic' culture.  As shown in Fig. 1A, a large
percentage of cells is labeled in the absence of TGF-β1.
However, addition of  TGF-β1 to the cultures for a 48 h
period leads to a 94% decrease in labeling.

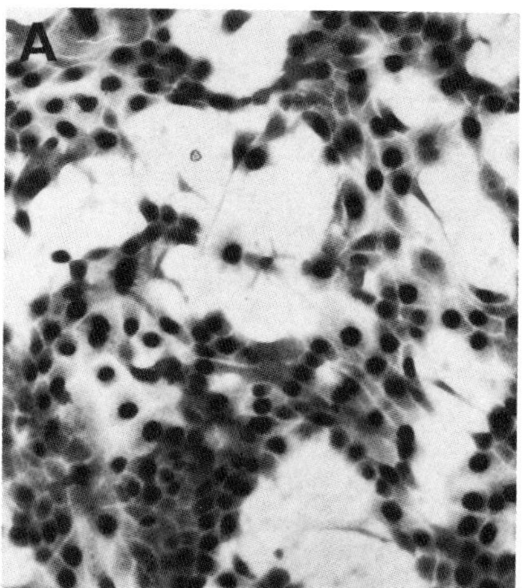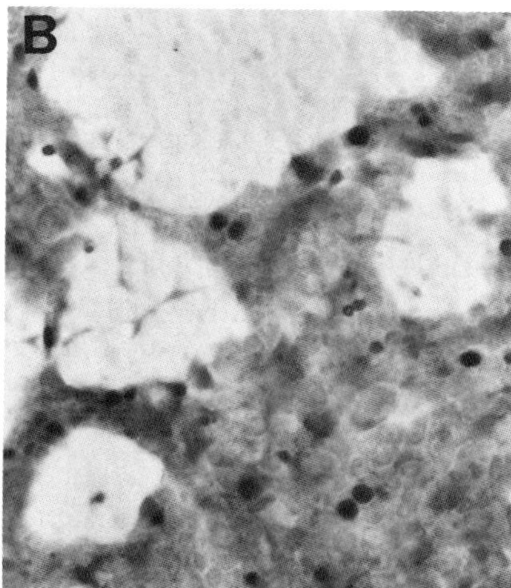

Fig. 1:  Inhibition of DNA synthesis by TGF-β1 in HPKIA
cells grown in three-dimensional (organotypic) culture.
HPKIA cells were grown as described in Methods in the
presence (A) or absence (B) of TGF-β1 (10 ng/ml for 48 h).
Since cells were densely packed the number of labeled
nuclei/cm2 was counted.

A comparison of the response of HPKIA cells grown in
monolayer cultures, co-cultured with 3T3s or grown in
three-dimensional cultures is shown in Table 2.  We found
that TGF-β1 was more inhibitory to the growth of HPV 16-
immortalized cells in three-dimensional cultures than in
either monolayer culture or co-culture with 3T3s, supporting the idea that TGF-β1 may be inhibitory to keratinocytes
*in vivo*.

Table 2:   Comparison of response of HPKIA cells to TGF-$\beta$1 under different growth conditions[a]

|                              | Labeling Index (%) | |
|------------------------------|---------------------|---------------------|
|                              | -TGF-$\beta$1(% control) | +TGF-$\beta$1(% control) |
| monolayer culture[b]         | 97(100)             | 29(30)              |
| co-culture[b]                | 73(100)             | 38(52)              |
| 3-dimensional culture[c]     | 65(100)             | 4.2(6)              |

[a]Subconfluent cultures were treated with 10 ng/ml TGF-$\beta$1 for 48 h and labeled with [$^3$H]-thymidine for 24 h in medium containing 10% FBS (10); [b]Labeling index was calculated as labeled cells/total number of cells counted in at least four low power fields (500-1000 cells counted); [c]Labeling index was calculated as labeled cells/cm$^2$ in at least four low power fields.

*Effects of TGF-$\beta$1 on HPV 16 mRNA expression.*

We have previously shown that HPV 16 mRNA expression is suppressed by TGF-$\beta$1 in HPKIA cells but not in HPV 16-positive carcinoma cells (10).  The growth inhibitory effect of TGF-$\beta$1 on HPKIA cells occurs in a dose-dependent manner and is completely reversible within 48 h after removal of TGF-$\beta$1 from the culture medium (10).  To determine if the suppression of HPV 16 mRNAs by TGF-$\beta$ is also reversible in HPKIA cells, we exposed cultures to TGF-$\beta$1 for 24 h, after which time the cells were fed fresh medium without TGF-$\beta$1.  As shown in Fig. 2A, the inhibitory effect of TGF-$\beta$1 on HPV 16 mRNA expression in HPKIA cells is dose-dependent and is almost completely reversed within 48 h after removal of the protein.  These results are in agreement with previous work by Woodworth *et al.* (11) and indicate that continuous exposure to TGF-$\beta$1 is required to sustain the suppressive effects on both growth and papillomavirus gene expression.

To determine if HPV 16 expression was also modulated in other HPV 16-immortalized lines, we analyzed the effects of TGF-$\beta$1 on steady-state levels of HPV 16 mRNA transcripts

in two additional cell lines established by independent
transfections.  As shown in Fig 2B, high levels of HPV 16
mRNAs are detected in all cell lines.  After a 24 h exposure to TGF-β1, a marked decrease in steady state levels of
HPV 16 mRNAs is observed in each cell line with the magnitude of suppression highest in HPK IA cells and lowest in
the HPKIII line.  On the other hand, TGF-α and TGF-β1 mRNA
transcripts are induced in each line, although the levels
of TGF-α transcripts in HPKIA cells are low in comparison
to HPKII, HPKIII cells or normal keratinocytes (Fig. 2C).

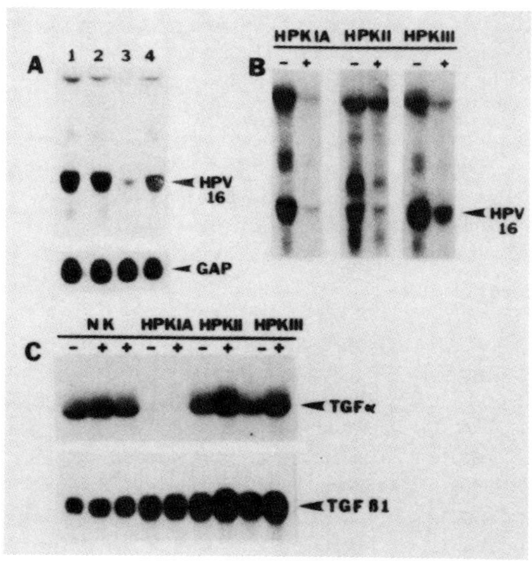


Fig. 2:   TGF-β1 suppression of HPV 16 mRNA production in
HPV 16-immortalized keratinocytes.    A.  Reversibility of
TGF-β1 inhibition of HPV 16 mRNA expression.  TGF—β1 was
added to HPKIA cells for 24 h.  In parallel dishes TGF-β1
containing medium was removed and cultures were incubated
with fresh medium without TGF-β1 for an additional 48 h;
lane 1, control cells grown in the absence of TGF-β1; lane
2, TGF-β1 1 ng/ml; lane 3, TGF-β1 10 ng/ml; lane 4, removal
of TGF-β1.  Northern hybridization using full length HPV 16
as a probe. B.  Subconfluent cultures of HPKIA, HPKII and
HPKIII cells were exposed to TGF-β1 (10 ng/ml) for 24 h and
RNA was analyzed by Northern hybridization.  C.  Filters
used in B were washed and rehybridized with TGF-α  and TGF-
β1 cDNA probes.  NK, normal keratinocytes; HPK, HPV 16-
transfected keratinocytes.

*Differentiation resistance and TGF-β1 sensitivity.*

The hallmark of cervical intraepithelial neoplasia is the unregulated proliferation of cells in the basal layer of the epithelium which display aberrant patterns of squamous cell differentiation. Recent work by Pietenpol *et al.* (13) has shown that HPV 16- and HPV 18-immortalized keratinocytes, selected for resistance to serum-induced differentiation, were resistant to TGF-β1 inhibition. Since altered differentiation is thought to be a cellular manifestation of the premalignant state, this suggested to us that resistance to terminal differentiation may be accompanied by resistance to growth inhibition by TGF-β1. To explore this possibility, we have transfected secondary passage keratinocytes with HPV 16 and HPV 18 DNAs in serum-free, growth factor supplemented medium (L. Braun, M. Dürst, R. Mikumo, manuscript in preparation) and selected for differentiation-resistant subpopulations in two ways: a) by growth in serum-containing medium; and b) by treatment of cultured cells with the phorbol ester, TPA.

When HPV-immortalized cells were sparsely in medium containing either serum or TPA, they enlarged and became squamous in appearance. Most of the population then ceased to proliferate. After about a month of regular feeding, however, nests of small, cuboidal cells emerged which had a shorter population doubling time and a higher labeling index than the unselected, parent population. This process was quite dramatic in the case of TPA exposure; no viable cells were detectable for 10 days to two weeks. Thus, HPV-immortalized keratinocytes selected by chronic exposure to TPA represent a very minor population of cells present in the parent population. Because of their rapid growth rate, we anticipated that this differentiation-resistant cell line might have escaped from TGF-β1-mediated growth inhibition. Interestingly, a comparison of the effects of TGF-β1 on HPV 18 -transfected cells (PK-18) grown in serum-free medium to that of PK-18 cells grown in serum free medium to which TPA (10 ng/ml) had been added (PK-18/TPA), shows that the proliferation of both cell lines is inhibited by TGF-β1 (Fig. 3). Whether the increased sensitivity of the PK-18/TPA line to TGF-β1 is due to induction of biologically active TGF-β1 by TPA remains to be established. Serum-selected cell lines were more heterogeneous morphologically and slightly less sensitive to TGF-β1 than the TPA-selected lines (unpublished data). These results suggest that resistance to differentiation *per se* is not associated with loss of negative growth regulation by TGF-β1. Therefore, if resistance to TGF-β1 is a key biological event in HPV-associated carcinogenesis, it is likely that the growth of cells which are resistant to TGF-β1 is a relatively late step in the progression of HPV-positive epithelial cells to malignancy.

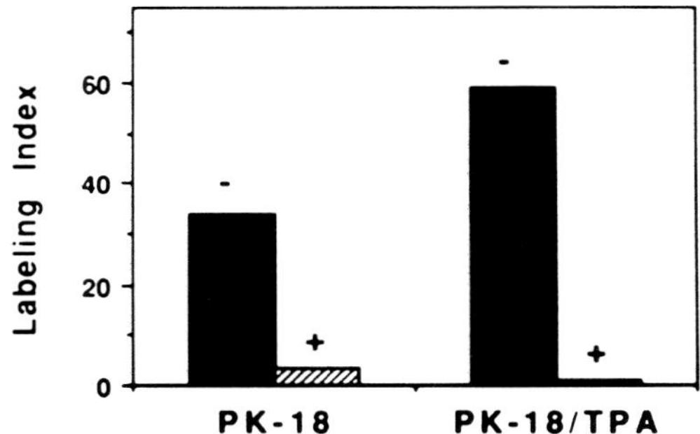


Fig. 3: Proliferative response of PK-18 and PK-18/TPA cells cultured in the presence (+) or absence (-) of TGF-β1 (10 ng/ml). Subconfluent monolayers were exposed to TGF-β1 as described in the legend to Fig. 2. Results are expressed as % labeled nuclei.

## DISCUSSION

We have used an *in vitro* model of HPV-associated carcinogenesis to compare the effects of the epithelial inhibitor TGF-β1 on the growth of HPV-positive cells prior to and after acquisition of the malignant phenotype. Previous work from our laboratories (8-10) as well as that of Woodworth *et al.* (12) has shown that TGF-β1 is inhibitory to the growth of HPV-immortalized keratinocytes but not to that of tumor-derived cervical epithelial cell lines. In normal and immortalized keratinocytes as well as other cell types, growth inhibition by TGF-β1 is preceded by induction of c-*jun* (14) and c-*fos* and inhibition of c-*myc* whereas in malignant cervical cell lines c-*myc* is unaffected by TGF-β1.

A major limitation of these studies, however, is that when cells are isolated from their normal tissue environment and placed in culture, cell-cell and cell-matrix interactions are disrupted, often drastically altering the physiologic response of the cells to extracellular signals, including that of growth factors. Thus, an important concern in generalizing from *in vitro* model systems to human cancer is whether cultured cells adequately reflect the *in vivo* situation. Our first priority was, therefore, to establish that the growth response of cells in monolayer culture to TGF-$\beta$1 could be replicated in a more physiologic, 'organotypic' culture system. This is particularly important when studying human papillomavirus-induced diseases since the high species specificity of HPVs, for the most part, prevents their replication in non-human tissues. We found that when HPV-immortalized cells were grown on a matrix of collagen into which metabolically active fibroblasts were incorporated, their sensitivity to TGF-$\beta$1 was similar to that in monolayer culture, supporting the concept that TGF-$\beta$1 is an important regulator of keratinocyte growth and differentiation *in vivo*.

Expression of HPV E6 and E7 proteins is required for high efficiency transformation of keratinocytes and maintenance of the transformed phenotype (15). Our findings that TGF-$\beta$1 suppresses the steady-state levels of HPV 16 E6 and E7 mRNA transcripts in nontumorigenic but not tumorigenic cells suggest that loss of responsiveness to TGF-$\beta$1 may lead to constitutive expression of the E6 and E7 oncoproteins of high risk HPVs. Unregulated expression of these proteins may select for a population of preneoplastic cells which are more susceptible to malignant transformation by subsequent exposure to tumor promoting agents. Contrary to our expectations, cell lines that were selected for differentiation-resistance with two different keratinocyte differentiation agents, fetal bovine serum and TPA, remained growth inhibited by TGF-$\beta$1. On the basis of these studies we conclude that loss of sensitivity to TGF-$\beta$1 is a late step in HPV-associated transformation, perhaps related to malignant conversion or tumor progression.

## Acknowledgements

We thank Carol White and Ann Baxter for their help in preparing this manuscript. This work was supported by USPHS Grant CA46617 (LB) and Deutsche Forschungsgemeinschaft Du 162/1-1 (MD).

## REFERENCES

1. zur Hausen H, Cancer Res. 49:4677-4681, 1989.
2. Howley PM. In: BN Fields and DM Knipe (eds.), Virology, 1625-1650, Raven Press, LTD., New York, 1990.
3. McCance DJ, Kopan R, Fuchs E and Laimins LA, Proc. Natl. Acad. Sci., 85:7169-7173, 1988.
4. Werness BA, Levine AJ, Howley PM, Science, 248:76-79, 1990.
5. Dyson N, Howley PM, Munger K, Harlow E, Science, 243:934-937, 1989.
6. Laiho M, DeCaprio JA, Ludlow JW, Livingston DM and Massague J, Cell, 63:175-185, 1990.
7. Dürst M, Dzarlieva-Petruseska RT, Boukamp P, Fusenig NE and Gissmann L, Oncogene 1:251-256, 1987.
8. Braun L, Lauchlan S, Mikumo R, Gomez M, J. Cell Biochem Supplement 13C:181, 1989.
9. Braun L, Lauchlan S, Mikumo R, Gomez M. In: PM Howley and TR Broker (eds.), Papillomaviruses, 157-167, Wiley-Liss, Inc., 1990.
10. Braun L, Dürst M, Mikumo R and Gruppuso P, Cancer Res., 50:7324-7332, 1990.
11. Rollins BJ, O'Connell TM, Bennett G, Burton LE, Stiles CD and Rheinwald JC, J. Cell. Phys., 139:455-462, 1989.
12. Woodworth CD, Notario V and DiPaolo JA, J. Virol., 64:4767-4775, 1990.
13. Pietenpol JA, Stein RW, Moran E, Yaciuk P, Schlegel R, Lyons RM, Pittelkow MR, Munger K, Howley PM and Moses HL, Cell 61:777-785, 1990.
14. Kim, S-J, Angel P, Lafyatis R, Hattoic K, Kim KY, Sporn MB, Mol. Cell Biol. 10:1492-1497, 1990.
15. Munger K, Phelps WC, Bubb V, Howley PM and Schlegel R, J. Virol., 63:4417-4421, 1989.

# CELL GROWTH TRANSFORMATION BY EPSTEIN BARR VIRUS

Elliott Kieff, Fred Wang, Mark Birkenbach, Jeffrey Cohen, Jeffrey Sample, Blake Tomkinson, Sankar Swaminathan, Richard Longnecker, Andrew Marchini, Joan Mannick, So-fai Tsang, Clare Sample, Ken Kaye and Michael Kurilla

Departments of Medicine, Microbiology and Molecular Genetics, Harvard University
BWH, Thorn Building, 75 Francis Street, Boston, MA   02115

Epstein-Barr Virus (EBV) was discovered 25 years ago during a search for an etiologic agent in human Burkitt lymphoma (BL), a remarkably unusual, geographically restricted, tumor. In vitro infection of primary B lymphocytes acutely and efficiently resulted in persistent latent infection and lymphocyte growth transformation (for a review of biological properties and for relevant references prior to 1989 see 1). The latently infected, growth transformed, lymphocytes are not only immortal in culture, but also are tumorigenic when inoculated into the brain of nude mice or into the peritoneum of SCID mice. Large virus innocula also induce rapidly fatal lymphoproliferative disease in cotton top tamarinds. In some genetically predisposed or severely immune deficient humans, EBV infection can also evolve into rapidly fatal lymphoproliferative disease. Aside from these direct effects on cell proliferation, EBV infection is also closely associated with nasopharyngeal carcinoma (NPC) and African BL, tumors which occur long after primary EBV infection; even among populations with a relatively high incidence of these tumors. The uniform presence of EBV in all malignant cells of endemic BL or NPC and the molecular biologic evidence that these tumors grow from an EBV infected cell, link EBV etiologically to these late onset malignancies. However, the delayed onset and low incidence of these malignancies amoung EBV infected people worldwide favors the hypothesis that endemic BL and NCP evolve as multi step processes. Environmental and host genetic cofactors are important in endemic BL and NPC,

respectively. EBV associated BL is endemic only in African
native populations with malnutrition and holoendemic malaria
and not in related populations elsewhere. In fact, Burkitt
originally described changes in disease incidence in tribes
with migration. In contrast, nasopharyngeal cancer is endemic in southern chinese populations even after emigrating to
distant sites. Dysregulated c-myc expression is a critical
step in BL evolution. The dependence on c-myc translocation
partially explains the long interval between EBV infection
and the malignant outgrowth of these infected cells. Less is
known about the changes in the EBV infected epithelial cell
which are associated with evolution into NPC.

Over the past 20 years, a great deal has been learned
about the molecular processes by which EBV latently infects
and growth transforms normal human lymphocytes ( for review
and for relevant references prior to 1989, see 2). The first
two steps in delineating these processes were the characterization of the EBV genome and the analysis of EBV gene
expression in latently infected growth transformed B lymphocytes. EBV "latent" infection in B lymphocytes is clearly
not quiescent as is characteristic of herpes simplex or
varicella zoster virus latent infection in dorsal root
ganglia.  The EBV genome is quite active in latent lymphocyte infection. In growth transformed B lymphocytes
virtually the entire 172 kb is transcribed.  Nine highly
spliced mRNAs and two non-polyadenylated small RNAs (EBERs)
result. The EBV genes characteristically expressed in
latent, growth transforming, infection encode nuclear
proteins, EBNA-1, -2, -3a, -3b, -3c and -LP,  membrane
proteins, LMP -1, -2a and -2b, and the two EBERs. After the
initial characterization of these genes and their products,
analyses of the effects of the EBNAs or LMPs in murine
fibroblast cell lines or in non EBV infected BL cell lines
provided important indications of the role of these genes in
maintaining latent infection or in lymphocyte growth transformation. Most recently, recombinant EBV molecular genetics
has been developed to assess the role of each EBV latent
infection gene in transformation of primary human lymphocytes.

EBNA-2 and EBNA-LP are the first EBV genes expressed
in lymphocytes following EBV infection (3,4). EBNA-2 transactivates cell genes such as CD23, CD21 and cfgr and virus
genes such as LMP-1 and LMP-2 (5-8).  EBNA-2 also affects a
regulatory element upstream of its own promoter and may be

responsible for a promoter shift which takes place in some
cells after EBNA-2 expression (9,10). After the first 24-36
hours of infection all of the EBNAs and LMPs are expressed.
Cell DNA synthesis ensues and, with a slight delay, the
EBERs are expressed. The EBNAs, LMPs and EBERs are then
persistently expressed throughout latent infection. The
first approach to a functional analysis of the EBV genes
which are expressed in latent infection and growth transformation was to study the effects of these genes in fibroblasts or lymphoblasts. The results of these studies are
summarized in figure 1. Heterologous promoters were required
because EBV promoters were inactive or less active than in
the context of the EBV genome. The effects of the EBV genes
proved to be dependent on expression beyond a minimum
threshold, usually near the level expressed in latent infection. High level expression was usually cytotoxic.

EBNA-1 is necessary for EBV DNA persistence in cells
as an episome. The effect is cell species restricted and
requires a specific cis acting EBV DNA segment, ori p. The
essential features of the cis acting DNA segment are 21
directs repeats of a 30 bp palindromic oligonucleotide, a kb
of largely unrelated DNA and a dyad symmetry consisting of
four partial copies of the 30 bp palindrome. The 30 bp
palindrome specifically binds EBNA-1 (11-13). EBNA-1 binding
to the direct repeats is cooperative and highly sequence
specific. The dyad symmetry functions as a DNA replication
origin in the presence of EBNA-1; while the direct repeats
terminate replication (14). Thus, in the context of the EBV
episome, DNA synthesis proceeds almost entirely from ori p
clockwise, following the direction of EBNA gene transcription (15). EBNA-1 binding to ori p has transcriptionally
activating effects on heterologous promoters (16-18);
although effects on nearby latent infection promoters appear
to be minimal. Two cell proteins can also specifically and
competitively bind to ori p. Their physiological significance is not established; although their existence in cells
raises the expectation that there may be patho-physiolog-
ically significant EBNA-1 cognate sequences in cell DNA.
EBNA-1 and ori p are efficient in assuring episome
persistence in primate and some non primate cells. The
episome is usually maintained in low copy number and may
integrate. EBNA-1 is unique among the EBNAs in associating
with chromosomes (19). EBNA-1 binds randomly to metaphase
chromosomes and may thereby mediate metaphase episome
transmission to progeny cells. The EBNA-1 domains necessary

for chromosome association have not been identified;
although initial genetic evidence suggests that the carboxy
terminal domain may be important (18).

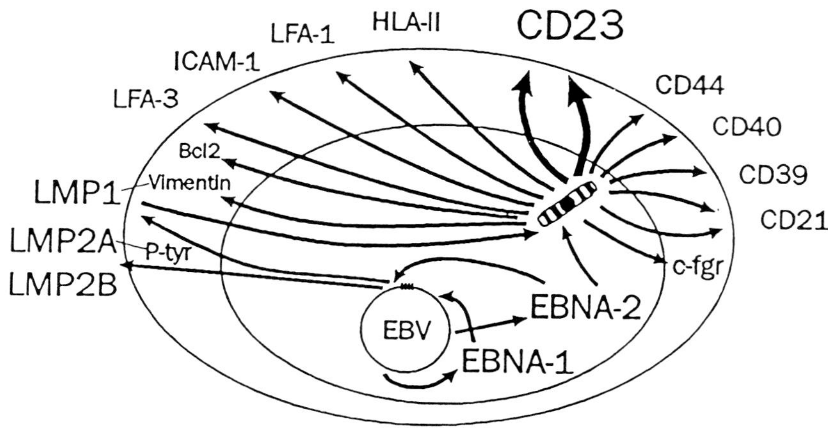


Figure 1: Effects of EBV genes on B lymphocytes

EBNA-2 expression in Rat-1 cells enables the cells to
grow in media supplemented by lower serum than is required
by control vector transfected cells. The most dramatic
effects are evident in B lymphoma cells where EBNA-2
expression induces higher levels of CD21, CD23 and cfgr
mRNAs (5-7). EBNA-2 transactivates the CD23 promoter which
ordinarily functions at a very low level in primary B
lymphocytes (6). A DNA fragment upstream of this promoter
conveys EBNA-2 responsiveness to heterologous promoters
(20). CD23 also has a cryptic promoter within its second
intron which is activated by LMP-1 (6). EBNA-2 synergizes
with LMP-1 and markedly increases CD23 mRNAs transcribed
under control of both promoters (6). EBNA-2 also upregulates
the LMP-1 and LMP-2 promoters which are near each other and
share EBNA-2 responsive elements (5,8,21,22). Stable or
transient transfection of an EBNA-2 expression vector into
lymphoblasts with EBV DNA fragments containing the LMP-1
gene and its upstream promoter and regulatory elements
results in higher level LMP-1 mRNA and protein expression
than cells transfected with the control expression vector
lacking EBNA-2. As with CD23, the LMP-1 upstream DNA can
convey EBNA-2 responsiveness to heterologous promoters (8).

These observations are compatible with the hypothesis that
EBNA-2 is a transactivator of virus (LMP) and cell (CD23,
CD21 and cfgr) gene expression through effects on upstream
regulatory elements. The LMP-1 responsive DNA element has
been narrowed to a -104 to -234 sequence relative to the
LMP-1 transcriptional initiation site. At least part of the
required element for EBNA-2 responsiveness is between -204
and -234 (8).

The other EBNAs may also activate cell gene
transcription. The EBNAs have acidic domains similar to
known transactivators, bind non specifically to DNA, and
associate with chromatin. Transfection of EBNA-3c into
lymphoblast under control of heterologous promoters results
in induction of CD21 (6).

Of all EBV genes expressed in latent infection, LMP-1
has the most dramatic effects on cell growth. LMP-1 consists
of a short amino terminus, six markedly hydrophobic
transmembrane domains separated by short reverse turns, and
a long acidic carboxy terminus. In Rat-1 cells, an immortalized rat cell line, LMP-1 expression under control of
heterologous promoters results in increased ability of the
cells to grow in media supplemented with low serum, markedly
decreased contact inhibition, anchorage independence and
increased tumorigenicity in nude mice. In murine NIH 3T3
cells, LMP-1 also increased the ability of the cells to grow
in media supplemented with low serum. In Balb C 3T3 cells,
LMP-1 caused loss of anchorage dependence. In non EBV
infected human Burkitt tumor B lymphoblasts, LMP-2
expression induced many of the phenotypic changes characteristic of EBV infection of primary B lymphocytes or
Burkitt tumor cells. LMP-1 caused cells to grow in clumps by
activating adhesion molecules and inducing LFA1, LFA3, and
ICAM1 expression (6). LMP-1 also caused down regulation of
CD10 and upregulation of CD23 (6).

LMP-1 is an integral membrane protein which post
translationally inserts into membranes. Nascent LMP-1 has a
half life of 6 h. The protein undergoes serine and threonine
phosphorylation. LMP-1 aggregates in a patch in the cells
plasma membrane, oriented with the amino and carboxy termini
in the cytoplasm. The LMP-1 patch colocalizes with a patch
of vimentin, an intermediate filament protein which is not
ordinarily organized in a plasma membrane patch. Once
associated with vimentin, LMP-1 follows vimentin as vimentin

forms rings around the nucleus in response to treating cells
with colcemid or as cells are extracted with non ionic
detergent leaving cytoskelatal residues. Association with
the cytoskeleton extends LMP-1's half life. LMP-1 expression
also induces vimentin mRNA (23). Surprisingly, association
with vimentin is not central to many of LMP-1's effects
since LMP-1 exhibits the same effects in lymphoblasts
lacking vimentin (24). Thus, the effects on vimentin may be
downstream of the central effects of LMP1 in activating
cells. The effects of LMP-1 in both lymphocytes and
fibroblasts are consistent with LMP-1 associating with a key
plasma membrane mediator of cell growth; and, thereby,
conveying a constitutive activating signal.

LMP-2 is a complex gene with multiple exons spanning
the EBV genome termini (25,26).  There are two promoters,
the LMP-2A promoter 3' to the LMP-1 gene and the LMP-2B
promoter, immediately 5' to the LMP-1 promoter. LMP-2B
transcription initiates in an LMP-2A intron after the first
encoding exon. The LMP-2A exon 5' to the LMP-2B transcriptional initiation site encodes an amino terminal cytoplasmic
domain which LMP-2B lacks. Both proteins have 12 transmembrane domains and a carboxy terminal cytoplasmic domain.
LMP-2A or LMP-2B expression in rodent fibroblasts or lymphoblasts has little apparent effect on cell growth or serum
dependence. However, LMP-2 colocalizes with LMP-1 in a
plasma membrane patch in latently infected lymphocytes
(26,27). Expression of LMP-2A alone in lymphoblasts is
sufficient to cause it to patch in the plasma membrane
(26,27). LMP-2A alters plasma membrane tyrosine phosphorylation. LMP-2A is a major tyrosine kinase substrate in
transiently transfected lymphoblasts and induces the
phosphorylation of a 70 kda cell protein (27). LMP-2A also
diminishes the intracellular free Ca increase associated
with surface Ig cross linking. The data indicate that LMP-2A
and B are likely to be modulators of LMP-1 effects on cell
growth.

The definitive demonstration of the role of each latency and growth transformation cycle associated gene in
growth transformation has recently been made possible by the
development of EBV recombinant molecular genetics. Since EBV
replicates, in vitro, in latently infected B lymphocytes in
which virus replication is induced, recombinant genomes can
be obtained by transfecting latently infected lymphocytes
with mutant recombinant EBV DNA fragments which had been

cloned and amplified in E. coli. When virus replication is
induced immediately following transfection, replicating
viral DNA undergoes homologous recombination with the transfected cloned viral DNA. Parental and recombinant virus can
be passaged into primary B lymphocytes or into B lymphoma
cells (28-30). Primary B lymphocytes are dependant on virus
infection for their ability to grow, in vitro. B lymphoma
cells can be made dependent on recombinant virus for their
growth by including a linked positive selection marker in
the transfected recombinant viral DNA and by plating the infected cells in selective media (30). The frequency of
recombinant versus parental non recombinant virus varies
considerably among different sites in the EBV genome, making
it more difficult to obtain some mutants.

Initial studies exploited a non transforming virus
strain, P3HR-1, which is deleted for a DNA fragment that
includes the last two encoding exons of EBNA-LP and the
EBNA-2 open reading frame (28, 29). Recombination with a
wild type EBV derived cosmid DNA fragment which spans the
deletion restores transformation. This opened the possibility of examining the effect of specific mutations within
the EBNA-LP or EBNA-2 open reading frames to establish which
of these is essential for growth transformation. Some
deletion, linker insertion or stop codon mutations within
the EBNA-2 open reading frame resulted in no transforming
recombinants, formally demonstrating that EBNA-2 is
essential for lymphocyte growth transformation (28,29).
Further studies demonstrated the importance of EBNA-2 in the
type specific differences in growth transformation noted
among EBV isolates  (29). Two EBV types circulate in nature.
These two types differ in their ability to initiate growth
transformation and in their EBNA-2 and -3 genes (31).
Recombinant virus with a high transforming type 1 virus
derived EBNA-2 gene exhibited a high transforming phenotype;
while, an isogenic recombinant with a type 2 EBNA-2 gene
exhibited a low transforming phenotype (29). Thus, type
specific differences in EBNA-2 are the principal determinant
of type specific differences in lymphocyte growth
transformation.

Analysis of the phenotype of 11 linker insertion and
15 deletion mutations within the EBNA-2 open reading frame
revealed four separable domains which are essential for
transformation of primary B lymphocytes (32). All mutations
which inactivated transformation also inactivated the

ability of EBNA-2 to transactivate LMP-1 in a transient
transfection assay. Thus, these data are consistent with the
hypothesis that transactivation is the principal mechanism
for EBNA-2's action in transformation. Surprisingly, the
last twenty amino acids of EBNA-2 were fully dispensable for
transactivation or for transformation. The penultimate
carboxy terminal domain is however one of the four domains
essential for transformation and transactivation. This
latter domain is a strong acidic transactivator in B lymphocytes when directed to a promoter by fusion to a site
specific DNA binding protein such as gal 4 and by inserting
gal 4 recognition sites upstream of the promoter (33).

EBNA-LP has a very different intranuclear localization
than the other EBNA's in that it localizes to discrete
intranuclear particles. The last two exons encode for an
acidic domain likely to be important in transcriptional
activation. Although initial studies suggested that recombinant EBV containing an EBNA-LP gene without the last two
encoding exons had almost normal transforming activity (28),
subsequent experiments with deletion or stop codon insertion
mutants reveal a markedly reduced transformation efficiency,
an unusual dependence on fibroblast feeder layers for
outgrowth of infected cells as long term cell lines, and, an
inability of LP mutant recombinant EBV infected  cells to
proliferate when seeded at low density (34). The expression
of other EBNAs and LMPs was unaffected by the LP mutation.
These data are compatible with the hypothesis that EBNA-LP
regulates a cell growth factor or growth factor receptor
which is critical for LCL outgrowth.

Other studies are using recombinant EBV molecular
genetics to investigate the essentiality of the EBNA-3s,
LMPs and EBERs in growth transformation. Deletion of both
EBERs had no effect on EBV gene expression, on B lymphocyte
growth transformation or on EBV replication in lymphocytes
in response to inducers of the EBV replicative cycle (35).
These data are inconsistent with a role for the EBERs in RNA
processing but are consistent with a role in mediating
resistance to interferon effects on transformation or
replication.

In summary, EBV latent infection and B lymphocyte
growth transformation involve EBNA-1 in episome maintenance,
EBNA-2 and possibly EBNA-3s and EBNA-LP as transactivators
of virus and cell gene expression, LMP-1 as a plasma

membrane activator of cell growth, and LMP-2 as a mediator
of plasma membrane activation.  Cellular targets of  EBNA
and LMP action have been identified such as CD21 and CD23;
although, their role in mediating EBV effects on cell growth
is not established. Because of the similarity between EBV's
and Ig cross linking's effects on B lymphocytes the EBNAs
and LMPs are likely to be interacting with regulators of
normal B lymphocyte growth. Similar mechanisms mediate early
onset EBV associated lymphopro-liferative disease or EBV
infected cell proliferation in SCID mice which are
characterized by the full repertoire of EBNA and LMP
expression, low CD10 and high CD21 and CD23 expression
(36,37). The role of EBNA and LMPs in malignancies which
appear long after EBV infection is substantially less
certain. In many Burkitt lymphomas, EBV gene expression is
largely confined to EBNA-1; the cells expressing high level
CD10 and low level CD23 (38). The lack of expression of the
other EBNAs and of the LMPs may be in part in response to
selective pressure against EBNA-2, EBNA-3 or LMP1 expression
because these genes render B lymphocytes susceptible to
immune T lymphocyte cytotoxicity (39-41). EBNA-2, EBNA-3 and
LMP1 include target epitopes and LMP1 induces conjugation of
EBV transformed B lymphocytes with immune T lymphocytes. In
Burkitt lymphoma, other genes including c-myc have
supplanted the need for EBNAs and LMPs as mediators of B
lymphocyte proliferation. Still, the EBV genome is
maintained in these cells and EBNA-1 is expressed. This is
the first direct evidence of a less active state of EBV
latency characterized by EBNA-1 expression without the other
EBNAs and LMPs. The existence of a similar state in B
lymphocytes or B lymphocyte precursors, in vivo, could
explain EBV's ability to persist in the face of a strong T
cytotoxic response. Recent analysis of Burkitt lymphoma
cells expressing only EBNA-1 indicate that EBV gene
expression is trans-criptionally regulated in such cells and
that a previously unrecognized promoter in Bam F is the only
active EBV promoter in these cells (42).

Nasopharyngeal carcinoma appears to be a third type of
latent EBV gene expression. EBNA expression may be confined
to EBNA-1 (43,44). Despite the absence of EBNA-2, LMP-1
seems to be frequently expressed. LMP-2 has not been
investigated. LMP-1 has effects on epithelial cell growth
and differentiation (45,46). Thus, at some stage, LMP-1 may
contribute to the growth abnormalities of nasopharyngeal
carcinoma cells. The low frequency of NPC and the long delay

in tumor onset, even among southern chinese in whom
nasopharyngeal carcinoma is endemic, indicates that several
steps beyond EBV infection are involved in the evolution of
this tumor.

## Acknowledgements

Our research program is supported by grant no.: CA47006 from
the National Cancer Institute of the USPHS.

REFERENCES


1.    G. Miller. <u>Virology.</u> 2nd Ed., B. Fields, D. Knipe et
      al. Eds., Raven Press, N.Y. p1921 (1990).
2.    E. Kieff and D. Liebowitz. <u>Virology</u>, 2nd Ed.,
      B. Fields, D. Knipe et al., Eds., Raven Press, Ltd., New
      York, p1889 (1990).
3.    C. Rooney, G. Howe, <u>et al.</u> <u>J. Virol.</u> 63, 1531 (1989).
4.    C. Alfieri, M. Birkenbach, <u>et al.</u> <u>Virology</u>, 181, 595
      (1991).
5.    F. Wang, S. Tsang, <u>et al.</u> <u>J. Virol.</u> 64, 3407 (1990).
6.    F. Wang, C. Gregory, <u>et al.</u> <u>J. Virol.</u> 64, 2309 (1990).
7.    J. Knutson. <u>J. Virol.</u> 64, 2530 (1990).
8.    S. Tsang, F. Wang, <u>et al.</u> <u>J. Virol.</u> submitted, (1991).
9.    M. Woisetschlager, X. Jin, <u>et al.</u> <u>Proc. Natl. Acad. Sci.</u>
      88, 3942 (1991).
10.   N. Sung, S. Kenney, <u>et al.</u> <u>J. Virol.</u> 65, 2164 (1991).
11.   C.H. Jones, S.D. Hayward, <u>et al.</u> <u>J. Virol.</u> 63, 101
      (1989).
12.   R. Ambinder, W. Shah, <u>et al.</u> <u>J. Virol.</u> 64, 2369 (1990).
13.   R. Ambinder, M. Mullen, <u>et al.</u> <u>J. Virol.</u> 65, 1466
      (1991).
14.   T. Gahn, C. Schildkraut, <u>et al.</u> <u>Cell</u>, 58, 527 (1989).
15.   J. Sample and E. Kieff. <u>J. Virol.</u> 64, 1667 (1990).
16.   B. Sugden and N. Warren. <u>J. Virol.</u> 63, 2644 (1989).
17.   D. Wysokenski, J. Yates. <u>J. Virol.</u> 63, 2657 (1989).
18.   J. Yates, S. Camiolo. <u>Cancer Cells</u>, 6, 197 (1988).
19.   L. Petti, C. Sample, <u>et al.</u> <u>Virology</u>, 176, 563 (1990).
20.   F. Wang, H. Kikutani, <u>et al.</u> <u>J. Virol.</u> 65, 4101 (1991).
21.   U. Zimber-Storb, K. Suentzenich, <u>et al.</u> <u>J. Virol.</u> 65,
      415 (1991).
22.   R. Fahraeus, A Jansson, <u>et al.</u> <u>Proc. Natl. Acad. Sci.</u>
      87, 7390 (1990).
23.   M. Birkenbach, D. Liebowitz, <u>et al.</u> <u>J. Virol.</u> 63, 4079
      (1989).
24.   D. Liebowitz and E. Kieff. <u>J. Virol.</u> 63, 4051 (1989).
25.   J. Sample, D. Liebowitz, <u>et al.</u> <u>J. Virol.</u> 63, 933
      (1989).

26. R. Longnecker and E. Kieff. <u>J. Virol.</u> 64, 2319 (1990).

27. R. Longnecker, B. Druker, <u>et al.</u> <u>J. Virol.</u> 65, 3681 (1991).

28. W. Hammerschmidt and B. Sugden. <u>Nature</u>, 317, (1989).

29. J. Cohen, F. Wang, <u>et al.</u> <u>Proc. Natl. Acad. Sci.</u> 86, 9558 (1989).

30. F. Wang, A. Marchini, <u>et al.</u> <u>J. Virol.</u> 65, 1701 (1991).

31. J. Sample, L. Young, <u>et al.</u> <u>J. Virol.</u> 64, 4084 (1991).

32. J. Cohen, F. Wang, <u>et al.</u> <u>J. Virol.</u> 65, 2545 (1991).

33. J. Cohen and E. Kieff. <u>J. Virol.</u> Submitted (1991).

34. J. Mannick, J. Cohen, <u>et al.</u> <u>J. Virol.</u> Submitted (1991).

35. S. Swaminathan, B. Tomkinson, <u>et al.</u> <u>Proc. Natl. Acad. Sci.</u> 88, 1546 (1991).

36. L. Young, C. Alfieri, <u>et al.</u> <u>N.E. J. Med.</u> 321, 1080 (1989).

37. M. Rowe, L. Young, <u>et al.</u> <u>J. Exp. Med.</u> 173, 147 (1991).

38. C. Gregory, D. Rowe, <u>et al.</u> <u>J. Gen. Virol.</u> 71, 1481 (1990).

39. S. Burrows, T. Sculley, <u>et al.</u> <u>J. Exp. Med.</u> 171, 345 (1990)

40. S. Burrows, I. Misko, <u>et al.</u> <u>J. Exp. Med.</u> 171, 345 (1990a).

41. R. Murray, M. Kurilla, <u>et al.</u> <u>Proc. Natl. Acad. Sci.</u> 87, 2906 (1990).

42. J. Sample, L. Brooks, <u>et al.</u> <u>Proc. Natl. Acad. Sci.</u> 88, 6343 (1991).

43. K. Gilligan, H. Sato, <u>et al.</u> <u>J. Virol.</u> 64, 4948 (1990).

44. M. Hitt, M. Allday, <u>et al.</u> <u>EMBO J.</u> 8, 2639 (1989).

45. J. Wilson, W. Weinberg, <u>et al.</u> <u>Cell</u>, 61, 1315 (1990).

46. C. Dawson, A. Rickinson, <u>et al.</u> <u>Nature.</u> 344, 777 (1990).

From: *Neoplastic Transformation in Human Cell Culture,*
Eds.: J. S. Rhim and A. Dritschilo ©1991 The Humana Press Inc., Totowa, NJ

ISOLATION AND CHARACTERIZATION OF A TRANSFORMATION-

ASSOCIATED GENE FROM HUMAN NASOPHARYNGEAL CARCINOMA CELLS

Y. Sun[1], S. Poirier[2], Y. Cao[2], G. Hegamyer[2], and
N.H. Colburn[2]
[1]BCDP, Program Resources Inc./DynCorp, NCI-
FCRDC, Frederick, MD 21702, USA, [2]Cell Biology
Section, Laboratory of Viral Carcinogenesis,
National Cancer Institute-FCRDC, Frederick, MD
21702, USA

Nasopharyngeal carcinoma (NPC) is a common disease
in Southern China and Southeast Asia that also develops
elsewhere (1). It has been well documented that NPC is
associated with Epstein-Barr virus (EBV) infection (2,3) as
well as with certain dietary and environmental factors,
such as salted fish, some medicinal herbs, and vegetables
(4-7). It has been proposed that initiation of NPC
requires EBV expression, but induction of preneoplastic
events and maintenance of tumor cell phenotype require
critical cellular genes (8-12). We previously found that
DNA sequences from a human NPC cell line, $CNE_2$, could confer
sensitivity to TPA-induced transformation when transferred
to promotion-insensitive (P⁻) mouse JB6 cells (13,14). In
addition, $CNE_2$ DNA sequences, when introduced, can produce
neoplastic transformation of promotion-sensitive (P⁺) mouse
JB6 cells (15). Both the NPC-DNA associated promotion
sensitivity and the oncogenic activity function were found
to act independently of concurrent EBV gene expression
(15). To isolate the DNA sequence(s) that are responsible
for transforming activity, we initiated the present
investigation that yielded a cloned transformation-associated gene from $CNE_2$ A15 cells, a clonal line of $CNE_2$ (16).
Our strategy for cloning is shown in Figure 1, and
the assay for DNA-mediated transfer of transforming
activity is shown in Figure 2. After three cycles of
transfection accompanied by selection for both induced
anchorage independent transformation and the presence of
human Alu sequences, two independent clonal tertiary
CNE/JB6 transfectants, 6-2-5 and 14-1-1, were isolated.
Their neoplastic phenotypes, as tested by anchorage
independent growth and tumorigenicity in nude mice, is

**FIGURE 1**

**Strategy for Cloning a Transformation-Associated Gene
from a Human Nasopharyngeal Carcinoma Cell Line**

Transfect sheared $CNE_2$ A15 DNA into mouse C141P$^+$ cells
↓
Pluck largest colonies from soft agar
↓
Grow as clonal transfectants
↓
Extract DNA
↓                          ↓
Human <u>Alu</u> detection     Transforming activity
↓                          ↓
Human <u>Alu</u> positive DNAs    TX DNAs
↓
Second cycle transfection
↓
Third cycle transfection
↓
Make genomic library from tertiary transfectant
↓
Screen the library with Human <u>Alu</u> (Blur 8)
↓
Three cycles of library screening
↓
Pick up 8 single positive plaques
↓
Characterize isolated clones

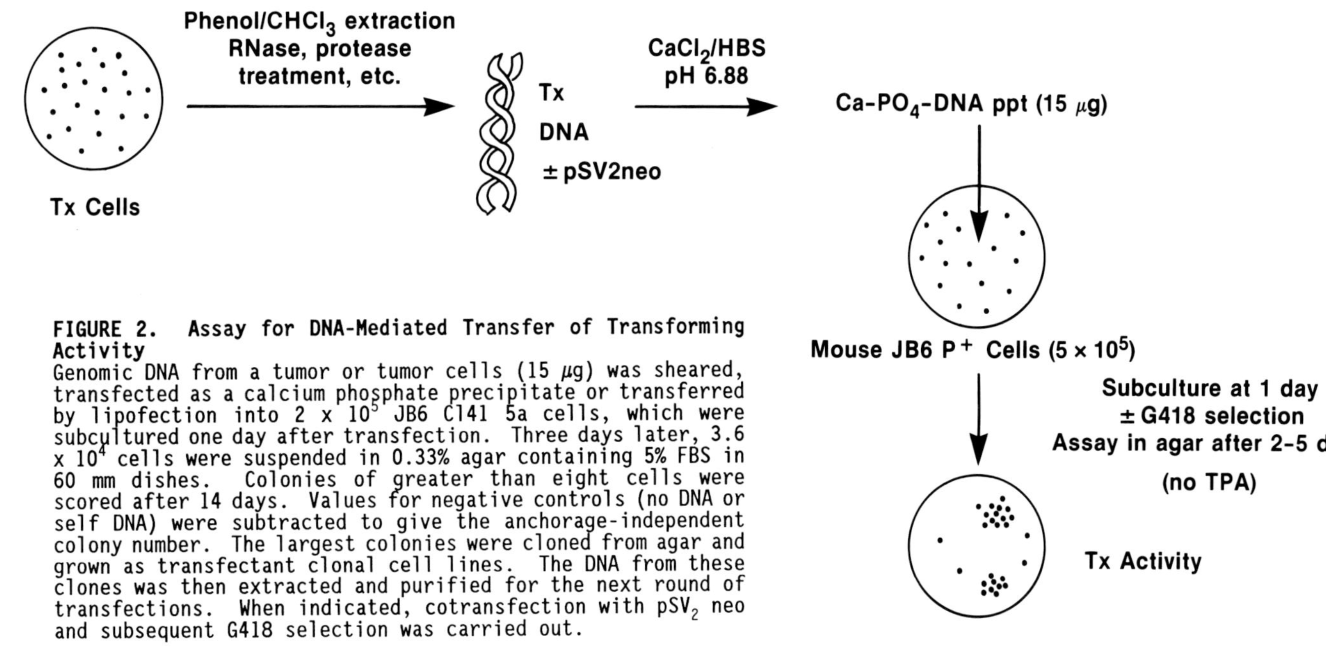



**FIGURE 2.** Assay for DNA-Mediated Transfer of Transforming Activity

Genomic DNA from a tumor or tumor cells (15 µg) was sheared, transfected as a calcium phosphate precipitate or transferred by lipofection into $2 \times 10^5$ JB6 Cl41 5a cells, which were subcultured one day after transfection. Three days later, $3.6 \times 10^4$ cells were suspended in 0.33% agar containing 5% FBS in 60 mm dishes. Colonies of greater than eight cells were scored after 14 days. Values for negative controls (no DNA or self DNA) were subtracted to give the anchorage-independent colony number. The largest colonies were cloned from agar and grown as transfectant clonal cell lines. The DNA from these clones was then extracted and purified for the next round of transfections. When indicated, cotransfection with pSV$_2$ neo and subsequent G418 selection was carried out.

shown in Table 1.  Since the 6-2-5 transfectant was more tumorigenic and showed a stronger <u>Alu</u> signal than 14-1-1 (Table 1 and not shown), it was used as the DNA source to construct a genomic library in the λ dash vector.  Three cycles of screening of this genomic library with human <u>Alu</u> (Blur 8) probe yielded 8 single positive clones that originated from independent first-screen plaques.  All of the eight clones showed identical human <u>Alu</u> hybridization patterns after various restriction enzyme digestions.  One of the clones, 3-2-3, was selected for further characterization.  Figure 3 shows restriction and hybridization mapping of the isolated NPC clone 3-2-3.  The human <u>Alu</u> containing sequence was mapped to a 3.3-kb Xho I/Sal I fragment at one end of the insert.  Two human <u>Alu</u>-negative internal fragments, a 2.8-kb Eco RI fragment and a 3.0-kb Eco RI/Xho I fragment, as shown in Figure 3, were used as hybridization probes in Southern analysis.  The results demonstrated the same size hybridization bands in the original $CNE_2$ cell line, the nude mouse tumors derived from them, and in tertiary transfectant 6-2-5, but not in JB6 Cl41 recipient cells (not shown), indicating the preservation of genomic structure in the cloned 3-2-3 sequence as it existed in the original $CNE_2$ cells.

To test for transforming activity of the isolated clone 3-2-3, we co-transfected λ3-2-3 or clone 3-2-3 insert only with $pSV_2$ neo into JB6 Cl41 recipient cells with lipofectin reagent followed by G418 selection.  Neo-resistant cells were then tested for anchorage independent growth.  The results from two independent experiments are summarized in Table 2, and representative areas of soft agar colonies are shown in Figure 4.  The clone 3-2-3 showed a measurable transforming activity (4-fold as compared with neo-control); however, the transforming activity was much less than that of known oncogenes, such as H-ras, when introduced into JB6 P[+] cells (not shown).  We reason that the low biological activity of clone 3-2-3 could be due to the lack of a complete promoter region in the sequence, to the presence of inhibitory intron sequences, or to the truncation of the coding regions.  Since the 2.8-kb <u>Alu</u>-negative internal fragment in clone 3-2-3 (Figure 3) can detect a 1.3-kb transcript in the original $CNE_2$ cells by Northern analysis (not shown), we sequenced the entire 2.8-kb fragment from the genomic clone.  Computer analysis did not show homology to any known oncogenes. Using this 2.8-kb fragment as a probe, we screened a cDNA library generated from the C15 tumor, an EBV[+], nude mice-carried nasopharyngeal carcinoma (gift of Dr. N. Raab-Traub at University of North Carolina). Tertiary screening of the library yielded 12 positive clones.  Nine of them had an insert with a size of 0.7-kb.

**TABLE 1.** Phenotypes of the Tertiary CNE/JB6 Clonal Transfectant Used for Construction of a Genomic Library

| Cell Line | Anchorage Indep. Transforming Activity of DNA (colonies per $5 \times 10^4$ cells) | Anchorage Indep. Growth of cell line (colonies per $10^4$ cells) | Tumorigenicity in nude mice of cell line (# with tumor/total) | (Min. latent period in wks). |
|---|---|---|---|---|
| Mouse JB6 Cl41 | 6 | 35 | 0/48 | >9 |
| Human CNE$_2$ A15 | 102 | 1010 | 14/15 | 2 |
| CNE/JB6 14-1-1 | 125 | 550 | 1/32 | 7 |
| CNE/JB6 6-2-5 | 105 | 225 | 8/31 | 4 |

Transfer of anchorage independence was assayed as described in the legend to Figure 2. Tumorigenicity is shown as the tumor yielded at eight weeks following injection of $2 \times 10^6$ cells subcutaneously and intrascapularly. The anchorage independence assays were reproduced at least 3 times with standard errors of about 15%.

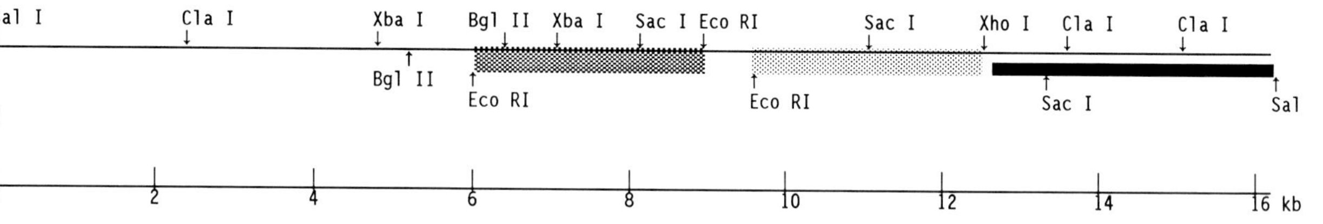



**FIGURE 3.  Restriction and Hybridization Mapping of the Isolated NPC Clone 3-2-3**
A human <u>Alu</u> positive clone, designated as 3-2-3, was digested to completion with
Sal I.   The 16kb insert was gel-purified then mapped by cutting with various
restriction enzymes or pairs of enzymes.  Restriction sites were assigned, based
upon the agarose gel banding pattern of the enzyme digests.  To more accurately
define the restriction sites, the insert was $^{32}$P end labeled using polynucleotide
kinase, cut with restriction enzyme(s), run on an agarose gel, dried, and exposed
directly to X-ray film.  This provided us with accurate placement of the end sites
for each enzyme used.  A human <u>Alu</u> probe (Blur 8) was used to localize the position
of the <u>Alu</u> positive fragment by Southern hybridization.

**TABLE 2.** Transforming Activity of the Isolated $CNE_2$ $\lambda$3-2-3 Clone

| DNA transfected into JB6 $P^+$ cells | Number of soft agar colonies per $3.6 \times 10^4$ cells |
|---|---|
| $pSV_2$ neo (2 $\mu$g) | 9 |
| $pSV_2$ neo + Cl 41 up to 10 $\mu$g | 15 |
| $\lambda$ 3-2-3 16 kb insert + Cl 41 up to 10 $\mu$g | 60 |
| $\lambda$ 3-2-3 uncut + Cl 41 up to 10 $\mu$g | 56 |

The genomic clone $\lambda$ 3-2-3 or clone 3-2-3 insert only were co-transfected with 2 $\mu$g of $pSV_2$ neo into JB6 Cl 41 recipient cells by lipofectin, followed by G418 selection. The neo-resistant cells ($3.6 \times 10^4$) were seeded in 0.33% agar to be tested for their ability to grow in soft agar. DNA amount used for transfection was equimolar for the two forms of NPC gene at 1.5, 2.9, 5.8 $\mu$g for the $\lambda$3-2-3 16 kb insert and 4.1, 8.2, 16.4 $\mu$g for uncut $\lambda$3-2-3. Since no dose dependency was observed in the ranges listed above, the soft agar numbers shown are the average from two independent soft agar assays with three different doses of DNA.

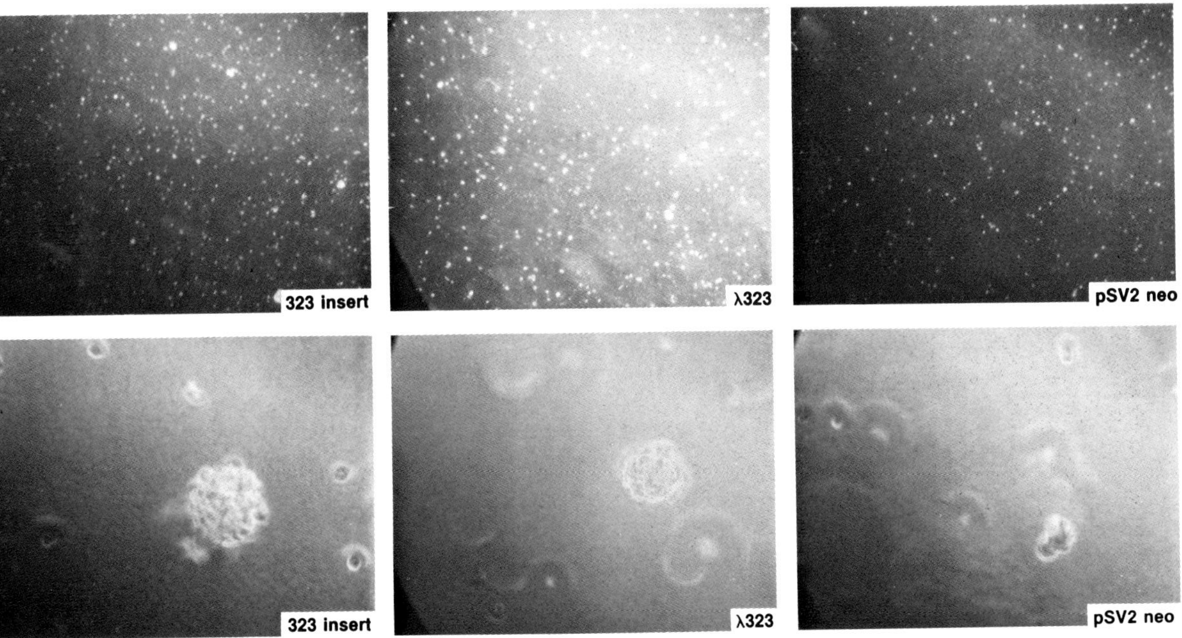



**FIGURE 4.** Formation of Anchorage-Independent Colonies After Transfection of the JB6 Cells with a Cloned NPC 3-2-3 Sequence

Genomic clone λ3-2-3 or cloned 3-2-3 insert only was co-transfected with $pSV_2$ neo into JB6 C141 recipient cells by lipofectin as recommended by the supplier (BRL), using recipient cell DNA as a carrier. Neo-resistant cells were selected by growing in 5% EMEM medium containing G418 (500 µg/ml) for 2 weeks with medium change every 3 days. $3.6 \times 10^4$ resistant cells were seeded in 0.33% agar to test their ability to grow anchorage-independently. A representative area was shown.

Four out of the nine clones were sequenced, and all were
verified to be identical. The potential AATAAA
polyadenylation signal, followed by a poly A tail, was
found in the 3'-end of these cDNA clones. Computer
analysis revealed that about 0.5-kb of the sequence was
identical with part of the 2.8-kb fragment, but no sequence
homology to any known oncogenes was found, thus promising
a novel oncogene in NPC. Our current effort is to identify
the remaining 0.6-kb sequence at the 5'-end. Our long term
goal is to construct this 1.3-kb cDNA sequence into an
expression vector and test its biological activity for
neoplastic transformation. The isolation of a potentially
novel oncogene and the elucidation of its role in NPC
etiology will lead us to a better understanding of
multistage human carcinogenesis.

"This project has been funded in part with Federal funds
from the Department of Health and Human Services under
contract number NO1-CO-74102 with Program Resources, Inc.
The content of this publication does not necessarily
reflect the views or policies of the Department of Health
and Human Services, nor does mention of trade names,
commercial products, or organizations imply endorsement by
the U.S. Government."

REFERENCES

1. De The, G., Ho, J.H.C. & Muir, C.S. (1982) in *Viral Infections of Humans. Epidemiology and Control*, ed. Evans, A.S. (Wiley, New York) pp. 126-144.
2. Klein, G., Giovanella, B.C., Lindahl, T., Fialkow, P.J., Singh, S., and Stenlin, J.S. (1974) *Proc. Natl. Acad. Sci. USA.* 71, 4737-4741.
3. Klein, G. (1977) in *The Epstein-Barr Virus*, eds. Epstein, M.A. & Achong, B.G. (Springer-Verlag, Berlin) pp. 339-346.
4. Zeng, Y., Zhong, J.M., Mo, Y.K. & Miao, X.C. (1983) *Intervirol.* 19, 201-204.
5. Yu, M.C., Mo, C.C., Chong, W.X., Yeh, F.S. & Henderson, B.E. (1988) *Cancer Res.* 48, 1954-1959.
6. Zeng, Y. (1985) *Adv. Cancer Res.* 44, 121-138.
7. Zeng, Y., Miao, X.C., Jaio, B., Li, H.Y., Ni, H.Y. & Ito, Y. (1984) *Cancer Lett.* 23, 53-59.
8. Shao, Y.M., Poirier, S., Ohshima, H., Malaveille, C., Zeng, Y., De The, G. & Bartsch, H. (1988) *Carcinogenesis*, 9, 1455-1457.
9. Ho, J.H.C., Huang, D.P. & Fong, Y.Y. (1978) *Lancet*, 2, 626.

                                                            

10. Armstrong, R.W., Armstrong, M.J., Yu, M.C. & Henderson, B.E. (1983) *Cancer Res.*, **42**, 2967-2970.
11. Ho, J.H.C. (1971) in *Recent Advances in Human Tumor Virology and Immunology*, eds. Nakahara, W., Nishioka, K., Hirayama, T. & Ito, Y. (University of Tokyo Press, Tokyo) pp. 275-295.
12. Hirayama, T. & Ito, Y. (1981) *Prev. Med.*, **10**, 614-622.
13. Lerman, M.I., Sakai, A., Yao, K.T. & Colburn, N.H. (1987) *Carcinogenesis*, **8**, 121-127.
14. Dowjat, W.K., Ya, C., Nagashima, K., Sakai, A., & Colburn, N.H. (1988) *Mol. Carcinogenesis*, **1**, 33-40.
15. Colburn, N.H., Raab-Traub, N., Becker, D., Winterstein, D. & Cao, Y. (1989) *Int. J. Cancer*, **44**, 1012-1016.
16. Cao, Y., Sun, Y., Poirier, S., Winterstein, D., Hegamyer, G., Seed, J., Malin, S., & Colburn, N.H. (1991) *Mol. Carcinogenesis*, in press.

# Molecular Pathogenesis of Lung Cancer

## Mutations in Dominant and Recessive Oncogenes, and the Expression of Opioid and Nicotine Receptors in the Pathogenesis of Lung Cancer.

D. Carbone, R. Maneckjee, D. D'Amico, S. Bader, S. Bodner, I. Chiba, J. Fedorko, I. Linnoila, , T. Mitsudomi, M.Nau, H. Pass, H. Oie, E. Russell, T. Takahashi, T. Unger, J. Whang-Peng, A. Gazdar, J. Minna. NCI-Navy Medical Oncology Branch, National Cancer Institute & USUHS, Bethesda, MD 20814

## Mutations in Dominant and Recessive Oncogenes:

Lung cancer is the leading cause of cancer deaths in the United States for both men and women in 1991. It is also unique among the common cancers in that most cases can be associated with a single environmental exposure, namely cigarette smoke. Cigarette smoke contains many substances that can damage DNA and act as carcinogens or mutagens in *in vitro* systems. It is presumed that this ability to directly damage DNA in lung cells is a primary event in lung cancer carcinogenesis.

This damage is manifested at the level of whole chromosomes by the abnormal karyotypes of lung cancer cells. Gross deletions and translocations are frequent occurences in these cells. Such loss of genetic material is thought to be one mechanism by which point mutations are uncovered in tumor suppressor genes residing on the remaining allele. For this reason, we undertook a systematic study designed to look for regions of chromosomes which are frequently deleted in lung cancer (1). This and other studies using karyotype and RFLP analysis point to several regions of the genome including 1, 3p, 11p, 13q (the location of the retinoblastoma gene) and 17p (location of p53) as being involved more frequently than others. Several potential recessive oncogene sites appear located on the 3p chromosome arm at 3p14, 3p21, and 3p24-25. These regions are being intensively studied for specific genetic lesions associated with lung cancer.

## Lesions in dominant oncogenes

Lung cancer cells exhibit several genetic lesions involving mutations activating the dominant cellular proto-oncogenes as well as an even greater number inactivating the recessive or "tumor suppressor" genes. Dominant oncogenes *myc* and *ras* have been the best studied in lung cancer. Overexpression of the *myc* family of genes is common in small cell lung cancers (SCLC), and especially high in tumors recurring after therapy and variant forms (2), but coding sequence mutations have not been observed. *Ras*, on the other hand, is found to be activated by point mutations, most frequently involving K-*ras* and most frequently at codon 12. Mutations in *ras* are frequently involved in non-small cell lung cancer (NSCLC) but have never been seen in SCLC. Table 1 summarizes these results. Thus there seems to be a different pattern in the molecular lesions seen in dominant oncogenes in the different types of lung cancer.

| Cancer type | K-ras 12 | 13 | 61 | H-ras 61 | N-ras 61 | Total | (%) |
|---|---|---|---|---|---|---|---|
| **NSCLC** | 14 | 5 | 3 | 1 | 2 | 25/77 | (32) |
| **Adenoca** | 6 | 4 | 0 | 0 | 1 | 11/44 | (25) |
| **Squamous** | 3 | 0 | 0 | 0 | 0 | 3/8 | (38) |
| **Large Cell** | 4 | 0 | 3 | 1 | 1 | 9/15 | (60) |
| **Carcinoid** | 1 | 0 | 0 | 0 | 0 | 1/5 | (20) |
| **Other** | 0 | 1 | 0 | 0 | 0 | 1/5 | (20) |
| **Small Cell Ca** | 0 | 0 | 0 | 0 | 0 | 0/42 | (0) |
| **SCLC** | 0 | 0 | 0 | 0 | 0 | 0/37 | (0) |
| **Expul SC** | 0 | 0 | 0 | 0 | 0 | 0/5 | (0) |

Table 1. Incidence of mutations in H- N- and K-*ras* in the different lung cancer histologic types (3).

## Lesions in tumor suppressor genes

The *rb* gene was first discovered by virtue of its universal inactivation in retinoblastoma tumors. It is also altered in nearly all SCLC (4) and at least some NSCLC. In retinoblastoma, nearly all tumors completely lack the Rb protein, but in lung cancer, while complete lack of protein expression is common, there are many examples of tumors which produce normal levels of Rb protein of normal size. Upon evaluation, however, many of these are found to be abnormal in phosphorylation as the result of point mutations (5).

The nuclear phosphoprotein *p53* appears mutant in at least 50% of NSCLC (highest in squamous cell cancer) and nearly 100% of the cases of SCLC(6, 7). This different incidence is another example of the molecular specificity of these lesions found in different histologic types of lung cancer. Mutations of all types are found (deletions, splicing

and nonsense mutations) but the most common lesion is a
nonsense mutation leading to the production of an abnormal
protein product.  The lesions found in lung cancer are
scattered over the open reading frame, but are concentrated
in the regions of highest evolutionary conservation and those
involved in binding with the SV40 virus oncoprotein large T
antigen.  Figure 1 shows the locations of a number of these
mutations.

Table 2 shows the type of base changes seen in p53
point mutations from lung cancer as compared to colon and
breast cancer.  As can be seen, G to T transversions are by
far the most frequent alteration in lung cancer, in contrast to
G to A transversions in others.  This may be due to a
different spectrum of carcinogens involved in the production
of lung cancer and the other cancers, and/or differences in
carcinogen metabolizing enzymes found in the different
tissues.  The symmetric mutation involving the other strand,
C to A, is also not seen, implying that there is a strand
specificity to the mutagenic process in lung cancer.  This
may be due to selective repair of the coding strand or it
selective protection by proteins from the effects of activated
carcinogens.

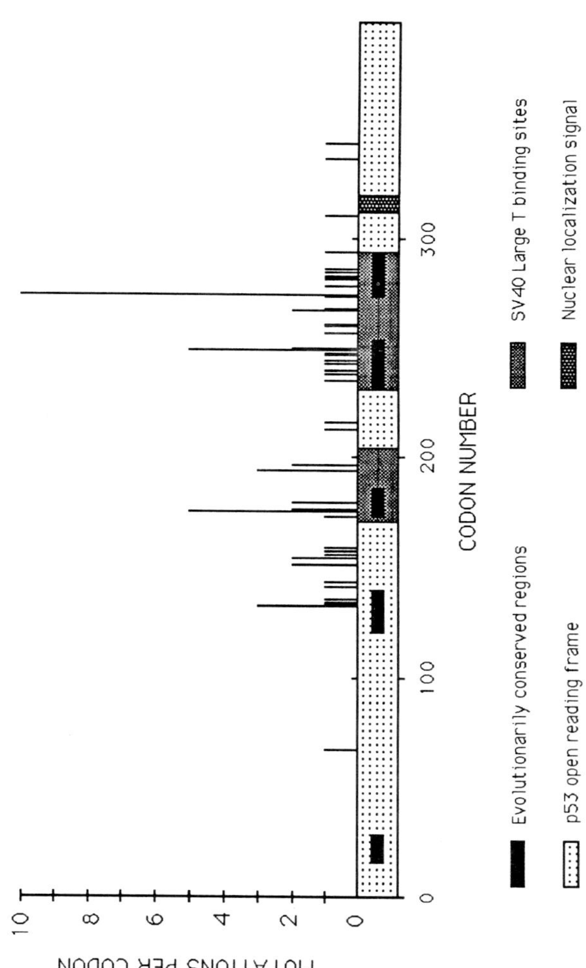


Figure 1. Histogram showing the open reading frame of p53 with the locations of 70 point mutations found in human tumors. Regions that are highly conserved through evolution and those thought to be important in binding to SV40 T antigen are marked.

| Base | SCLC | NSCLC | Lung | Other |
|---|---|---|---|---|
| G to T | 9 | 26 | 35 | 0 |
| C to T | 3 | 10 | 13 | 6 |
| G to C | 2 | 8 | 10 | 2 |
| A to C | 2 | 1 | 3 | 1 |
| T to G | 2 | 0 | 2 | 0 |
| G to A | 1 | 4 | 5 | 11 |
| A to G | 1 | 4 | 5 | 2 |
| C to A | 1 | 0 | 1 | 0 |
| T to A | 1 | 0 | 1 | 0 |
| C to G | 0 | 0 | 0 | 0 |
| A to T | 0 | 4 | 4 | 1 |
| T to C | 0 | 2 | 2 | 1 |

Table 2.  Summary of base changes found in lung cancer compared to those in other cancers (Mitsudomi, D'Amico, Carbone, unpublished data).

The number of genetic lesions (10-20 per cancer cell) required for tumors to become clinically evident raises the possibility of Mendelian inheritence or acquistion of mutations during embryonic development as well as from carcinogen exposure in adult life.  The recent finding of inherited p53 mutations as the basis of the Li-Fraumeni familial cancer syndrome is an example of this.  Lung cancer is not a part of the syndrome definition but no study has yet evaluated the relative risk of patients carrying one of these alleles for lung cancer.  A study evaluating carriers of a mutant *rb* gene, however, found these patients to have a 10 fold increased risk for lung cancer, and SCLC in particular (8), the type most strongly associated with abnormal Rb from previous studies.  There is some evidence from family studies that relatives of lung cancer patients have an increased risk of lung cancer that cannot be accounted for by lesions in these genes or other known risk factors (9) suggesting the involvement of as yet undescribed genes.

## Opioids and Nicotine Represent a Novel Type of Growth Regulatory System in Lung Cancer:

We have identified new autocrine/paracrine regulatory systems involving opioid and nicotine receptors which affect the growth of lung cancer cells. Using specific radiolabeled ligands we find that lung cancer cell lines of all histologic types express multiple, high affinity membrane receptors (Kd = $10^{-9}$ to $10^{-10}$ M) for $\mu$, $\delta$, and $\kappa$ opioid agonists and for nicotine and $\alpha$-bungarotoxin. These receptors are biologically active since cyclic AMP (cAMP) levels decreased in lung cancer cells after opioid and nicotine application. Nicotine at concentrations (~100 nM) found in smokers had no effect on *in vitro* lung cancer cell growth while $\mu$, $\delta$, and $\kappa$ opioid agonists at low concentrations (1-100 nM) inhibited lung cancer growth *in vitro* . We also found that lung cancer cells expressed various combinations of immunoreactive opioid peptides ($\beta$-endorphin, enkephalin, or dynorphin), suggesting the participation of opioids in a negative autocrine loop or tumor suppressing system. Since patients with lung cancer are exposed to nicotine, we tested whether nicotine affected the response of lung cancer cell growth to opioids and found that nicotine at concentrations of 100-200 nM partially or totally reversed opioid induced growth inhibition in 9/14 lung cancer cell lines. The finding that lung cancer cells express opioid receptors and produce endogenous opioid peptides, yet have their growth inhibited by exogenously added opioids represents a paradox. We would like to explain this paradox by proposing that expression of opioid peptides and their cognate receptors represent a new system of "tumor suppression" whose function can be inactivated in cancer cells.

## Order of Events

With the many known, and undoubtedly many as yet unknown lesions involved in the pathogenesis of lung cancer, it is important to attempt to establish whether a particular order of events is required, and which are fundamental to tumor growth and which are associated with tumor progression.as is postulated for colon cancer, or rather simply the accumulated number.  For SCLC, even the rare small resectable stage I cancers appear to have universal 3p and p53 abnormalities, suggesting these events are "early" in the carcinogenesis pathway.  For NSCLC, there is no apparent correlation of frequency of p53 mutations with tumor size or whether the lesion is primary or metastatic, again suggesting that these abnormalities are involved in tumor initiation rather than progression.
Part of the difficulty with establishing an order for the known molecular lesions in lung cancer is the absence of a well defined clonal premalignant lesion similar to the villous adenoma and colon cancer.  No somatic lesions have yet been reported in metaplastic bronchial epithelium, or bronchial epithelium with mucous gland hyperplasia, though they are changes that are frequently associated with smoking.  It will be interesting to see if such lesions are found with the ever-increasingly sensitive molecular techniques.

Together, our findings suggest that there are many molecular lesions associated with the pathogenesis of lung cancer and that detection of molecular genetic abnormalities in these genes should be applied in studies of prevention, early diagnosis, prognosis, and familial inheritence of lung cancer.

# References

1.	Whang-Peng, J., T. Knutsen, et al. (1991). <u>submitted</u> :

2.	Johnson, B. E., D. C. Ihde, et al. (1987). <u>J Clin Invest</u> **79**: 1629-1634.

3.	Mitsudomi, T., J. Viallet, et al. (1991). <u>Oncogene</u> **submitted**.

4.	Harbour, J. W., S.-L. Lai, et al. (1988). <u>Science</u> **241**: 353-357.

5.	Kratzke, R., J. Gerster, et al. (1990). 81st annual meeting of the AACR, Washington, D.C.,

6.	Chiba, I., T. Takahashi, et al. (1990). <u>Oncogene</u> **5**: 1603-1610.

7.	D'Amico, D. and J. Minna (1991). <u>submitted</u> :

8.	Sanders, B., M. Jay, et al. (1989). <u>Br J Cancer</u> **60**: 358-365.

9.	Sellers, T. A., W. J. Bailey, et al. (1990). <u>J Natl Cancer Inst</u> **82**(15): 1272-9.

From: *Neoplastic Transformation in Human Cell Culture,*
Eds.: J. S. Rhim and A. Dritschilo ©1991 The Humana Press Inc., Totowa, NJ

Molecular Control of Expression of Plasticity of

Tumorigenic/Metastatic Phenotypes

George E. Milo and Hakjoo Lee

The Ohio State University, Columbus, OH 43210

ABSTRACT

Several anchorage independent cell lines that are
nontumorigenic (AIGNT) have been isolated from spontaneous
squamous cell carcinoma (SCC) tumors. The tumorigenic SCC
phenotype (AIGT) has also been isolated. The AIGNT phenotype treated with either methylmethane sulfonate (MMS) or
N-methyl-N'-nitro-N-nitrosoguanidine (MNNG) converts the
AIGNT phenotype to a progressively growing tumor and
subsequently to a metastatic phenotype. Treatment of the
AIGT phenotype with the same chemicals does not convert
that phenotype to a metastatic phenotype. The AIGNT
phenotype yields evidence for a mutation in codon 12 of
the Ha-*ras* gene. This activated gene also is routinely
overexpressed in the MMS or MNNG converted AIGNT $T_1$ tumors
but not in the converted AIGNT cells *in vitro*.
Administration of 1-5.0 mM benzamide (BZ) *in vitro* to the
MMS-converted AIGNT phenotype delays the onset of
tumorigenesis from 4 to 14 weeks. At 10 mM no tumors were
formed in the host receiving the BZ treated MMS-SCC.
Administration of BZ to a 2.0 cm $T_1$ tumor bearing nude
mouse has no effect on regression of the tumor that
eventually kills the animal. It is our opinion that events
leading to the expression of a tumorigenic phenotype and

---

$T_0 \longrightarrow T_4$ designation has to do with our notation for
passage of tumors in nude mice (14). This notation should
not be confused with $T_{24}$ bladder carcinomas.

subsequently to a metastatic phenotype are phenotype
specific and can be reversed. The AIGT tumorigenic
phenotype appears to be a terminal stage in this system.


## INTRODUCTION

For many years we (1-3) and others (4-7) have pursued
the goal to transform human epithelial cells to an
aggressive malignant phenotype. Rarely, have we (8,9)
observed such a change. We have routinely been able to
transform the cells to an anchorage independent growth
(AIG) phenotype. This AIG phenotype when isolated from
soft agar, reseeded onto a substratum, expanded the cell
population we observed the expression of a cell surface
membrane SCC tumor associated epitope. While the
population doublings of these AIG positive phenotypes were
extended, they did not exhibit an infinite life span (8).
We have identified these populations as $AIG^{term}$ (2).
Subsequently, we transfected the DNA from the $AIG^{term}$
positive populations into NIH 3T3 cells (9) and the foci
isolated and expanded *in vitro* when injected into a nude
mouse produce a progressively growing tumor (9). We,
therefore, are able to produce chemical carcinogen
transformed cells that exhibit definite early stages of
progression consistently, but not late stages.

Different phenotypes also were observed in the
spontaneous tumors, they are: 1) local limited growth at
the site of injection into a nude mouse which may or may
not be followed by regression (1), 2) progressive tumor
growth (2), and 3) metastasis (2). Recently (2), these
patterns of growth were clearly identifiable and may
reflect the expression of specific critically activated
genes. It appears that a premalignant AIGNT (8) phenotype
found in $T_0$ tumors (14) and chemical carcinogen induced
transformed cells contain malignant DNA when evaluated by
transfection into the NIH 3T3 recipient cell. Moreover,
the continued expression of the tumor phenotype of
chemically treated AIGNT cells was not related to the
persistent overexpression of either c-*myc* or Ha-*ras* genes
(8).

It has been interesting to note that the use of the DNA
polymerase chain reaction (PCR) analysis of DNA prepared
from surgical tumor slices of SCC tumors that a mutation

in the 12th codon of the Ha-*ras* has been detected (10).
Recently we found a mutation in the 12th codon region in
the MMS-converted AIGNT tumorigenic phenotype, and the CA
clones from the $T_1$ tumors by PCR analysis.  It has been
recognized that activated *ras* has been found in 10-15% of
the malignant tumors analyzed (11). Other percentages are;
40% of the colon carcinomas contain mutations in the K-*ras*
gene;  90% of all pancreatic tumors contain activated
K-*ras*, (12,13). To date we have no evidence by PCR for the
presence of other activated genes (3,8).  Others (14) have
reported that in approximately 40% of the tumors and >95%
of the progressively growing tumors in mice the presence
of other activated *ras* genes.

We have selected to investigate the role of carcinogen
conversion of the AIGNT phenotype to a tumorigenic stage
in these cells.

## MATERIALS AND METHODS

<u>Tumorigenicity evaluation.</u>  Prior to evaluating the
tumorigenic potential of cells, four to six week old
gnotobiotic male NCr/sed (nu/nu) nude mice were
splenectomized and treated with 0.1 ml of mouse
antilymphocyte serum (ALS) (1:1 dilution of HBSS:ALS)
twice weekly.  The animals were allowed to recover and
used as xenogenic hosts for the transformed cells 4 weeks
after splenectomy (15,16).

<u>Growth in soft agar.</u>  Anchorage independent growth of
spontaneous SCC tumor cells was determined by the capacity
of the cells for growth in soft agar.  Cells isolated from
squamous cell carcinomas, by mincing the tumor tissue and
filtering the minced tissue through a sieve, were seeded
in soft agar as described by Milo *et al.* (8).  Cell
colonies which developed to greater than 60 $\mu$m in diameter
were removed from the soft agar after 14 days and seeded
*in vitro* to establish monolayer cultures (15,16).

<u>Cell culture.</u>  Tumor cells prepared in culture from
colonies that previously had expressed AIG were grown in
Eagle's minimum essential medium (MEM) supplemented with
essential amino acids, 1.0 mM sodium pyruvate, 2.0 mM
glutamine, 0.1 mM nonessential amino acids and 50 $\mu$g/ml of
gentamycin. This complete growth medium was supplemented
with 10% FBS and designated as growth medium (GM), (18).

    <u>MMS or MNNG treatment.</u> To convert AIGNT phenotype to a progressively growing tumor phenotype cells *in vitro* were treated either MMS or MNNG. Twenty-four hours after seeding the cells, 50 $\mu$g/ml MMS was added to the GM and the cultures were incubated for 24 hr at 37°C in a 4% $CO_2$ enriched air atmosphere. MMS was freshly prepared in spectrar grade acetone. The final concentration of acetone in the GM of both MMS-treated and control cultures was $\leq$0.02%. The treatment regimen and time of treatment with MMS followed a schedule described by Kerbel *et al.* (18). The other cultures were fed with GM containing 0.01 $\mu$g/ml MNNG in a final concentration of 0.5% dimethyl sulfoxide (DMSO). Control cultures were treated with 0.5% DMSO. The concentration of MNNG and time of treatment followed a schedule described by Rhim *et al.* (7). Thereafter, the cultures were rinsed with three volumes of GM minus FBS to remove the residual treatment medium and then the treated cells were allowed to grow in GM to 90% confluency (3-4 weeks). Cultures were then split 1 to 4 for 3 passages (1:4 split ratio = 2 population doublings) after which 5 x $10^6$ cells were injected subcutaneously into the flank of each nude mouse (8).

    <u>Re-establishment of cells *in vitro* from progressively growing tumors: cell culture.</u> To establish *in vitro* cell cultures of SCC-83-01-82 or other cell lines from progressively growing tumors produced in different nude mice, tumor $\geq$ 2.0 cm in size will be minced into ~1x1 mm sections digested with 0.5% collagenase in growth medium supplemented with an additional 5% (vol/vol) FBS at 37°C in a 4% $CO_2$-enriched air atmosphere for 4 hr (8,19,20).

    <u>Benzamide (BZ) treatment.</u> Fourty eight to 72 hr following completion of treatment with either MMS or MNNG the cells were allowed to grow under GM to 75% confluent density in a 4% $CO_2$ enriched air atmosphere at 37°C. At that time BZ was added to the GM. The treatment was repeated every 5 days for 2 weeks. At that time, the 5 x $10^6$ treated and untreated cells were injected subcutaneously into the mice as described above.

    <u>PCR expansion of DNA from transformed cells and direct DNA sequencing.</u> Genomic DNA from anchorage independent cells bearing the sarcoma associated cell surface antigen were amplified at *ras*-specific regions with the Onco-Lyzer core kit (Clontech Laboratories, Inc., Palo Alto, CA).

Each PCR mixture contained genomic DNA (0.5 $\mu$g), specific primers (0.6 $\mu$M each), all for dNTPs (0.2 mM each), 1X reaction buffer (with 1.5 mM $MgCl_2$) and Ampli Taq polymerase (1.25 U, Perkin-Elmer Cetus, Norwalk, CT). The genomic DNA was amplified in 30 cycles whereby each cycle included a 1 min denaturation step at 94°C, a 1 min primer annealing step at 65°C, and 1 min primer extension step at 74°C. The amplified products were then purified by centrifugation through a Ventricon 100 microconcentrator (Amicon) and an aliquot was used in an asymmetric PCR assay to generate single-stranded DNA that was directly sequenced. The asymmetric PCR process was carried out exactly as above, except that one primer was limiting (0.6 $\mu$M vs 0.06 $\mu$M), (21).

The amplified products were purified by centrifugation through a Centricon 100 microconcentrator (Amicon) and then sequenced with the Sanger dideoxy method. First, an equimolar amount of the limiting primer in the asymmetric PCR process was annealed to the amplified DNA in a 10 $\mu$l reaction volume by heating to 70°C for 3 min, then to 42°C for 10 min in the presence of a 5X annealing buffer (35 mM $MgCl_2$ and 250 mM Tris, pH 8.8). To begin the synthesis of DNA chains, 0.5 $\mu$l of ($\alpha$-[$^{35}$S]thio)dATP (>1000 Ci/mmol), 2 $\mu$l of labeling mix (1.5 $\mu$M each of dCTP, dGTP and dTTP), 2 $\mu$l of Sequenase (2 U) and 3 ml of $dH_2O$ was added to the annealed DNAs and incubated at 42°C for 5 min, then cooled to room temperature. The 4 $\mu$l aliquots of this mixture were added to 4 $\mu$l of the A, C, G or T termination mixes (20 $\mu$M of all four dNTPs and 60-800 $\mu$M of the particular ddNTP) and incubated at 70°C for 5 min. The sequencing products were then run out on an 8% urea-polyacrylamide gel which was exposed to Kodak X-omat AR film overnight at room temperature (22).


## RESULTS

We have isolated lines from different body sites that represent the AIGNT phenotype. When these AIGNT cells, SCC-83-01-82, (Table 1) and other AIGNT lines or clones of each line from the same body site or other sites (4) were treated with MMS or MNNG, the tumor frequency was found to be 7 nude mice formed progressively growing tumors out of 22 nude mice receiving the MMS/MNNG treated cells. One to 5 months later we obtained evidence that $T_1$ tumors (14)

### Table 1:  SCC Cell Lines That Exhibit Anchorage Independent Growth and Are Tumorigenic

| Cell Line | Anchorage Independence |
|---|---|
| SCC-83-01-82 | + |
| SCC-83-01-82 CA | + |
| SCC-83-01-82 CA $C_1$ | + |
| SCC-83-01-82 CA $C_2$ | + |
| SCC-83-01-82 CA $C_3$ | + |
| SCC-89-08-28 | + |
| SCC-83-01-175 | + |
| SCC-89-05-109 | + |

See Figure 1 for explanation of SCC and CA.

produced metastatic multiple foci of MMS/MMNG converted AIGNT cells. None of the untreated AIGNT phenotypes produced progressively growing $T_1$ tumors (2), i.e. 0 tumors out of 8 nude mice receiving the AIGNT cells. Other phenotypes, i.e. AIGT penotype, the frequency of tumor formation was 6 progressively growing tumors out of 6 nude mice receiving the AIGT cells (2). Treatment with either MMS or MNNG did not alter the time of 4 wk required for the progressively growing tumor to reach $\geq$ 2.0 cm in size. When these mice were evaluated 2 months later for the presence of metastatic foci of tumor cells, none were detected. Reversal of expression of a tumorigenic phenotype was achieved upon treatment of the MMS converted AIGNT phenotype with BZ.

Treatment of the MMS converted AIGNT phenotype *in vitro* with BZ from 1.0 mM to 5 mM delayed the time of appearance of the progressively growing tumors from 1 wk to 10 wk and the time necessary to grow $\geq$ 2.0 cm progressively growing tumors was delayed from 4 wk to 14 wk. However, if the progressively growing tumors were permitted to grow to $\geq$ 2.0 cm in size in the mice before administration of twice weekly injections of 5 mM BZ, no reduction in tumor size or delay in the onset of death of the mice was observed. At the time of death of these specific tumor bearing nude mice, metastatic foci of malignant cells were observed.

To date we have found mutations in the 12th codon of Ha-*ras* in SCC, CA, CA clones and SCC $T_0$ tumors. This point mutation results in a change in the glycine-coding triplet

GGC to GTC. GTC codes for valine. The mutation is the same as the $T_{24}$ bladder carcinoma cell line.

A typical autoradiogram of Ha-*ras* with mutations in the 12th codon region (Fig. 1) indicated that there was a mutation in that region of that gene. A summary of the results of the PCR experiments using different amplimers for Ha-*ras*/12,13, Ha-*ras*/61, K-*ras*/12,13, K-*ras*/61 and N-*ras*/12,13 codons were negative for both 5′ and 3′ sequences.

Other data, using RNA (Northern) blot hybridization and *in situ* hybridization, we detected overexpression of the gene in $T_0$ and $T_1$ tumors. Moreover, there was a spatial localization of expression of these mRNA population in both $T_0$ and $T_1$ tumors (3,8). Interestingly, the overexpression of the Ha-*ras* mRNA population was not uniformly distributed over the tumor population (9) and attentuated to a non-detectable level as the $T_1$ to $T_4$ in the nude mice. It is interesting also to note that a mutation in the 12th codon of the Ha-*ras* gene converting the proto-oncogene to the activated oncogene in and by itself results in the expression of an unstable tumorigenic and metastatic phenotype. The $T_1$ tumor derived cell line, designated as the CA cell line, was evaluated for the presence of human chromosomes and ploidy. These cells were found to be of human origin and a human diploid to pseudodiploidy composition (2).


## DISCUSSION

Several years ago we (1,5,7) recognized that an environmental insult of a human epithelial cell in early S phase with a direct acting xenobiotic could induce the expression of a transformed AIG phenotype. Furthermore, we (1), found that on the surface of these carcinogen transformed cells we discovered the presence of an antigen that was associated with the plasma membrane of the SCC $T_0$ tumor phenotype. When we examined frozen cross-sections of spontaneous human SCC tumors for the presence of antigens associated with normal cellular phenotypes and tumor associated phenotypes, it was interesting to note that $T_0$ tumors contained subpopulations in the tumor matrix that expressed either tumor antigen or normal/tumor antigen on different subpopulations in the tumor matrix (1). $T_1$-$T_4$ tumors exhibited predominately the cell surface tumor

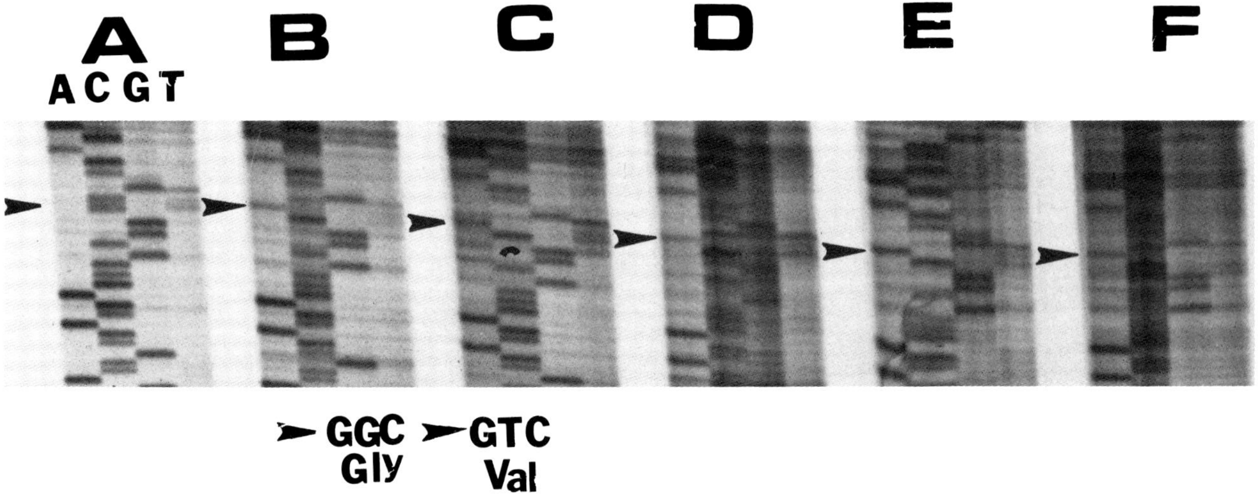

Autoradiogram of a polyacrylamide-urea gel comparing sequences of the Ha-ras[14] 12th codon region. DNA templates for the sequencing were prepared by conventional PCR amplification of genomic DNA. Asymmetric PCR was carried out using the amplified DNA using specific primers for the codon region (Clontech). Sequencing reactions were labeled by incorporation of {[$^{35}$S]thio}dATP and one of the primers used for the sequencing reactions. The products were resolved on a sequencing gel. The reaction sets were loaded from left lane to right lane in sets of 4 from A-F in the sequence A,C,G,T nucleotides.
A: normal human fibroblast cells;  B: CA clone 1;  C: CA clone 2;  D: CA clone 3; E: CA cells; and F: SCC AIGNT cells.

antigens. It was interesting to note that of the $T_0$ tumors received from the surgical suite(s), 40% of the $T_0$ tumors formed progressively growing $T_1$ tumors in the nude mouse. Many investigators have recognized in 50% of the $T_0$ tumors, mutations in the 12th/13th codons of the Ha-*ras* oncogene. This reversible expression, we observed, of the malignant $T_1$ phenotypic CA cell line suggests to us that the intervention in expression of these phenotypes that suppressor gene-oncogene interaction is controlled by a yet another unexplained regulatory mechanism. Just the activation of the oncogene and deletion or specific mutations in a suppressor gene is insufficient to explain this reversibility.

Conversion of the AIGNT to an AIGT phenotype and subsequently to a metastatic phenotype and comparing these phenotypes with the presence of a fixed AIGT phenotype that could not be converted to a metastatic phenotype was of interest. Reversal of the conversion of the AIGNT to a metastatic phenotype with BZ treatment suggests to us that these stages of progression are also under molecular control and reversible.

Although most human tumors are assumed to be clonal in origin, each tumor contains subpopulations of cells which differ in their pattern of cellular differentiation (23). We conclude that it appears that several different pathways exist to achieve either an AIGNT or AIGT phenotype. Each of these different phenotypes may exhibit a different potential for subsequent conversion to a tumorigenic-metastatic phenotype after chemical treatment.

These results suggest that the AIGNT phenotype may be the result of several types of heritable alterations, some of which predispose the treated cells to the tumorigenic-metastatic phenotype and some of which do not. These results also suggest that epigenetic, rather than genetic factors may play a role in the conversion of tumorigenic cells to metastatic cells. Clearly, additional studies are required to delineate those molecular events involved in the conversion of premalignant -> tumorigenic -> metastatic cells and that the events leading to expression of a tumorigenic phenotype and subsequently to a metastatic phenotype are phenotype specific and not pathway specific.

ACKNOWLEDGMENTS

The work was supported in part by NIH-NCI RO1CA25907-09 (G.E.M.) and NIH-NCI P30CA16058-15 (OSUCCC).

REFERENCES

1. G.E. Milo, J. Yohn, *et al.* <u>J. Invest. Dermatol.</u> 92, 848 (1989).
2. G.E. Milo, C.F. Shuler, *et al.* In preparation (1991).
3. G.E. Milo, C.F. Shuler, *et al* . <u>Proc. Natl. Acad. Sci. USA</u> 87, 1268 (1990).
4. M. Namba, K. Nishitami, *et al.* <u>Japanese J. Exptl. Med.</u> 48, 303 (1978).
5. S.Chang. <u>Biochimica et Biophysica Acta</u> 283, 161 (1986).
6. C.A. Reznikoff *et al.*, D. Kaufman, *et al.*, J. Rhim, *et al.* Different chapters In: G.E. Milo, B. Casto, and C. Shuler (eds), Transformation of Human Epithelial Cells: Molecular and Oncogenetic Mechanisms, CRC Press, Boca Raton, 1991, in preparation.
7. J. Rhim, J. Fuita, *et al.* <u>Science</u> 232, 385 (1986).
8. C. Shuler, P. Kurian, *et al.* <u>Teratogenesis Carcinog. Mutagen.</u> 10, 53 (1990).
9. H.L. Kumari, C. Shuler, *et al.* <u>Carcinogenesis</u> 10, 401, (1990).
10. M. Corominas, *et al.* <u>Proc. Natl. Acad. Sci. USA</u> 86, 6372 (1989).
11. J.L. Bos. <u>Mutation Res.</u> 95, 255 (1988).
12. C. Almogiera, *et al.* <u>Cell</u> 53, 549 (1988).
13. V.T. Smith, *et al.* <u>Nucleic Acids Res.</u> 16, 7773 (1988).
14. J-C. Chen, C.F. Shuler, *et al.* <u>J. Oral Surg.</u> 71, 457 (1991).
15. J. Donahoe, I. Noyes, *et al.* <u>In Vitro</u> 18, 429 (1982).
16. G.E. Milo, B. Casto, *et al.* <u>Mutation Res.</u> 199, 387 (1987).
17. J. Huttner, G.E. Milo, *et al.* <u>In vitro</u> 14, 854 (1978).
18. R.S. Kerbel, P. Frost *et al.* <u>J. of Cellular Physiology Supplement</u> 3, 87 (1984).
19. P. Rose, A. Koolemans-Beynen, *et al.* <u>Amer. J. Obstet. Gynecol.</u> 156, 730 (1987).
20. G.E. Milo, J. Oldham, *et al.* <u>In Vitro</u> 17, 719 (1981).
21. Step by Step Protocol for DNA Sequencing with Sequenase, 5th Edition, U.S. Biochemical Corp. (1989).
22. R. Frye, P. Cogswell, *et al.* <u>Newsletter Clon Tech Labs</u> 1, 1 (1990).
23. G.H. Heppner. <u>Cancer Res.</u> 44, 2259 (1984).

# IV. Multistep Models

# ALTERED REGULATION OF GROWTH AND DIFFERENTIATION AT DIFFERENT STAGES OF TRANSFORMATION OF HUMAN SKIN KERATINOCYTES

N. E. Fusenig, P. Boukamp, D. Breitkreutz, A. Hülsen. Division of Differentiation and Carcinogenesis In Vitro, Institute of Biochemistry, German Cancer Research Center (DKFZ), D-6900 Heidelberg, Germany

Neoplasia is a collective term for a number of exceptionally complex disturbances in the regulation of cellular proliferation and differentiation in multicellular organisms. Cancer development is generally understood as a progressive multistage process in which cells pass through different stages of phenotypic and genotypic alterations and gradually acquire abnormal growth characteristics usually associated with malignancy. The step by step evolution of premalignant lesions and their further progression to malignant tumors reflect different degrees of dysregulation of endogenous growth control mechanisms on one side and on the other increasing autonomy of transformed cells of local and systemic factors regulating growth and differentiation. Malignancy, the final stage of this process (the same applies to most premalignant stages), describes different and heterogeneous endpoints identified solely by histopathology and clinical experience. Due to this complexity, our understanding of the biological characteristics of tumors is still insufficient to adequately characterize malignancy at the cellular and molecular level.

The understanding of the cellular and molecular events involved in the process of transformation of normal cells to carcinoma cells has been greatly improved by the use of *in vitro* systems. However, the known phenotypic changes associated with different stages of neoplastic transformation are tissue phenomena and only discernible in organized multicellular systems. Thus, it has been impossible up to now to identify molecular changes at the single cell level, which are directly (and causally)

correlated to the onset of malignant cell transformation
or to any of the intermediate stages.

In transformation studies *in vitro* (using mainly
rodent cell cultures), various endpoints of the
transformation process have been used as parameters for
malignancy, but were often not correlated to alterations
in cells isolated from carcinomas induced in animal
experiments (1). Since no generally accepted and reliable
*in vitro* criteria for malignant epithelial cells exist at
present, the endpoints of cell transformation have to be
defined in every experimental system for the cell type
used and their significance for the carcinogenesis process
*in vivo* proven by comparison with appropriate *in vivo*
criteria.

Histopathologic observation suggested that, as a
common phenotypic feature, tumor cells are characterized
by defects in their differentiation program, although the
significance of these alterations for the carcinogenesis
process is still unclear (2). It has been hypothesized
that preneoplastic cells by the acquisition of a selective
resistance to inducers of differentiation (due to defect
or altered controlling pathways) may have a clonal growth
advantage over normal cells (3, 4, 5, 6). Although these
and other data strongly support the hypothesis that
uncoupling of differentiation and proliferation pathways
is involved in the generation of neoplasms, it is also
clear that aberrations in the pathways of differentiation
*per se* are insufficient to cause tumorigenesis. Moreover,
it is not possible to decide at present, whether tumor
cells bear genetic defects in their differentiation
program or exhibit only incomplete expression due to
altered external signals and/or modified signal transduction pathways. Proliferation and differentiation of
normal cells are usually controlled by different signal
transduction pathways. The well-regulated interactions of
these controlling mechanisms ensure the homeostatic
balance between cell proliferation and terminal differentiation. Uncoupling of this normal balance by either
genetic or epigenetic changes is thought to be a critical
step in the generation and further progression of the
malignant cell phenotype.

With human cells the problems encountered in
transformation studies at the cellular level are even more
pronounced. In contrast to rodent cells, human cells have
been found to be rather resistant to transformation *in
vitro* using chemical, physical or viral agents including
cellular oncogenes (7, 8, 9). The basis for this

discrepancy in transformation sensitivity is not known,
but several explanations have been postulated such as
differences in natural life span, degree of inbreeding
and, to the most part, to different genetic stability (10,
11). Up to now, immediate malignant transformation of
normal human epithelial cells to fully developed carcinoma
cells has not been reproducibly achieved so far in cell
culture systems with any oncogenic agents. In most cases,
human cells in culture could only be partially transformed
to a stage called "immortality" (indicating escape of *in
vitro* senescence) when oncogenic viruses or their DNA
(predominantly Simian Virus 40 (SV 40) and human papilloma
virus (HPV type 16 and 18) were used (Table 1) (11, 12).
All these immortalized cell lines were non-tumorigenic
following subcutaneous injection into nude mice but
exhibited aneuploid karyotypes with progressive
chromosomal rearrangements and showed altered growth
properties in culture. Although spontaneous progression
of SV 40-immortalized human cell lines to tumorigenicity
has been observed after long-term propagation of cells *in
vitro* (13), these cell lines are usually considered rather
stable intermediate stages. The immortalized cell lines
showed higher sensitivity to transforming agents and
represent at present the generally used and only efficient
human cell systems for studying tumor progression by
oncogenic agents such as viral DNA, chemical, and
radiation (see this volume). As postulated for rodent
fibroblasts and keratinocytes (1, 14), immortalization
seems to be an obligatory premalignant state at least for
conversion of human cells to malignancy *in vitro*.

**Table 1:   Immortalization of human skin keratino-
           cytes**

| Tissue | Immortalizing agents | Reference |
|---|---|---|
| Foreskin | SV40 virus | Steinberg & Defendi, 1979 |
| Foreskin | SV40 virus | Taylor-Papa-dimitrion *et al.*1982 |
| Foreskin | SV40 DNA | Banks-Schlegel & Howley, 1983 |

**Table 1:   Immortalization of human skin keratino-
            cytes (continued)**

| | | |
|---|---|---|
| Foreskin | Ad12-SV40 virus | Rhim *et al.*, 1985 |
| Foreskin | HPV16 DNA | Pirisi *et al.*, 1987 |
| Foreskin | HPV16 DNA | Dürst *et al.*, 1987 |
| Foreskin | HPV18 DNA | Kaur & McDougal, 1988 |
| Trunk skin | SV40 DNA | Fusenig *et al.*, 1987 |
| Foetal skin | V40 DNA | Brown & Parkinson, 1985 |
| Foreskin | spontaneous | Baden *et al.*, 1987 |
| Trunk skin | spontaneous | Boukamp *et al.*,1988 |

In the past immortalization of human epidermal
keratinocytes has been generally considered to have a
massive impact on their differentiation properties.  This
is certainly true for many virally transformed cells,
which are often only capable of expressing an irregular
differentiation program at best (2, 12).  Based on these
observations, the hypothesis seemed to be verified that
immortalization unequivocally leads to a dramatic loss of
differentiation potential (3, 15, 16, 17).  After we had
shown that this was not necessarily the case with murine
cell lines (1, 18), we also succeeded in developing a
human keratinocyte cell line (HaCaT) which had
spontaneously developed immortality *in vitro* and
maintained a virtually normal differentiation potential
(19).  This cell line could be stably transfected with the
human cellular Harvey *ras*-oncogen (c-Ha-*ras*) and several
derived cell clones established which exhibited different
stages of neoplastic progression coincident with
alterations in cellular growth control, while their

differentiation potential was not drastically reduced (20, 21, 22).

## Stages of transformation of human keratinocytes

Comparable to rodent cells, different stages of transformation of human cells can be induced and distinguished by alterations in their growth capacity *in vitro* and *in vivo*, although the significance of these changes for the carcinogenesis process *in vivo* and their relevance for different neoplastic stages are still unclear (Fig. 1). Immortalization, *i.e.*, loss of senescence or self reproductive capacity *in vitro* is usually considered an early or the first stage of transformation of human cells for the following reasons: (i) This change in cell behaviour was the first and in most cases also the final stage of transformation of human cells observed after infection with oncogenic viruses or transfection of viral oncogenes (Table 1 and ref. 23). (ii) In contrast to normal human cells, the immortalized lines were sensitive to most carcinogenic agents (chemical, physical or viral) for induction of tumorigenic stages and further progression to malignancy. (iii) Immortalized human cell lines exhibit improved, often clonogenic growth behavior *in vitro* and are characterized by chromosomal alterations with pronounced genetic instability, features usually associated with transformed cells.

**Stages of Keratinocyte Transformation**

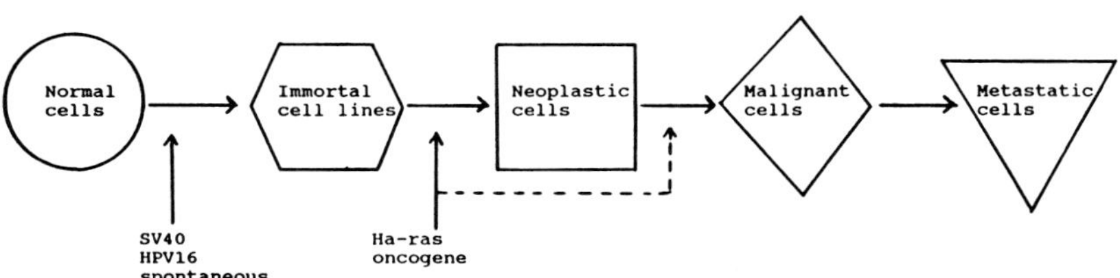


Figure 1: Schematic description of different stages of transformation of human skin keratinocytes.

Thus, immortalized cell lines must be considered transformed cells, although they have not reached the final stage of malignant transformation. Whether the state of immortalization, which is only operationally defined *in vitro* and cannot be correlated to known premalignant lesions *in vivo* so far, is an obligatory biological, intermediate stage between normal and tumor cells or even prerequisite for tumorigenicity, is still a matter of debate. The observation that cells from benign tumors or premalignant lesions (*i.e.*, of the colon) usually did not give rise to permanent cell lines *in vitro* (without further manipulation) has been interpreted in that immortalization is not an early event in tumorigenesis (24). However, the fact that most premalignant lesions do not give rise to immortal cell lines should be considered to be rather due to insufficient culture conditions then used as an argument against the importance of immortalization as an early step in the carcinogenesis process. Not so long ago, potential immortality *in vitro* as a general characteristic of malignant cells was questioned with similar arguments. However, these have lost much of its logic in the meantime when improved culture methods led to the successful growth and long-term propagation of most malignant tumor cells. On the other hand, as long as there is no further characterization of the stage of immortalization with defined cellular and molecular criteria replacing or complementing the operational term of "indefinite growth *in vitro*", the significance of this stage for tumorigenicity remains a matter of debate. Irrespective of whether immortalization can be associated with a critical stage in tumor development *in vivo* or remains an operational definition for abnormal cell phenotypes *in vitro*, those cells having "escaped *in vitro* senescence" are at present the most sensitive (and so far only suitable) target cells for inducing malignant progression *in vitro*.

By treatment of immortal cell lines with chemical carcinogens or by introducing viral or cellular oncogenes, tumorigenic phenotypes could be induced. The tumors formed by these altered cells after subcutaneous injection in nude mice were usually not discriminated whether they belonged to different tumor phenotypes. However, by careful observation, a distinction between progressively enlarging and infiltrating tumors (carcinomas) and slowly growing or stationary (encapsulated cystic/benign) tumors could be made (20, 25). Whether these different tumor phenotypes represent different stages in transformation,

are due to varying mixtures of heterogenous tumor cell
populations or result from different microenvironmental
conditions in the nude mouse, cannot be explained at
present. Further *in vitro* propagation of tumorigenic
cells and/or additional manipulations with carcinogenic or
promoting agents may eventually lead to metastatic
variants forming metastasis either after subcutaneous
(spontaneous) or intravenous (experimental) injection.

## The immortal keratinocyte cell line HaCaT

In contrast to rodent cells, the establishment of
immortal cell lines that arose spontaneously from mortal
normal human cell cultures, without viral or chemical
intervention, has only been seldom reported (19, 26, 27).
Comparable to the rapidly increasing number of human
carcinoma cell lines established by improved cell culture
methodology, a similar increase of spontaneously
immortalized human cell lines may be expected in the
future. The cell lines established so far exhibit
chromosomal alterations with a tendency to adopt further
changes with continued passaging (19, 23, 28) indicating
that cytogenetic changes are prerequisite or causal for
immortalization either due to activation of "immortalizing
genes" or to loss or inactivation of "senescence genes"
(29). It may be hypothesized that such genetic changes
leading to immortality occur at very low frequency and
their probability depends on the number of cell
replications under favorable growth conditions and will
hence increase with extended culture life time and
proliferative activity of cells. Thus, improved culture
conditions favouring rapid and long-term growth of normal
human cells will favour both cytogenetically visible
genetic changes and the development of potentially
immortal cell lines, comparable, although at a much lower
probability level, to earlier observations with mouse
cells (1). At present, the role of (unspecific) genetic
damages due to *in vitro* growth and propagation conditions
(*e.g.*, trypsin), the significance of preexisting
subpopulations with genetic predispositions in the initial
cell pool, or both cannot be ruled out as major factors in
the process of spontaneous immortalization. The lack of
immunologic or other types of surveillance in vitro (which
may detect and eliminate aberrant cell clones *in vivo*) and
a certain adaptation of these aberrant clones to growth in
culture will then eventually lead to the emergence of such
immortalized cell clones.

The spontaneous emergence of the human skin keratinocyte cell line HaCaT in a culture of normal adult skin keratinocytes occurred gradually through different stages of adaptation to culture conditions accompanied and probably caused by genetic changes visible as chromosomal alterations (19) (Table 2). The concomitant acquisition of different growth properties and cytogenetic alterations throughout the first 20 passages indicated that, following the first translocations in a hypodipoid population, a hypotetraploid cell clone emerged with improved growth potential in culture (23). With further passages cells acquired growth capacity in soft agar and showed reduced dependency on serum concentration and growth factors, although the mean population doubling time did not decrease significantly. With continued propagation cells acquired multiple additional cytogenetic alterations which so far could not be associated with altered growth or differentiation behaviour nor led to tumorigenicity even after 300 passages. The persistence of the initial marker chromosomes up to highest passages indicates that the original cell clone was maintained and that these alterations were essential for permanent growth of these cells *in vitro* (Fusenig *et al.*, manuscript in preparation).


**Table 2: Growth and differentiation properties of the immortalized HaCaT cells *in vitro* and *in vivo***

- Continued proliferation (>300 passages)
- Accumulation of cytogenetic alterations (with passages)
- Maintained differentiated keratinocyte phenotype
- Expression of epidermal keratins (*e.g.*, K1/K10)
- Preserved sensitivity to inducers ($Ca^{2+}$, retinoids, density)
- Decreased stratification *in vitro*
- Increased proliferative activity
- Increased cloning efficiency (on plastic and in agar)
- Decreased serum dependency
- Preserved capacity for tissue regeneration *in vivo*
- Retained non-tumorigenicity (s.c. injection)
- Absence of invasion (surface transplants)


The HaCaT cells exhibit epithelial morphology with typical differentiation features such as stratification, a phenomenon that was maintained at earlier but lost at later passages (see Table 2). Moreover, these cells are capable of expressing an unusually broad spectrum of keratins, not observed so far in epithelial cells. This expression is modulated by environmental conditions including cell density and retinoids (21, 22, 30). The cells constitutively expressed the keratins K5, K6, K14, K16, K17, which are also common in cultures of normal keratinocytes. In addition, keratins K7, K8, K18 and K19, generally associated with simple epithelia, were synthesized (to a most pronounced extent in sparse cultures), while keratins K4, K13 and K15 appeared at confluence presumable with the onset of stratification. Moreover, the epidermal "suprabasal" keratins, K1 and K10 were expressed in conventional, submerged cultures, rising with cell density, but not strictly correlated with the degree of stratification. However, there was a significant delay in the appearance of K10 compared to K1, as visible in cross sections of cell sheets, an alteration which might be related to altered growth control of these cells. In surface transplants on nude mice, HaCaT cells formed well-differentiated stratified epithelia with the expression of specific differentiation products such as keratins K1 and K10, filaggrin and involucrin as detected by immunofluorescence and 2D-gel electrophoresis (19, 22, 30). In transplants of HaCaT cells, in contrast to those of normal keratinocytes, K1 appeared prematurely already in basal cells, while K10 localized rather normally in suprabasal position. Up to highest passage levels, HaCaT cells essentially maintained this high degree of differentiation and cells did not grow invasively in these surface transplants, as typically seen with carcinoma cell lines (31).

Thus, the immortalized cells although exhibiting improved growth potential in vitro and some minor but probably critical alterations in the regulation of differentiation, their overall expression of differentiation parameters, both histotypic and cytotypic, their overall differentiation features were largely maintained and responded typically to external signals.

## Tumorigenic and malignant progression following *ras* oncogene transfection

At passages 29 and 33, the HaCaT cell line was transfected with a plasmid containing the cellular Harvey *ras* oncogene giving rise to several individual cell clones selected by their resistance to neomycin. these clones expressed a morphology very similar to the untransfected HaCaT cells, did not form visible foci nor exhibited major phenotypic changes at normal culture conditions (Table 3).

The randomly selected clones showed unique patterns of
integration of the *ras* oncogene which remained unchanged
at later passages and did not reveal a loss of the protooncogene allele (20, 23). Comparable to the variations in
the integration pattern, the different clones varied in
their levels of expression of Ha-*ras* mRNA, ranging from
levels commensurate with that of the parental HaCaT cells
to an approximately three fold higher expression. This
was similarly reflected at the level of protein expression
of the mutant *ras* p21 (20). When tested for tumorigenicity (by subcutaneous injection into nude mice), the
clones expressing the mutated *ras* at the RNA and protein
level formed nodules, however with different growth rates
and histological appearance. One group formed nodules
which enlarged slowly and either persisted over several
months or slowly regressed. Histologically, these nodules
were benign cysts with dysplastic epidermis-like
epithelium surrounding areas of extensive keratinization.
The other group gave rise to progressively enlarging solid
tumors which were classified as highly differentiated
squamous cell carcinomas with local invasion into the
muscle fascia (Fig. 2). These two types of tumorigenic
clones could be more readily and unmistakably distinguished in surface transplants on nude mice. Both formed
differentiating well-organized surface epithelia, similar
to the parental HaCaT cells. While the benign (cyst-
forming) clones remained as surface epithelia, comparable
to the parental HaCaT cells, the malignant (carcinoma-
forming) clones elicited angiogenesis within a few days
transplantation and later grew invasively into the mouse
mesenchyme, forming large tumor masses (20). Thus,
clearly two different tumorigenic phenotypes could be
distinguished by their growth behavior under in vivo
conditions. Both types of clones had acquired additional
structural chromosomal alterations in addition to the
maintained stable HaCaT marker chromosomes, but so far no
specific genetic differences between the benign and
malignant clones could be identified. However, the common
chromosomal rearrangements a documented that both clones
originated from the same HaCaT subclone, thus indicating
that no selection of preexisting malignant or benign
clones had occurred (unpublished results).


**Table 3: Characteristics of tumorigenic (benign
and malignant) HaCaT-*ras* clones**

- Common chromosomal alterations
- Maintained differentiated keratinocyte phenotype

- Improved stratification in vitro
- Serum- and growth factor-independent growth
- Loss of anchorage-independent clonal growth
- Decreased sensitivity to TGFβ (malignant clones)
- Tumorigenicity after s.c. injection (cyst/carcinomas)
- Preserved tissue regeneration in surface transplants
- Induced angiogenesis and invasion by malignant clones
- Experimental metastasis (malignant clones)

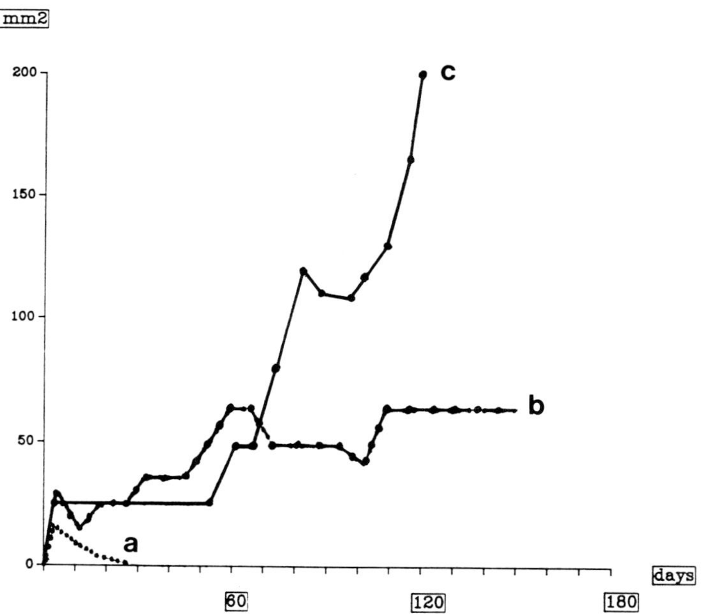


Fig. 2: Typical growth behavior of different stages of transformation of human skin keratinocytes a) the immortalized HaCaT cell line, b) benign tumor-forming clones and c) malignant clones. (Fictive size obtained by multiplication of two diameters).


As far as the differentiation potential is concerned, none of the tumorigenic *ras* clones showed significant reduction in keratinization. Whether benign

or malignant, the HaCaT *ras* clones had maintained their
capacity to synthesize differentiation specific keratins
(K1 and K10) in culture, particularly at high cell
densities.  In contrast to the parental HaCaT cell line,
which had gradually lost the ability to stratify in
culture, most of the HaCaT *ras* clones had retained this
ability and could form multilayered sheets on plastic and
in organotypic cultures on collagen gels (21).  Similarly,
in surface transplants, the HaCaT *ras* clones expressed
keratin K1 and K10, initially exhibiting a rather normal
localization with some delay for K10.  However, staining
for both keratins persisted in a typical suprabasal
localization even in invasive tissue masses and solid
carcinomas (22).  Thus, not withstanding some minor
variations, differentiation potential was not
significantly reduced in the tumorigenic HaCaT-*ras* clones
nor was their response to differentiation inducers
irrespective of the level of *ras* oncogene expression and
the tumorigenic growth behavior in vivo (Table 3).

Growth capacity under normal culture conditions
(with 10% or 5% fetal calf serum) was not significantly
altered in the *ras*-transfected tumorigenic clones compared
to HaCaT cells as population doubling time and cloning
efficiency on plastic are concerned.  The tumorigenic
HaCaT-*ras* clones, however, showed significantly decreased
dependency on serum concentration, which was particularly
evident at cloning cell densities.  The tumorigenic clones
had a reasonable cloning efficiency on plastic (15%-20%)
in serum- and growth factor-free medium (23).  However,
there was no difference in the growth capacity of the
benign as compared to the malignant clones.  Surprisingly,
all HaCaT-*ras* clones had lost or drastically reduced their
ability to grow in soft agar, while HaCaT cells and clones
transfected with the neomycim gene only grew reasonably
well in an anchorage-independent way.  These observations
indicated that the *ras*-oncogene had caused significant
alterations in growth control of the HaCaT cells.  The
growth capacity at cloning densities in serum- and growth
factor-free medium indicated improved growth autonomy
possibly caused by an autocrine loop of growth regulation,
while the altered growth behavior in soft agar is still
unexplained.  The various *ras*-clones did not differ
considerably in their response to stimulatory growth
factors, compared to the parental HaCaT cells. However,
the malignant clones exhibited a significantly altered
sensitivity towards the growth inhibitory activity of
TGFβ.  Both at normal and clonal cell densities, the
malignant clones were significantly less inhibited by TGFβ
or even slightly stimulated at concentrations below 1

ng/ml, while both the HaCaT cells and the benign HaCaT-*ras*
clones were inhibited (Hülsen *et al.*, manuscript in
preparation). The decreased sensitivity to TGFβ of the
malignant clones was somehow correlated to a decreased
receptor density and TGFβ production, although it is not
clear whether the produced TGFβ was present in an active
or latent form (Prime *et al.*, in preparation).

These results demonstrate that ras-transfection of
the immortalized keratinocyte cell line had induced two
types of tumorigenic clones, i) benign or premalignant
non-invasive tumor-cells and ii) progressively growing,
invasive carcinoma cells. We hopothesize that the
prolonged growth capacity under in vivo conditions (in the
nude mouse), visible by the ability to form tumors, was
induced by the ras-oncogene by altering cellular growth
control and providing the cells with a higher degree of
growth antonomy, either by autocrine growth factor
production or altered signal transduction. Whether the
non-invasive, benign tumor-forming clones represent a
stable intermediate state or are premalignant and progress
towards malignancy with time, has not yet been firmly
established. Within several in vitro passages, however,
the benign clones did not progress to malignancy. The
significantly induced resistance of the malignant clones
concerning growth inhibition by TGFβ may be critical for
their improved growth capacity in vivo, although its
relevance for malignancy, i.e. invasion and angiogenesis
is not yet clear.

## Conclusions

The spontaneously immortalized human keratinocyte
line HaCaT and the derived c-Ha-ras oncogene transfected
tumorigenic clones represent a unique system to study
different stages of transformation of human cells and the
mechanisms underlying tumor progression. By comparing
cell growth and differentiation characteristics in
conventional as well as organotypic cultures with those
expressed in a surface transplantation assay (allowing
full expression of the normal and malignant cell
phenotype) crucial features of distinct transformation
stages could be analyzed (19, 21, 22, 11, 23). Particular
interest of future studies is focussed on the role of
mesenchymal interaction for the expression of the normal
differentiated as well as the malignant, invasive
phenotype in both in vitro and in vivo systems (32).

Among all human keratinocyte cell lines we have examined so far, the HaCaT cells and the HaCaT-ras clones provide an optimum concerning their differentiation potential and their maintained response to external regulators, in particular to still undefined mesenchymal signals. The expression of specific features of differentiation including morphogenesis and keratin synthesis, are still induced in all transformed stages by mesenchyme under in vivo conditions in surface transplants, comparable to normal keratinocytes. Thus, concerning the major differentiation characteristics, the potential to keratinize in a rather ordered fashion was not affected in any stage of transformation and no correlation whatsoever between tumor progression and differentiation can be established in the HaCaT cell system.

As far as growth regulation is concerned, the altered interaction with mesenchymal control mechanisms is most pronounced at advanced states of tumor development. Although tumorigenic clones revealed increased growth autonomy in normal culture conditions (by their independence of serum-derived growth factors), their altered sensitivity to mesenchymal growth control in vivo seems to be more crucial for their oncogenic potential. Both the immortal HaCaT cells and the benign clones can transiently grow at ectopic sites in vivo (subcutaneously) but with clearly longer growth periods for the benign tumor cells (Fig. 2). This indicates a partial escape of early tumor stages (benign cysts) from mesenchymal growth control, which is further reduced or even lost in the malignant, progressively growing clones.

Whether this escape of local growth restraint at the injection site is due to reduced sensitivity of malignant cells for controlling negatively regulating mesenchymal signals (e.g. TGFβ) or to factors produced by the malignant cells that interfere with mesenchyme control mechanisms, or to both, is at present not understood. The reduced sensitivity of malignant cells to the growth inhibitory effect of TGFβ could well play a role in this context, but also not yet defined factors secreted by the malignant HaCaT-ras cells inducing angiogenesis and fibroblast activation in surface transplants may be important for invasion. These as well as other obser- vations strongly indicate that disturbances in the epithelial-mesenchymal interactions (regulating epithelial cell growth and differentiation) are crucial for the induction and maintenance of progressive growth of a neoplasm. The analysis of the regulating factors

controlling normal epithelial growth and of the
alterations in malignancy are not only important for the
understanding of malignancy, but may eventually be of
therapeutic value for controlling the growth of cancer
cells.

## Acknowledgements

We would like to acknowledge the work of our
colleagues Drs. Petrusevska, Pascheberg and Thiekötter, as
well as of the students M. Mappes, S. Altmeyer, J. Gäbler
and P. Tomakidi which was discussed in the context of this
paper. The technical assistance of E. Tomakidi, H.
Steinbauer, G. Haffner and S. Heid is gratefully
acknowledged.

## References

1.  Fusenig, N.E, et al., In: Barrett, J.C. and Tennant,
    R.W. (eds), Carcinogenesis Vol. 9 pp. 293-327 New
    York: Raven Press (1985).
2.  Fusenig, N.E., Breitkreutz, D., et al, In: J.R.W.
    Masters (ed.): Human Cancer in Primary Culture A
    Handbook. Kluwer Academic Publishers The Netherlands
    (1991).
3.  Rheinwald, J.G., and Beckett, M.A. Cell 22:629
    (1988).
4.  Harris, C.C. Cancer Res 47:1 (1987).
5.  Parkinson, E.K. Br J Cancer 52:479 (1985).
6.  Willie, J.J., Pittelkow, M.R., Shipley, G.D. and
    Scott, R.E. J Cell Physiology 121:31 (1984).
7.  DiPaolo, J.A. J Natl Cancer Inst 70:3 (1983).
8.  Barrett, J.C. and Tennant, R.W. (eds.) Carcino-
    genesis Compr Surv 9:1 (1985).
9.  Christian, B.J., Loretz, L.J. Cancer Res 47:6066
    (1987).
10. Sager, R., Tanka, K., et al. Proc Natl Acad Sci USA
    80:7601 (1983).
11. Fusenig, N.E., Boukamp, P., et al. In: K.H. Chadwick,
    C. Seymour, B. Barnhard (eds.) Cell Transformation and
    Radiation-induced Cancer. Adam Hilger, Bristol, New
    York (1989).
12. Rhim, J.S. Anticancer Res. 9:1345 (1989).
13. Brown, K.W. and Gallimore, P.H. Br J Cancer 56:545
    (1987).
14. Newbold, R.F. and Overell, R.W. Nature 304:648
    (1983).

15. Winter, H., Schweizer, J., *et al.* <u>Carcinogenesis</u>
    1:391  (1980).
16. Yuspa, S.H., Kilkenny, A.E., *et al.* <u>Nature</u> (Lond.)
    314:459  (1985).
17. Roop, D.R., Krieg, T.M., *et al.* <u>Cancer Res</u>  48:3245
    (1988).
18. Breitkreutz, D., <u>et al</u>. <u>Eur J Cell Biol</u>  42:255
    (1986).
19. Boukamp, P., Petrusevska, R.T., *et al.* <u>J Cell Biol</u>
    106:761  (1988).
20. Boukamp, P., Stanbridge, E.J., *et al.* <u>Cancer Res</u>
    50:2840  (1990).
21. Ryle, C.M., Breitkreutz, D., *et al.* <u>Differentiation</u>
    40:42  (1989).
22. Breitkreutz, D., Boukamp, P., *et al.* <u>Canc Res</u>  (in
    press)  1991.
23. Fusenig, N.E., Boukamp, P., *et al.* <u>Toxic In Vitro</u>
    4:627  (1990).
24. Paraskeva, C., Finerty, S., *et al.* <u>Int J Cancer</u>
    41:908  (1988).
25. Williams, A.C., Harper, S.J., *et al.* <u>Cancer Res</u>
    50:4724  (1990).
26. Baden, h.P., Kubilus, J., *et al.* <u>In Vitro Cell Dev</u>
    <u>Biol</u>  23:25  (1987).
27. Soule, H.P., Maloney, T., *et al.* <u>Cancer Res</u>  50:6087
    (1990).
28. Raddel, R.R., Yang, K., *et al.* <u>Cancer Res</u>  48:1904
    (1988).
29. Boyd, J.A. and Barrett, J.C. <u>Pharmac Ther</u>  46:469
    (1990).
30. Breitkreutz, D., Boukamp, P., *et al.* Reichert, U,
    Shroot, B (eds) <u>Pharmacol Skin</u>. Vol 3, Karger Verlag
    Basel, pp 8-14  (1989).
31. Boukamp, P., Rupniak, H.T., *et al.* <u>Cancer Res</u>
    45:5582  (1985).
32. Fusenig, N.E., Breitkreutz, D., *et al.* In: Johnson,
    N.W. (ed.) <u>Risk Markers of Oral Disease</u>. <u>2. Oral</u>
    <u>Cancer</u>. Cambridge University Press  in press  (1991a).

Neoplastic Transformation and Suppression of
Transformation of Human Bronchial Epithelial Cells <u>In
Vitro</u>

Teresa A. Lehman and Curtis C. Harris

Laboratory of Human Carcinogenesis, National
Cancer Institute, National Institutes of
Health, Bethesda, MD  20892

We have taken the following strategy to investigate
the role of oncogenes in the neoplastic transformation of
human bronchial epithelial cells.  First, activated proto-
oncogenes that are associated with human lung cancer are
identified.  Next, these oncogenes are transferred into
the progenitor epithelial cells of broncheogenic
carcinoma.  The preneoplastic and neoplastic cells are
then selected out from the putative suppressive normal
cells.  The tumorigenicity of the cells containing the
transfected oncogenes is then determined using the athymic
nude mouse assay system.  If the transfected or infected
cells show increased tumorigenicity, the dysregulation in
the molecular controls of growth and terminal
differentiation are then investigated.  The methods used
to investigate tumor suppressor genes involves several
different methodologies including production of somatic
cell-cell hybrids with tumorigenic and non-tumorigenic
cells, and analysis of mutational events in known tumor
suppressor genes in human lung carcinoma cell lines and
tumors.

Seven families of activated proto-oncogenes have
been correlated with lung cancer.  These gene families are
the following:  <u>ras</u> (1-3), <u>raf</u> (4,5), <u>myc</u> (6-8), <u>myb</u> (9),
<u>jun</u> (10), erb-B2 (<u>neu</u>) (11), and <u>fms</u> (12).  We have
performed extensive analysis of several of these genes by
either introducing them alone or in combination into

normal human bronchial epithelial (NHBE) cells and SV 40 T
antigen "immortalized" cells.  We have optimized the
growth of these cells by creating a chemically-defined
medium (13) which is free of serum and transforming growth
factor-$\beta_1$ (TGF-$\beta_1$) which inhibits cell growth and induces
terminal squamous differentiation in the cells grown at
clonal density (14).

To study the involvement of Ha-<u>ras</u> in human lung
carcinogenesis, we have transferred v-Ha-<u>ras</u> into NHBE
cells by protoplast fusion (15). These cells sustained
many phenotypic and genotypic events including decreased
responsiveness to inducers of squamous differentiation,
increased responsiveness to serum mitogens, increased
lifespan, aneuploidy, and rarely immortality and
tumorigenicity in athymic nude mice.

Normal human cells grown in culture are relatively
resistant to neoplastic transforming events (16-18).
Several studies have shown that the immortalization event
is the rate-limiting step in the multistage process of <u>in</u>
<u>vitro</u> human carcinogenesis (19-21).  To develop an
immortalized cell system, we have infected NHBE cells with
the SV 40 T antigen (22).  Unlike the precursor NHBE
cells, these BEAS-2B cells are immortalized, and in early
passages, they are non-tumorigenic.  The immortalized
BEAS-2B cell line has been used to define the conditions
under which several of the classes of oncogenes cause
neoplastic transformation.

Infection of BEAS-2B cells with a recombinant virus
containing v-Ha-<u>ras</u> produced BZR cells which were
tumorigenic in athymic mice (21).  Several cell lines were
developed from the tumors, all of which expressed abundant
21 kd protein immunoreactive to antibodies specific for
the codon 12 mutation present in the v-Ha-<u>ras</u> retroviral
vector (21).  BZRT33 was one such tumor-derived cell line
which exhibited a decreased tumor latency compared to BZR.
BEAS-2B, BZR and BZRT33 were examined for invasiveness,
metastatic potential, and the ability to repopulate
deepithelialized rat tracheal xenotransplants.  Studies of
tumorigenicity revealed that BEAS-2B cells were
nontumorigenic, a tumor latency of 1 to 3 weeks for BZR
cells, and a latency of less than 1 week for BZRT33 cells.
The incidence of spontaneous metastasis to the lung
following subcutaneous injection was negative for BEAS-2B,
intermediate for BZR (33%), and complete for BZRT33 (100%)
(21).  Analysis of cells in the xenotransplantation model

of the deepithelialized rat trachea transplanted to
athymic mice (23) revealed that BEAS-2B cells were able to
reconstitute a mucous-producing columnar epithelium.  BZR
cells were tumorigenic in this model and the tumor derived
cell lines were more malignant than the BZR cells.  The
increase in malignancy of the tumor-derived cell lines
corresponds with the increased type IV collagenase enzyme
activity and mRNA expression (23).

The role of Ki-<u>ras</u> in the multistep neoplastic
transformation of human bronchial epithelial cells was
investigated by transferring <u>ras</u> containing constructs
with mutations at codons 12 or 59.  Transfer of this
oncogene into BEAS-2B by either transfection or infection
resulted in neoplastic transformation (24).  These cells
were not sensitive to the squamous differentiation effects
of TGF-$\beta_1$ and they were mitogenically stimulated by serum
(25).  Tumors which were produced from these cells had
adenocarcinomatous elements (24).  This is an interesting
observation since most of the human lung carcinomas that
contain activation of a <u>ras</u> oncogene are lung
adenocarcinomas with an activated Ki-<u>ras</u> (1,26,27).

We have also investigated the functional role of the
<u>myc</u> and <u>raf</u> oncogenes both alone and in combination with
each other.  Two retroviral constructs, p-zip-<u>raf</u> and p-
zip-<u>myc</u>, containing the complete coding sequence of the
human c-<u>raf</u>-1 and the murine c-<u>myc</u> genes respectively were
constructed and transfected into BEAS-2B cells.  BEAS-2B
cells transfected with zip-<u>raf</u> or zip-<u>myc</u> alone were
nontumorigenic after 12 months, but BEAS-2B cells
transfected with zip-<u>raf</u> and zip-<u>myc</u> together formed large
cell subtype of small cell lung carcinomas (SCLC) in
athymic mice in 4 to 21 weeks (28).  BEAS-2B cells and
these tumors were analyzed for a variety of SCLC markers,
and large differences were present between the cell line
and the tumors derived from the transfected BEAS-2B (29).
BEAS-2B cell line was negative or extremely low for most
SCLC markers including gastrin releasing peptide,
serotonin, calcitonin, neuron-specific enolase, keratins
6, 9 and 11, and vimentin, and was positive for keratins 8
and 18.  The tumors derived from zip-<u>raf</u> and zip-<u>myc</u>
transfected BEAS-2B cells exhibited a very different
pattern of expression of these markers.  The tumors were
weakly to strongly reactive in assays for gastrin
releasing peptide, serotonin and calcitonin.  All tumors
were strongly positive for neuron-specific enolase,

vimentin, and keratins 6, 9 and 11 (29).  Since BEAS-2B
cells expressed very low levels of most of the markers of
small cell carcinoma, the neuroendocrine differentiation
induced in the tumors is directly related to the presence
of the zip-_raf_ and zip-_myc_ genes.

Suppression of tumorigenicity was first demonstrated
by Henry Harris and coworkers (30) who observed that cell-
cell hybrids made between cells of high and low
tumorigenic potential had transiently suppressed
tumorigenicity.  As these hybrids were propagated in
culture, tumorigenic segregants developed, and as
chromosomes in the hybrids were lost, the tumorigenicity
of the hybrids increased to that of the parent cell of
high tumorigenic potential (31).
Genetic analysis of somatic cell hybrids between
human cells has shown that suppressor activity of a normal
cell is functionally dominant over the tumorigenic cell
(32-34).  However, studies in which the tumorigenicity of
a cancerous cell type which is hybridized with its normal
epithelial progenitor cell have rarely been performed.  We
therefore created cell-cell hybrids between a
mucoepidermoid lung carcinoma HuT292DM and normal human
bronchial epithelial cells, non-tumorigenic but
immortalized BEAS-2B cells, and B39TL, a weakly
tumorigenic BEAS-2B derived cell line containing a 3p
deletion.  Hybrids formed between HuT292DM and normal
human bronchial epithelial cells had limited doubling
potential and senesced after 40 to 43 population
doublings, so no tumorigenicity assays could be done
(35).  Hybrids between BEAS-2B and HuT292DM cells have an
indefinite lifespan in culture (35).  Tumor latency was 27
days for the parental HuT292DM with 100% of all mice
developing tumors.  In B39TL-HuT292DM hybrids, the mean
tumor latency was 148 days with 50% occurrence, but none
of the BEAS-2B-HuT292DM hybrids were tumorigenic after one
year.  The tumorigenicity of the B39TL-HuT292DM cell
hybrids is comparable to the tumorigenicity of the
parental B39TL at 50% occurrence.  Cell lines were
isolated from tumors that arose from the BEAS-2B-HuT292DM
cell hybrids and the B39TL-HuT292DM hybrids.  On
reinjection of the lines, tumors were produced with
latency periods comparable to the HuT292DM parental cells.
These data support the hypothesis that reversion to
tumorigenicity may occur with the loss of one or more

chromosomes which harbor tumor suppressor genes.  From
these experiments, we can conclude that nontumorigenic or
weakly tumorigenic cells involved in a cell-cell hybrid
will dominate culture longevity and tumorigenicity of the
more tumorigenic cell type.  Further, genes other than
those involved in senescence can exhibit tumor suppressor
activity.

Recently, much attention has been focussed upon the
p53 gene as an example of a tumor suppressor gene that can
be inactivated by mutation in a wide variety of human
cancers (36).  We were interested in the p53 status in
human lung carcinoma cell lines and primary lung tumors,
and chose a number of parameters to examine to determine
this status.  While wild type 53 is capable of binding to
several viral proteins including SV 40 T antigen, some of
the mutant p53 proteins are capable of binding to the heat
shock proteins (hsc 70).  We  took advantage of this fact
to analyze cell lines for p53-hsc 70 coimmunoprecipitation
which implies the presence of mutated p53.  Additionally,
all cell lines were sequenced from exons 1 to 11, and all
were stained for the presence of p53 protein by
immunocytochemical techniques.  The results showed that of
9 cell lines assayed, 4 contained small amounts of wild
type p53, 3 had mutations which produced large amounts of
p53 protein capable of binding hsc 70, and 2 had mutations
which created a "null cell" phenotype where no p53 was
present (37).

Primary human non-small cell lung carcinoma samples
(11 squamous cell carcinomas, 11 adenocarcinomas and 2
large cell carcinomas) have been analyzed for mutations in
the evolutionary conserved region (exons 5 through 8,
codon 126 to 306) of the p53 gene.  Six p53 mutations have
been identified by DNA sequencing (4 in squamous cell
carcinomas and 2 in adenocarcinomas).  Immunohistochemical
staining for the presence of p53 protein in ethanol-fixed
samples of the same primary tumors with a polyclonal anti-
p53 antibody (CM-1) revealed the presence of p53 in 5 of
the 6 mutant cases.  Two other cases that were negative
for p53 mutations by DNA sequencing stained positive for
the presence of the protein.  These data confirm that p53
mutations are a frequent event in primary lung cancers,
but that mutation of p53 not absolutely required for the
development of lung cancer (unpublished results).

REFERENCES

1.   Rodenhuis, S., Van de Wetering, M.L., et al.,
     N.Engl.J.Med., *317*: 929-935, 1987.

2.   Yuasa, Y., Srivastava, S.K., et al. Nature, *303*:
     775-779, 1983.

3.   Yuasa, Y., Gol, R.A., et al.,
     Proc.Natl.Acad.Sci.USA, *81*: 3670-3674, 1984.

4.   Rapp, U.R., Huleihel, M., et al., Lung Cancer, *4*:
     162-167, 1988.

5.   Graziano, S.L., Cowan, B.Y., et al., Cancer Res.,
     *47*: 2148-2155, 1987.

6.   Little, C.D., Nau, M.M., et al., Nature, *306*: 194-
     196, 1983.

7.   Nau, M.M., Brooks, B.J.,Jr., et al.,
     Proc.Natl.Acad.Sci.USA, *83*: 1092-1096, 1986.

8.   Nau, M.M., Brooks, B.J.,Jr., et al., Nature, *318*:
     69-73, 1985.

9.   Griffin, C.A. and Baylin, S.B. Cancer Res., *45*: 272-
     275, 1985.

10.  Schuette, J., Nau, M., et al., Proc.Am.Assoc.Cancer
     Res., *29*: 1808, 1988.(Abstract)

11.  Weiner, D.B., Nordberg, J., et al., Cancer Res., *50*:
     421-425, 1990.

12.  Kiefer, P.E., Bepler, G., et al., Cancer Res., *47*:
     6236-6242, 1987.

13.  Lechner, J.F. and LaVeck, M.A. et al., J.Tissue
     Culture Meth., *9*: 43-48, 1985.

14.  Ke, Y., Reddel, R.R., et al., Differentiation, *38*:
     60-66, 1988.

15. Yoakum, G.H., Lechner, J.F., et al., Science, *227*: 1174-1179, 1985.

16. DiPaolo, J.A. JNCI, *70*: 3-8, 1983.

17. DiPaolo, J.A., DeMarinis, A.J. and Doniger, J. Pharmacology, *27*: 65-73, 1983.

18. Shamsuddin, A.K.M., Sinopoli, N.T., et al., Fed.Proc., *42*: 1042, 1983.(Abstract)

19. Rhim, J.S., Jay, G., et al., Science, *227*: 1250, 1985.

20. Namba, M., Nishitani, K., et al., Int.J.Cancer, *37*: 419-423, 1986.

21. Amstad, P., Reddel, R.R., et al., Mol.Carcinogenesis, *1*: 151-160, 1988.

22. Reddel, R.R., Ke, Y., et al., Cancer Res., *48*: 1904-1909, 1988.

23. Bonfil, R.D., Reddel, R.R., et al., J.Natl.Cancer Inst., *81*: 587-594, 1989.

24. Reddel, R.R., Ke, Y., et al., Oncogene Res., *3*: 401-408, 1988.

25. Masui, T., Wakefield, L.M., et al., Proc.Natl.Acad.Sci.USA, *83*: 2438-2442, 1986.

26. Rodenhuis, S., Slebos, R.J., et al., Cancer Res., *48*: 5738-5741, 1988.

27. Slebos, R.J., Kibbelaar, R.E., et al., N.Engl.J.Med., *323*: 561-565, 1990.

28. Pfeifer, A., Mark, G.E., et al., Proc.Natl.Acad.Sci.USA, *86*: 10075-10079, 1989.

29. Pfeifer, A.M.A., Jones, R.T., et al., Cancer Res., 1991. In press.

30.   Harris, H., Miller, O.J., et al., Nature, *223*: 363-368, 1969.

31.   Harris, H. Cancer Res., *48*: 3302-3306, 1988.

32.   Stanbridge, E.J. In: G. Klein (ed.), Advances in Viral Oncology, Volume 6, pp. 83-101. New York: Raven Press, 1987.

33.   Peehl, D.M. and Stanbridge, E.J. Int.J.Cancer, *27*: 625-635, 1981.

34.   Geiser, A.G., Der, C.J., et al., Proc.Natl.Acad.Sci.USA, *83*: 5209-5213, 1986.

35.   Kaighn, M.E., Gabrielson, E.W., et al., Cancer Res., *50*: 1890-1896, 1990.

36.   Hollstein, M., Sidransky, D., et al., Science, 1991. In press.

37.   Lehman, T.A., Bennett, W.P., et al., Cancer Res., 1991. In press.

From: *Neoplastic Transformation in Human Cell Culture,*
Eds.: J. S. Rhim and A. Dritschilo ©1991 The Humana Press Inc., Totowa, NJ

# AN IN VITRO HUMAN MAMMARY EPITHELIAL MODEL SYSTEM FOR STUDIES OF DIFFERENTIATION AND CARCINOGENESIS.

Martha R. Stampfer, Paul Yaswen, Gordon Parry, and Junko Hosoda

Lawrence Berkeley Laboratory, Cell and Molecular Biology Divison, Berkeley, CA 94720

Our laboratory has developed culture systems utilizing human mammary epithelial cells (HMEC) in order to facilitate studies on the normal mechanisms controlling growth and differentiation in these cells, and to understand how these normal processes may become altered as a result of immortal and malignant transformation. One aspect of this work has been to derive cell types which may represent different stages in the progression from normal cells to malignant cells. Another aspect has been characterize these various cell types for their synthesis of and responses to different growth factors, as well as their expresson of differentiated properties. We have additionally utilized our normal and malignant cultures to identify new gene products which may be differentially expressed in these cells. Underlying this work has been the assumption that carcinogenesis involves aberrations in the normal pathways of proliferation and differentiation, and that while in vitro model systems may still not fully reflect the in vivo situation, they will nevertheless prove useful in advancing our understanding of the mechanisms of human carcinogenesis.

In collaboration with other groups, we have developed culture conditions which support the long term growth of HMEC derived from reduction mammoplasty, mastectomy and benign tissues (1-3). These tissues are digested to yield small epithelial clumps, termed organoids, as well as single cell populations which preferentially contain mesenchymal cells. This material can be stored frozen in liquid nitrogen, permitting multiple experiments utilizing cells from the same individual. Two main types of medium have been used to support growth of the HMEC, a serum containing medium, designated MM (4), and a serum-free medium, designated MCDB 170 (2). Both media contain a variety of growth factors, including insulin, hydrocortisone, EGF, and a cAMP stimulator.  MM contains 0.5% fresh fetal bovine serum and 30% conditioned media from other human epithelial cell lines; MCDB 170 contains 70µg/ml bovine pituitary extract.

Cells grown in MM show active epithelial cell division for 3-5 passages before senescence.  In MCDB 170, there is initial active cell division for 2-3 passages of cobblestone appearing cells.  These cells gradually change morphology, becoming larger, flatter, striated, with irregular edges, and reduced proliferative capacity.  As these larger cells cease growth, a small number of cells with the cobblestone morphology maintain proliferative capacity and soon dominate the culture.  These cells continue growing with a fairly uniform cobblestone appearance for an additional 7-24 passages, depending upon the individual reduction mammoplasty specimen.  At senescence, the cells maintain the smooth-edged cobblestone appearance, but become larger and more vacuolated.  We have referred to this process, whereby only a small fraction of the cells grown in MCDB 170 display long-term growth potential, as "self-selection".

The post-selection HMEC have doubling times of 18-24 hrs, and will grow clonally with 15-50% colony forming efficiency.  Large batches of post-selection cells can be stored frozen, permitting repetition of experiments with cells from the same frozen batch, as well as from the same individual.  In order to relate the HMEC which maintain long-term growth in vitro to the different cell types identified in vivo, they have been examined for several phenotypes which have been studied using sectioned human breast tissues.  Northern blot analysis of mRNA expression and immunohistochemical analysis of protein expression for keratins 5, 14, 8, 18, 19, vimentin,  and the large polymorphic epithelial mucins have shown that the cells which initially proliferate in the serum-free MCDB 170 medium resemble mammary cells in the basal layer in vivo.  However, post-selection cells begin to express some properties associated with the luminal cell type.  Primary cultures of normal HMEC grown in MCDB 170 and early passage cultures grown in MM are heterogeneous.  From these results we have proposed that the cells which display long term growth in the serum-free medium represent a multipotent stem cell population present in the basal layer of the gland.  With increasing time in culture, these cells show a partial differentiation towards the luminal phenotype (5).  Tumor cells in vivo and in vitro generally express the phenotype of the mature luminal cell (5).

Normal HMEC from specimen 184 have been transformed to immortality following exposure to the chemical carcinogen benzo(a)pyrene (BaP) (6, 7).  Primary cultures were grown in MM and exposed 2-3 times to 2µg/ml BaP.  Selection for transformed cells was based on the ability of BaP treated cells to continue growing past the time that the control cells senesced. Treated cultures typically contained cells with an extended lifespan compared to controls, however, almost all of these cells eventually ceased growth. In only two instances have we observed escape from senescence, leading to cell lines with indefinite lifespan. The two resulting cell lines, 184A1 and 184B5, each show specific clonal karyotypic aberrations, indicating their independent origins from single cells (8). Upon continued passage in culture, these two lines show some genetic drift, but it is relatively minimal compared to that observed in most human breast tumor cell lines. Thus, the vast majority of the cell population would be expected to remain karyotypically stable when studied over the course of a few passages in culture, yet the presence of some genetic drift could give rise to rare variants in the cell population. Although 184A1 and 184B5 are immortally transformed, they do not have properties associated with malignant transformation. They do not form tumors in nude mice and they show very little or no capacity for anchorage independent growth (AIG) (6, 7).

Malignant derivatives of 184A1 and 184B5 have been obtained with the use of oncogene containing retroviral vectors and viruses. In the case a 184A1, a clonal derivative, A1N4, which showed reduced nutritional requirements, was exposed to the genes for SV40-T large antigen, v-H-ras, and v-mos singly and in combination (9). The combination of H-ras and SV40-T led to cells (designated A1N4-TH) which formed progressively growing tumors in nude mice and showed AIG. v-H-ras or v-mos alone gave cells that produced tumors with reduced frequency and longer latency. SV40-T alone did not yield tumorigenic cells, but did effect the growth factor requirements for anchorage dependent and independent growth (10). In all cases of oncogene exposure, the resultant cells were capable of proliferation in media that did not support the growth of the parental A1N4 cells.

The 184B5 cell line has been exposed to v-K-ras (designated B5-K). This gene alone was capable of producing cells which were 100% tumorigenic in nude mice, with a short latency. However, these tumors did not grow beyond approximately 5cm diameter (7). Most of our studies on these cells have utilized a tumor resected from a nude mouse and placed in culture, leading to the culture designated B5KTu. B5-K and B5KTu do not display AIG.

We have also conducted a series of experiments to attempt to obtain malignantly transformed derivatives of 184A1 and 184B5 following additional exposure to chemical carcinogens. To perform these experiments, we first determined the requirements of 184A1 and 184B5 for the various growth factors present in MCDB 170. Spontaneous variants of 184A1 and 184B5 could be obtained that showed active growth in the absence of EGF, insulin, hydrocortisone, or bovine pituitary extract, whereas normal HMEC grown without insulin, hydrocortisone, or bovine pituitary extract ceased growth after 1-3 passages. We next examined the effect of removal of multiple growth factors, and were able to define conditions which did not support the growth of any 184A1 or 184B5 populations.

Populations of 184A1 and A84B5 were then exposed to concentrations of N-nitroso-ethyl-urea (ENU) that yielded 80% growth inhibition, and the surviving cell populations were tested for their ability to grow in the restrictive media and for AIG. Under some conditions the ENU treated cells were capable of sustained growth whereas the untreated cell lines quickly ceased growth. However, none of the ENU treated cells showed an increase in AIG or formed tumors in nude mice. Thus, we have not yet been able to derive cells that showed tumorigenic properties following use of chemical carcinogens alone.

One main area of our research has been to study the effect of growth factors on normal HMEC proliferation, and compare these data with growth control of the transformed HMEC. In particular, we have examined the effects of TGFβ and EGF/TGFα. We have demonstrated that normal HMEC are growth inhibited by TGFβ, with the extent of inhibition increasing as cell are subcultured in vitro (11). All normal HMEC are ultimately growth arrested by TGFβ. In contrast, HMEC which have been transformed to immortality or malignancy may express sustained growth in the presence of TGFβ. However, even though TGFβ may not inhibit their growth, the immortalized HMEC lines retain receptors for TGFβ and, like the normal HMEC, express specific differentiated responses (12, 13). Synthesis of extracellular matrix associated proteins such as fibronectin, collagen IV, and plasminogen activator inhibitor 1 is increased upon TGFβ exposure.

Normal HMEC have a stringent requirement for EGF/TGFα for clonal growth. However, growth in mass culture proceeds without additional of exogenous EGF due to the significant level of endogenous production of TGFα (14). Addition of monoclonal antibody 225 IgG to the EGF receptor (MAb 225) prevents HMEC growth (15). Recent experiments have shown that MAb 225 produces a rapid, efficient, and reversible growth arrest in a Go or early G1 phase of the cell cycle. Protein synthesis remains depressed in the presence of the antibody, and DNA synthesis is sharply decreased by 24hr. Removal of MAb 225 leads to a rapid increase in protein synthesis. DNA synthesis increases only after 10hr and peaks around 18hr. A 1hr exposure to EGF after MAb 225 removal is sufficient to allow the majority of the competent cells to subsequently enter S phase. High levels of synthesis of mRNA for the early response genes c-myc, c-fos, and c-jun are observed within

1hr of antibody removal. Synthesis of TGFα mRNA, which is inhibited in the presence of MAb 225, is detected by 2hr after antibody removal. It thus appears that blockage of EGF receptor signal transduction is sufficient by itself to cause normal HMEC to enter a Go-like resting state. Further studies are now addressing possible differences between normal HMEC of finite lifespan and the immortally transformed HMEC cell lines with respect to their response to MAb225 and their cell cycle controls.

Our HMEC culture system has also been used to identify genes preferentially expressed in normal vs malignant HMEC. Subtractive hybridization was performed between the normal 184 parental cells and the malignantly transformed B5KTu cell line in order to identify genes preferentially expressed in the normal parental cells. Using this technique, a 1.4 kb mRNA, designated NB-1, was found to be expressed in the 184 cells but was barely detectable in the tumorigenic B5KTu (16). NB-1 mRNA has been thus far found only in normal epithelial cells and tissues from human breast, prostate, cervix, and skin. It has not been found in non-epithelial cells and tissues, or epithelial tumor cell lines. It's expression is decreased in the immortalized 184B5 cells and is undetectable in the immortalized 184A1 cells.

Sequence analysis of NB-1 revealed a 447 bp open reading frame with extensive similarity at the nucleic acid level to the three known intron containing human calmodulin genes. The NB-1 open reading frame displayed 70%, 71%, and 80% sequence identity with these three calmodulin mRNAs (17-19). The similarity between the translated amino acid sequence of NB-1 and human calmodulin was 85% over the length of the entire protein. The initial characterization of genomic DNA corresponding to the NB-1 transcript indicated the unexpected absence of introns. A literature search revealed the existence of a previously reported human calmodulin "pseudogene" hGH6, which shared identity with NB-1 cDNA (20). This gene was designated a pseudogene since the authors were unable to demonstrate the existence of a corresponding mRNA. Our evidence of expression of NB-1 at both the mRNA and protein levels suggests that NB-1 may be a rare example of an expressed retroposon (21).

Although NB-1 mRNA is easily detectable by Northern analysis in total RNA from cultured normal HMEC, it is less abundant in total RNA from organoids and unprocessed reduction mammoplasty tissue. Such differences are unlikely to be due to variations in proliferative state since expression of NB-1 mRNA is not significantly decreased when cells are growth arrested by exposure to anti-EGF receptor antibodies or in senescing cells where proliferation is minimal, and it is increased in cells growth arrested by TGFβ. One possible explanation is that, unlike calmodulin, NB-1 expression may be limited to a particular state of epithelial cell maturation, and thus be confined to certain subpopulations of epithelial cells in vivo. Since NB-1 mRNA levels are high in the post-selection normal HMEC population which displays active long-term growth in MCDB 170, and which has attributes of multipotent stem cells, it is possible that expression in vivo may be limited to a precursor stem cell population in the basal layer of the gland.

HMEC plated on EHS, an extracellular matrix preparation derived from the Englebreth-Holm-Swarm murine sarcoma, showed decreased levels of NB-1 mRNA synthesis while forming structures with striking resemblance to endbuds in intact mammary gland tissue. EHS has previously been shown to support increased differentiated functions of a variety of cell types. Additionally, the non-proliferative differentiated luminal cells sloughed off into milk during lactation were negative for NB-1 expression by Northern or PCR analysis. The findings are consistent with the hypothesis that NB-1 is only expressed during certain stages of epithelial differentiation.

We have recently produced polyclonal antisera which can distinguish the NB-1 protein from vertebrate calmodulin, using full length recombinant NB-1 protein as an immunogen. The recombinant NB-1 protein, like calmodulin, binds phenyl-Sepharose in the presence of calcium. Initial studies have indicated that the relative abundance of the 16kD protein reflects relative NB-1 mRNA levels in various cell types, being most highly expressed in normal HMEC, lower or undetectable in the immortally transformed cell lines, and virtually undetectable in tumorigenic breast and prostate cell lines as well as normal breast fibroblasts.

The discovery of a new gene product which is homologous to a regulatory molecule as pivotal as calmodulin offers exciting possibilities in efforts to understand calcium regulation of intracellular processes. The strong homology between NB-1 and calmodulin suggests that the NB-1 gene product is a calcium binding protein with signal transduction capabilities. The NB-1 product may compete with calmodulin for calcium and bind with different affinity to cellular substrates. The pattern of expression exhibited by NB-1 in cultured epithelial cells and tissues suggests that NB-1 plays a differentiation specific role. External calcium concentration has been shown to affect the proliferative potential and differentiated states of some cultured epithelial cells, including keratinocytes and mammary epithelial cells (22, 23). Loss of response to this calcium induced differentiation signal has been shown to correlate with the early stages of transformation in keratinocyte cultures (24). Downregulation of NB-1 expression observed after *in vitro* transformation of HMEC may reflect the fact that a particular state of differentiation may be required for transformation or that the transformed state is incompatible with high expression of NB-1. Changes in signal transduction of growth or differentiation factors and their associated intracellular second messengers are often implicated in neoplastic transformation. Further analysis of the NB-1 gene product; its expression, function, and regulation, will undoubtedly lead to a more complete understanding of normal and abnormal epithelial cell growth and differentiation.

## REFERENCES


1. Stampfer, M. R., Hallowes, R., Hackett, A. J., Growth of normal human mammary epithelial cells in culture. In Vitro, *16:* 415-425, 1980.
2. Hammond, S. L., Ham, R. G., Stampfer, M. R., Serum-free growth of human mammary epthelial cells: Rapid clonal growth in defined medium and extended serial passage with pituitary extract. Proc. Natl. Acad. Sci. USA, *81:* 5435-5439, 1984.
3. Stampfer, M. R., Isolation and growth of human mammary epithelial cells. J. Tissue Culture Methods, *9:* 107-116, 1985.
4. Stampfer, M. R., Cholera toxin stimulation of human mammary epithelial cells in culture. In Vitro, *18:* 531-537, 1982.
5. Taylor-Papadimitriou, J., Stampfer, M., Bartek, J., Lane, E. B., Lewis, A., Keratin expression in human mammary epithelial cells cultured from normal and malignant tissue: Relation to in vivo phenotypes and influence of medium. J. Cell Sci., *94:* 403-413, 1989.
6. Stampfer, M. R., Bartley, J. C., Induction of transformation and continuous cell lines from normal human mammary epithelial cells after exposure to benzo(a)pyrene. Proc. Natl. Acad. Sci. USA, *82:* 2394-2398, 1985.
7. Stampfer, M. R., Bartley, J. C., Human mammary epithelial cells in culture: Differentiation and transformation. *In:* R. Dickson, M. Lippman (eds.), Breast Cancer: Cellular and Molecular Biology, 1-24. Norwall, Kluwer Academic Publishers, 1988.
8. Walen, K., Stampfer, M. R., Chromosome analyses of human mammary epithelial cells at stages of chemically-induced transformation progression to immortality. Cancer Gen. Cyto., *37:* 249-261, 1989.
9. Clark, R., Stampfer, M., Milley, B., O'Rourke, E., Walen, K., Kriegler, M., Kopplin, J., Transformation of human mammary epithelial cells by oncogenic retroviruses. Cancer Res., *48:* 4689-4694, 1988.
10. Valverius, E. M., Ciardiello, F., Heldin, N., Blondel, B., Merlo, G., Smith, G., Stampfer, M. R., Lippman, M. E., Dickson, R. B., Salomon, D. S., Stromal influences on transformation of human

mammary epithelial cells overexpressing c-myc and SV40T. J. Cell. Physiol., *145:* 207-216, 1990.

11. Hosobuchi, M., Stampfer, M. R., Effects of transforming growth factor-β on growth of human mammary epithelial cells in culture. In Vitro, *25:* 705-712, 1989.

12. Valverius, E. M., Walker-Jones, D., Bates, S. E., Stampfer, M. R., Clark, R., McCormick, F., Dickson, R. B., Lippman, M. E., Production of and responsiveness to transforming growth factor β in normal and oncogene transformed human mammary epithelial cells. Cancer Res., *49:* 6407-6411, 1989.

13. Stampfer, M., Alhadeff, M., Prosen, D., Bissell, M., Hosoda, J., Effects of transforming growth factor β on human mammary epithelial cells in culture. J. Cell Biochem., *Supplement 13B:* 97, 1989.

14. Valverius, E., Bates, S. E., Stampfer, M. R., Clark, R., McCormick, F., Salomon, D. S., Lippman, M. E., Dickson, R., Transforming growth factor alpha production and EGF receptor expression in normal and oncogene tranformed human mammary epithelial cells. Mol. Endo., *3:*203-214, 1989.

15. Bates, S. E., Valverius, E., Ennis, B. W., Bronzert, D. A., Sheridan, J. P., Stampfer, M., Mendelsohn, J., Lippman, M. E., Dickson, R. B., Expression of the TGFα/EGF receptor pathway in normal human breast epithelial cells. Endocrin., *126:* 596-607, 1990.

16. Yaswen, P., Smoll, A., Peehl, D. M., Trask, D. K., Sager, R., Stampfer, M. R., Down-regulation of a calmodulin-related gene during transformation of human mammary epithelial cells. Proc. Natl. Acad. Sci. USA, *87:* 7360-7364, 1990.

17. SenGupta, B., Friedberg, F., Detera-Wadleigh, S. D., Molecular analysis of human and rat calmodulin complementary DNA clones. J. Biol. Chem., *262:* 16663-16670, 1987.

18. Wawrzynczak, E. J., Perham, R. N., Isolation and nucleotide sequence of a cDNA encoding human calmodulin. Biochem. Int., *9:* 177-185, 1984.

19. Fischer, R., Koller, M., Flura, M., Mathews, S., Strehler-Page, M.-A., Krebs, J., Penniston, J. T., Carafoli, E., Strehler, E. E., Multiple divergent mRNAs code for a single human calmodulin. J. Biol. Chem., *262:* 17055-17062, 1988.

20. Koller, M., Strehler, E. E., Characterization of an intronless human calmodulin-like pseudogene. FEB, *239:* 121-128, 1988.

21. Brosius, J., Retroposons - seeds of evolution. Science, *251:* 753, 1991.

22. Yuspa, S. H., Kilkenny, A. E., Steinert, P. M., Roop, D. R., Expression of murine epidermal differentiation markers is tightly regulated by restricted extracellular calcium concentrations in vitro. J. Cell Biol., *109:* 1207-1217, 1989.

23. Soule, H. D., McGrath, C. M., A simplified method for passage and long-term growth of human mammary epithelial cells. In Vitro Cell. & Dev. Biol., *22:* 6-12, 1986.
24. Yuspa, S. H., Morgan, D. L., Mouse skin cells resistant to terminal differentiation associated with initiation of carcinogenesis. Nature, *293:* 72-74, 1981.

From: *Neoplastic Transformation in Human Cell Culture,*
Eds.: J. S. Rhim and A. Dritschilo ©1991 The Humana Press Inc., Totowa, NJ

# TRANSFORMATION <u>IN VITRO</u> OF HUMAN UROEPITHELIAL CELLS


C.A. Reznikoff, C. Kao, E.A. Bookland,
A.J. Klingelhutz, C.I. Pratt, S.Q. Wu,
K.W. Gilchrist, and S. Swaminathan
University of Wisconsin
Department of Human Oncology
and Clinical Cancer Center,
Madison, Wisconsin 53792


## ABSTRACT


**Normal human uroepithelial cells can now be routinely cultured <u>in vitro</u>, immortalized by SV40 T antigen oncoprotein gene, and tumorigenically transformed after exposure to oncogenic agents including the human bladder carcinogen, 4-aminobiphenyl (ABP) and its metabolites and mutant EJ/<u>ras</u> to carcinoma phenotypes that resemble human bladder cancers. Neoplastic transformation of HUC <u>in vitro</u> is accompanied by chromosome changes that recapitulate many cytogenetic changes reported in clinical bladder cancers.**


## INTRODUCTION

In this report, I will briefly summarize challenges met and progress made in the last 10 years in our laboratory's efforts to develop an <u>in vitro</u>/<u>in vivo</u> transformation system to study the biochemical and molecular genetic mechanisms of human bladder carcinogenesis. I will also address our goals and hopes for progress in the next 5 years. First, let me briefly describe the nature of the disease bladder cancer and define the potential value of bladder cancer carcinogenesis studies.

## a.    Clinical bladder cancer characteristics

Bladder cancer is a significant health problem
in the USA, where it is the 2nd most prevalent
malignancy in men over 60 years of age (1).  Although
most (75%) bladder tumors are superficial and
indolent recurring papillomas or Grade I transitional
cell carcinomas (TCCs), invasive cancer is present in
10-20% of all recurrences (2).  However, there are no
sure markers to identify patients whose cancer will
progress.  In addition, 25% of bladder cancers are
high grade progressive invasive cancers at first
presentation, and 5% have already metastasized (2).

While most bladder cancers are TCCs, other
histopathological types are represented including
squamous cell carcinomas (SCC), adenocarcinomas
(AdC), and undifferentiated carcinomas (U)(3).  Thus,
bladder cancers represent a diverse spectrum of
biological and histopathological phenotypes.
Furthermore, bladder cancer incidence has not
decreased in the last 50 years (4), and the survival
rates for bladder cancer patients have not improved
significantly despite advances in therapy (4).  In
summary, bladder cancer is a heterogeneous, complex,
multistage, and unpredictable disease that is a
significant health problem in our society.

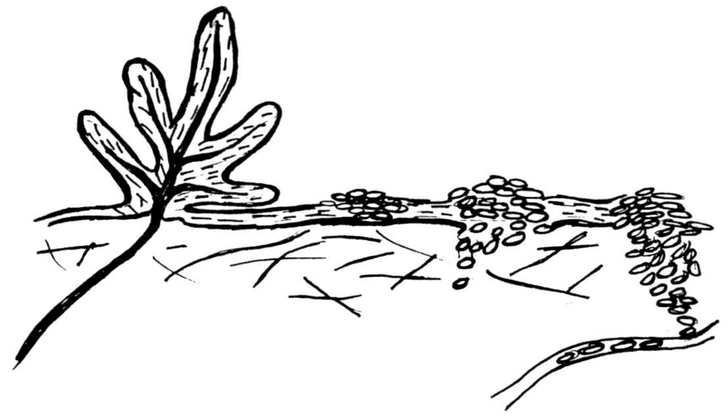



**Figure 1. <u>A schematic of bladder cancer stages</u>**

## b. Etiological agents in uroepithelial carcinogenesis

Increased risk for bladder cancers has been associated with exposure to chemical carcinogens (notably 4-aminobiphenyl) in the environment and industry, certain medicinal drugs, cigarette smoking and radiation therapy (5-7). In most of these situations, there is good evidence that the risk increases with higher doses and multiple exposures. Genetic studies suggest that individuals with a slow acetylator phenotypes may be at a greater risk to develop bladder cancer (8). At the present time, no tumor virus has been associated with bladder cancer.

## c. Molecular genetic changes in human bladder cancers

Many clinical cancers have been examined to identify activated _ras_ gene and to detect loss of putative cancer suppressor genes. Although the now famous mutant c-Ha-_ras_-1 oncogene was first isolated from the T24/EJ human bladder cancer cell line ten year ago, examination of human bladder cancers by many groups in the past decade have failed to demonstrate a role for _ras_ activation in the majority of human bladder cancers. Many investigators have demonstrated a role for activation of _ras_ by chemical carcinogens in rodent bladder uroepithelium (9), but the role of _ras_ mutations in human bladder carcinogenesis remains somewhat controversial (4).

In contrast, research to identify important genetic losses in human bladder carcinogenesis has revealed significant changes that probably apply to the majority of human bladder cancers. Some genetic deletions, including 9q and 11p losses were first observed as cytogenetic losses as reported by Sandberg and others (10-12). Common cytogenetic aberrations reported in bladder cancers include; t(3p14), -5q, -6q, +7, -8p, -9q, -10q, -11p, and -13q (12). Cytogenetic studies associate losses of 9q with indolent cancers and losses of 11p and alterations of chromosome 3 with higher grade cancers (11).

The laboratory of Peter Jones has reported a significant percent loss of heterozygosity (LOH) on chromosomes 9q (65%), 11p (40%), and 17p (63%) in human bladder cancers (13), and in a separate study also report that these 17p losses correlate with late stage bladder cancers (14). Earlier studies from the laboratory of Bert Vogelstein had also demonstrated similar losses of 11p in human bladder cancers and correlated these with a poor prognosis (15). More recently, Vogelstein's laboratory has reported frequent mutations in the remaining p53 alleles in bladder cancers that show 17p LOH (16). Loss of the RB gene are reported in about 33% of human bladder cancers (17). Finally, loss of 18q has now been reported for invasive TCCs (18).

These data are consistent with the hypothesis that chromosome homologue losses and/or functional mutational inactivation of both alleles of putative cancer suppressor genes in these specific chromosome regions may be required for transformation of HUC. It has been hypothesized that the genes whose loss is required in tumorigenesis are those that control normal growth and differentiation (19). This is consistent with observations indicating cell type specificity in the "sets" of genes lost in cancers.

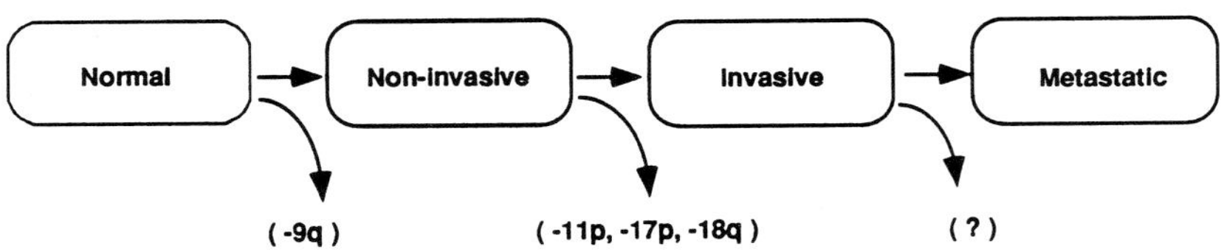


**Figure 2. <u>Genetic losses in multistage clinical TCC</u>**

## A GENETIC MODEL OF HUMAN BLADDER CARCINOGENESIS

Based on the above data collected from clinical observations, epidemiological studies, and genetic analysis of clinical bladder cancers, we propose the following updated model of human uroepithelial carcinogenesis.

> **Multiple genetic losses play a major role in uroepithelial carcinogenesis.  Certain gene losses are associated with more malignant phenotypes.  Genetic losses can result from chromosome homologue losses and/or mutational gene inactivation.  Chemical carcinogens contribute to bladder cancers by causing mutations in recessive and/or dominant cancer target genes.**

Put simply, individuals who are exposed to certain chemical carcinogens more frequently get bladder cancers than nonexposed persons.  Bladder cancers show mutational inactivations of specific target genes. Therefore, bladder carcinogens may cause mutations in these putative target genes.

> **However, this model is based on correlative data.**  It is not possible to fully test this hypothesis in humans.  Not only is it unthinkable to deliberately expose humans to known carcinogens, it is unreasonable to assume that patients can accurately identify the carcinogen that caused their cancer.  [One notable exception is, of course, smoking whose role in human cancer causation is unambiguous.]  It is also not possible with humans to passively observe the development of bladder malignancies.  Except in the most advanced cases, one must intervene by surgery, chemotherapy, and/or radiation.  Thus, opportunities to observe the natural evolution of low grade cancers to high grade cancers in patients are very limited.

## EXPERIMENTAL <u>IN VITRO/IN VIVO</u> HUC TUMORIGENESIS MODEL

A major goal of cancer researchers in the last 10 years has been the development of model systems to study the steps in human epithelial carcinogenesis. Our laboratory has been dedicated to the development of a system to study HUC tumorigenesis.

> **The development of an <u>in vitro/in vivo</u> model system that would allow tumorigenic transformation and neoplastic progression of HUC after exposure to relevant human bladder carcinogens would make it possible to associate genetic changes with the development and progression of uroepithelial cancers.**

As with the other human epithelial cell types, the
development of such a system has been a challenge at
every step of the way.  In this section, I will
briefly review the progress made in the last decade.

**a.    Growth and differentiation _in vitro_ of HUC**

        Our very first experience with HUC was that
specimens of human bladder uroepithelial cells (left
over from bladder surgery for noncancerous
conditions) had a low viability and did not
proliferate when placed on plastic culture dishes in
medium supplemented only with serum (20).  During the
next 5 years in our laboratory, residual pieces of
ureteral epithelium from kidney transplant surgery
were first identified as a routine source of viable
HUC (21),  the explant technique was adapted to
successfully initiate HUC cultures (20-22),  Type I
collagen-gels were defined as a substrate on which
HUC not only grew well but stratified and
differentiated resembling normal uroepithelium (20),
optimal concentrations of calcium and growth
supplements were established for the development of a
serum-free medium suitable for proliferation, passage
and expansion of HUC (22), conditions were defined
for low density clonal growth (23), and techniques
were developed to quantitatively assess cytotoxicity
(24).

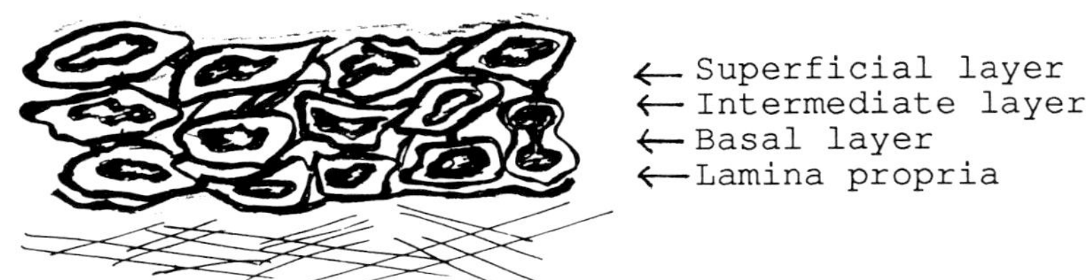


**Figure 3. HUC _Differentiation on collagen substrates._**

## b.    Immortalization of HUC

After numerous attempts to immortalize HUC by exposure to bladder carcinogens, including 4-aminobiphenyl and its reactive metabolites failed, we (like so many other investigators) turned to the use of a DNA tumor virus to immortalize cells. This was successful. HUC were reproducibly immortalized after infection with wild type Simian virus 40, SV40 (the SV-HUC system) (25) or after transfection with SV40 Tt antigen genes (the CK/SV-HUC system) (26). We of course, knew then and now that SV40 is not an etiological agent in human bladder cancers. *However, at that time we did not know in what way its presence in our transformation system might alter genetic results.*

SV40-immortalized SV-HUCs show cytogenetic abnormalities, as do essentially all SV40-immortalized human epithelial cells. One clonal cell line, SV-HUC-1 is special in that the chromosomal translocations that gave rise to rearrangements were balanced (27 ). In the CK/SV-HUC system, CK/clone-2 is special in that it shows cytogenetic losses; namely -3p, -11p, and -13q that mimic important losses seen in human bladder cancers (10-12). None of the 8 SV40 immortal lines established in our laboratory have formed tumors when inoculated into nude mice at early passage (25-26).

## c.    SV-HUC tumorigenic transformation by carcinogens

Exposure of the clonal and pseudodiploid nontumorigenic SV-HUC-1 cell line to the potent polycyclic hydrocarbon, 3-methylcholanthrene (MC) followed by a 6 week period of posttreatment proliferation reproducibly resulted in neoplastic transformation (28). Tumors (T-SV-HUCs) obtained after subcutaneous inoculation represented a spectrum of biological and histopathological phenotypes ranging from Grades I to III and representing TCCs, SCCs, AdCs, and U carcinomas, thus recapitulating the heterogeneity seen in clinical bladder cancers.

In the next series of experiments, tumorigenic transformation and neoplastic progression of SV-HUC by the relevant human bladder carcinogen, ABP and two of its reactive metabolites, N-hydroxy-4-amino-biphenyl and N-hydroxy-4-acetylaminobiphenyl (HAABP and HABP)) were achieved (29). In these experiments,

nontumorigenic cells exposed to ABPs were transformed
to tumorigenicity, and low grade T-SV-HUCs were
transformed to more progressed high grade cancers.
Some tumors also progressed spontaneously on
reinoculation.

     To date over 50 independent uroepithelial
cancers with heterogeneous carcinoma phenotypes have
been generated from these clonal SV40-immortalized
cells.

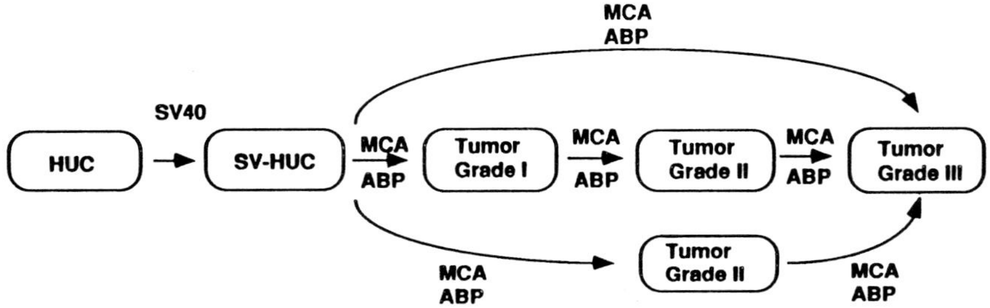


**Figure 4. <u>Multistep SV-HUC chemical transformation</u>**

## d.    Cytogenetic losses in transformation *in vitro*

     Early chromosomal analyses of MC-transformed
T-SV-HUCs indicated that losses of chromosome arms
3p and 6q were significant in SV-HUC transformation
(27).  Later detailed analyses of ABP-transformed
T-SV-HUC confirmed the significance of 3p (p=.0003)
and 6q (p=.01) losses and showed that 18q losses were
also nonrandom (p=.0003) (30-31).  Losses of 3p
associated with aggressive high grade carcinoma
phenotypes, losses of 6q associated with aggressive
cancer growth kinetics, and 18q losses accompanied
progression from noninvasive to invasive cancers
(30).  Losses of 11p and 13q were seen in about 33%
of T-SV-HUCs and losses of 11p were seen in about 40%
of high grade T-SV-HUCs.  Many of these same
cytogenetic losses were observed in association with
tumorigenic reversion of somatic cell hybrids between
SV-HUC and T-SV-HUCs (32).  Thus, most of the losses
observed in clinical bladder cancers were also
observed in SV40-immortalized cells after
transformation *in vitro*.

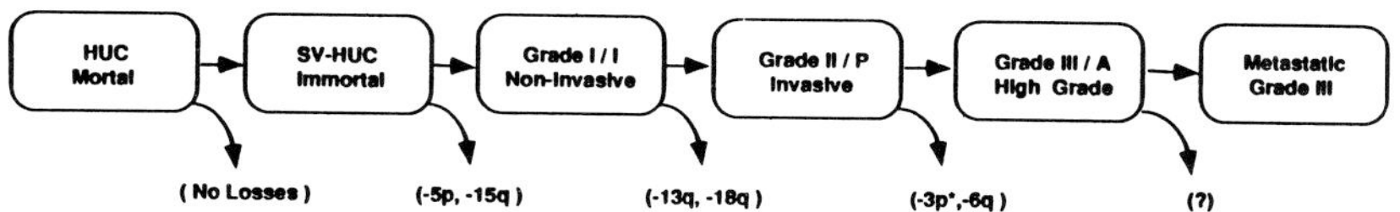


**Figure 5. <u>Chromosomal losses in HUC transformation</u>**

## e.     Tumorigenic transformation of SV-HUC by EJ/<u>ras</u>

Transfection of immortalized cytogenetically balanced SV-HUC with the oncogene EJ/<u>ras</u> did not result in tumorigenic transformation (33). In contrast, transfection of T-SV-HUC tumors at every stage of multistep transformation with mutant <u>ras</u> results in neoplastic progression (34). We proposed that the transforming action of mutant requires the prior loss of suppressor genes (33). Consistent with this hypothesis, somatic cell hybrids between tumorigenic and nontumorigenic mutant <u>ras</u>-expressing cells in this system are suppressed for tumorigenicity (35). Thus, in our hands at least, mutant <u>ras</u> plays a role in tumor progression of human bladder cancer cells, but was not by itself transforming. This result is similar to that obtained by Theodorescu and Kerbel, who showed that mutant <u>ras</u> upgraded cancer cells lines that were subsequently inoculated intravesicularly (36).

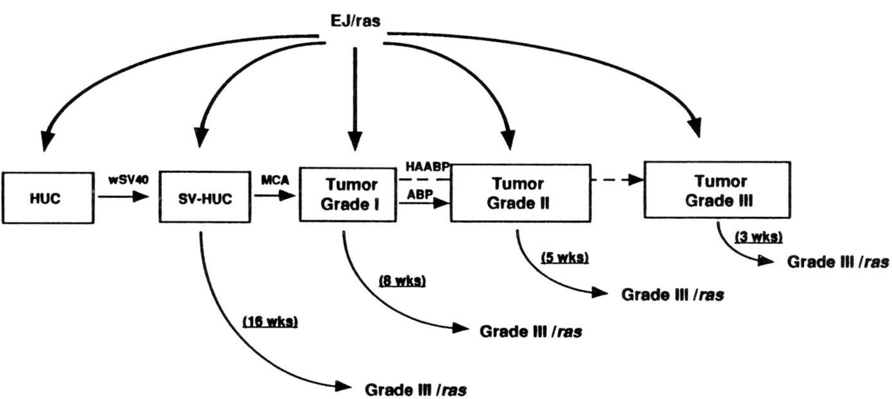


**Figure 6. <u>EJ/ras neoplastic progression of SV-HUC</u>**

## CONCLUSIONS AND FUTURE PERSPECTIVES

Thus, progress has been made in developing a system in which genetic changes associated with tumorigenic transformation and progression can be studied. Such a system will allow studies of mutational inactivation of putative cancer suppressor genes, as well as activation of oncogenes, including <u>ras</u> by relevant bladder carcinogens, such as the arylamines used in this study. Furthermore, this system should be very useful in testing the biological significance of genetic losses in tumorigenesis.

The histopathological phenotypes obtained after <u>in vitro</u> transformation recapitulated changes seen in clinical bladder cancers. However, there were some differences in the relative percentages of tumor types represented. More than 90% of clinical bladder cancers are TCCs, but in our study TCCs, SCCs, and U carcinomas were equally represented. This may reflect the "improper" site of inoculation, or perhaps the transforming agents used. To address the former problem, we in our laboratory are adopting the elegant intravesicular bladder inoculation technique developed by Peter Jones (37).

Uroepithelial cancers obtained after <u>in vitro</u> transformation also recapitulated most of the genetic losses seen in clinical cancers with one rather striking exception. While a high percent of clinical bladder cancers show  LOH 17p, none of the cancers obtained to date using the SV-HUC system showed 17p losses. This may be attributed to the presence of the SV40 viral T-antigen in the immortalized cells. SV40 T antigen binds the protein products of the p53 and RB genes, thus abrogating requirements for their losses in transformation. Therefore, mutational inactivation of the p53 gene by arylamines or other bladder carcinogens cannot be studied using an SV40-immortalized transformation system because these are not required in the presence of an oncoprotein that binds their products (38).

***This brings us to our future perspectives.  A major goal now is to develop a multistep HUC <u>in vitro</u> transformation system without using a viral gene.***

REFERENCES

1.   E. Silverberg, J.A. Lubera. Cancer 38, 5 (1988).
2.   W.F. Whitmore, Jr.  Urol. (Suppl.) 21, 5 (1988).
3.   F.K. Mostofi, C.J. Davis, Jr., I.A. Sesterhenn.
     In:  Advances in Urologic Oncology, pp. 1-20
     (1988).
4.   D. Raghavan, W.U. Shipley, M.B., Garnick, P.J.
     Russell, J.P, Richie. New Engl. J. Med. 322
     (1990).
5.   P.A. Schulte, K. Ringen, et al. J. Occupational
     Med. 27, 115 (1985).
6.   S.H. Moolgavkar, R.G. Stevens. J. Natl. Cancer
     Inst. 67, 15 (1981).
7.   E.J. Zingg, D.M.A. Wallace. Bladder Cancer,
     Springer-Verlag (1985).
8.   P. Vineis, N. Caproraso, et al. Cancer Res. 50,
     3002 (1990).
9.   T. Enomoto, J.M. Ward, A.O. Perantoni.
     Carcinogenesis 11, 2233 (1990).
10.  V.R. Babu, B.J. Miles, et al. Third Inter-
     national Workshop on Chromosomes in Solid
     Tumors, Abstract #27, 29 (1989).
11.  V.R. Babu, M.D. Lutz, et al. Cancer Res. 47,
     6800 (1987).
12.  A.A. Sandberg, C. Turc-Carel, R.M. Gemmill.
     Cancer Res. 48, 1049 (1988).
13.  Y.C. Tsai, P.W. Nichols, et al. Cancer Res. 50,
     44 (1990).
14.  A.F. Olumi, Y.C. Tsai, et al. Cancer Res. 50,
     7081 (1990).
15.  E.R. Fearon, A.P. Feinberg, et al. Nature 318,
     377 (1985).
16.  D. Sidransky, A. Von Eschenbach, et al. Science
     252, 706 (1991).
17.  J.M. Horowitz, S-H. Park, et al. Proc. Natl.
     Acad. Sci. 87, 2775 (1990).
18.  J. Presti, T. Galan et al. Proc. Amer. Assoc.
     Cancer Res. 32, 308 (1991).
19.  E.R. Fearon, B. Vogelstein. Cell 61, 759
     (1990).
20.  C.A. Reznikoff, M.D. Johnson, D.H. Norback,
     G.T. Bryan. In Vitro 19, 326 (1983).
21.  W.W. Schmidt, E.M. Messing, C.A. Reznikoff.
     J. Urol. 132, 1262 (1984).
22.  C.A. Reznikoff, L.J. Loretz, et al. J. Cell.
     Physiol. 131, 285 (1987).
23.  L.J. Loretz, C.A. Reznikoff. In Vitro Cell. &
     Develop. Biol. 24, 333 (1988).

24. C.A. Reznikoff, L.J. Loretz, M.D. Johnson, S. Swaminathan. Carcinogenesis 7, 1625 (1986).
25. B.J. Christian, L.J. Loretz, T.D. Oberley, C.A. Reznikoff. Cancer Res. 47, 6066 (1987).
26. C. Kao, S-Q. Wu, M. Bhatthacharya, L.F. Meisner, C.A. Reznikoff. Submitted.
27. L.F. Meisner, S-Q. Wu, B.J. Christian, C.A. Reznikoff. Cancer Res. 48, 3215 (1988).
28. C.A. Reznikoff, L.J. Loretz, B.J. Christian, S-Q. Wu, L.F. Meisner. Carcinogenesis 9, 1427 (1988).
29. E.A. Bookland, S. Swaminathan, K.W. Gilchrist, R. Oyasu, C.A. Reznikoff. Submitted
30. S-Q. Wu, B.E. Storer, E.A. Bookland, A.J. Klingelhutz, K.W. Gilchrist, L.F. Meisner, R. Oyasu, C.A. Reznikoff. Cancer Res., in press.
31. A.J. Klingelhultz, E.A. Bookland, Genes Chromosomes and Cancer, in press.
32. A.J. Klingelhultz, S-Q. Wu, C.A. Reznikoff. submitted.
33. B.J. Christian, C. Kao, S-Q. Wu, L.F. Meisner, C.A. Reznikoff. Cancer Res. 50, 4779 (1990).
34. C.I. Pratt, R. Oyasu, C.A. Reznikoff. Submitted.
35. C.I. Pratt, M. Bhattacharya, S-Q. Wu, C.A. Reznikoff. Submitted.
36. D. Theodorescu, I. Cornil, et al. Proc. Natl. Acad. Sci. USA 87, 9047 (1990).
37. T.E. Ahlering, L. Dubeau, P.A. Jones. Cancer Res. 47, 6660 (1987).
38. A.J. Levine, J. Momand. Biochim. et Biophys. Acta 1032, 119 (1990).

# MULTIPLE STEPS IN THE *IN VITRO* IMMORTALISATION AND NEOPLASTIC CONVERSION OF HUMAN COLONIC EPITHELIAL CELLS

A.C. Williams, A. Manning, S.J. Harper and C.Paraskeva

Department of Pathology and Microbiology, University of Bristol, School of Medical Sciences, University Walk, Bristol BS8 1TD, U.K.

The development of colorectal cancer is an excellent example of the complex multistep nature of carcinogenesis. A clear premalignant stage has been recognised, the adenoma, from which most colorectal cancers develop. There have been important recent developments in the cellular and molecular biology of colorectal cancer, in particular the mapping of the Familial adenomatous polyposis (FAP) gene to chromosome 5 (1,2) and the realization that both activation of dominantly acting oncogenes (*ras* gene in particular) and loss of tumour suppressor genes are involved in colorectal carcinogenesis. Common genetic alterations that occur during colorectal carcinogenesis include deletions on chromosomes 1, 5, 17, 18 and 22 (reviewed in 3,4). To study colorectal carcinogenesis we have previously isolated epithelial cell lines from  sporadic and FAP adenomas (5, 6) with the following objectives: (i) To develop markers to distinguish the different premalignant adenoma stages (ii) To establish an *in vitro* model for tumour progression by transforming premalignant human colonic adenoma cells to the malignant phenotype. This work is reviewed in this paper.

Complexity of the Precancer Stages: Parameters<br>to Study Tumour Progression

Although in colorectal carcinogenesis a clear premalignant stage, the adenoma, exists it is complicated by there being several histological states of adenomas representing different malignant

*281*

potentials (7).   To distinguish between the different malignant potentials of adenomas, Vogelstein et al. (1988) has classified the adenomas into three different classes, class 1, 2 and 3 (Class 1 having the lowest and Class III the highest malignant potential) and has identified specific molecular changes which occur from the normal through adenoma to carcinoma sequence (3).  One of our aims has been to develop an *in vitro* model system to study the sequential changes involved in the progression from colonic adenoma to carcinoma.  For these studies it is necessary to have markers to distinguish the different stages of progression.  For example, to convert *in vitro* an adenoma cell line with a low malignant potential (class I) to an adenoma cell line with a high malignant potential (class III) it is necessary to be able to identify and/or select for the malignantly more advanced cells.

Clear differences in *in vitro* and *in vivo* behaviour exists when comparing normal cells with cancer cells and the question arises as to the stage in tumour progression when the cells acquire their new characteristics (eg at the early or late precancer stage).   Markers to study tumour progression *in vitro* include: escape from senescence (*in vitro* immortalization), aneuploidy, clonogenicity (the ability to grow after single cell trypsinization), resistance to the inhibitory effects of the differentiation agent sodium butyrate, anchorage independent growth and tumorigenicity in athymic nude mice (8,9)   These markers have been used in our transformation experiments described below.

## Transformation of an Adenoma Cell Line to a Carcinoma in Multiple Steps

Clonal growth.   We have chosen a well characterized adenoma cell line designated PC/AA to study tumour progression in colorectal carcinogenesis the results of which are summarized in Fig 1.  (Figure 1 is taken from Reference 9).  Understanding the events involved in the conversion of the adenoma to carcinoma is important since only the carcinomas metastasize and are therefore often fatal.   PC/AA was originally derived from a single large adenoma of approximately 3-4 cm in diameter from a FAP patient (5)   This cell line, although normal diploid at early passage, had become immortal and shown signs of tumour progression with continuous *in vitro* passage (8) but remained anchorage dependent and non tumorigenic.   Taking advantage of our previous observation that colorectal cancer cell lines will grow clonally (after single cell trypsinization) but the majority of adenoma cultures will not (5,6) we isolated a clonogenic variant of late passage PC/AA designated AA/C1. We argued that a clonogenic variant of PC/AA may represent a later stage in tumour progression and that the AA/C1 adenoma cells are acquiring certain characteristics of cancer cells. AA/C1 remained, however, anchorage dependent and non tumorigenic (9).

Fig. 1.

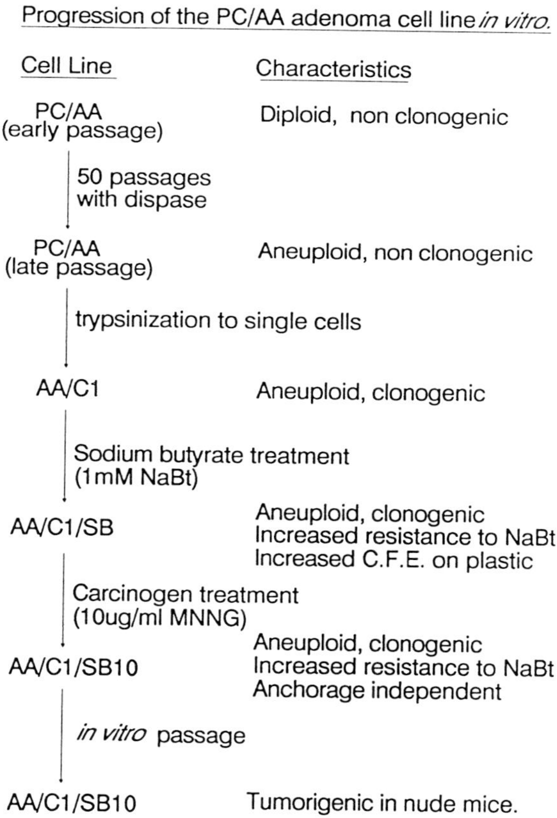


<u>Resistance to the differentiation agent sodium butyrate.</u> Sodium butyrate was investigated because it has been proposed to have a possible role in tumour promotion in human colorectal

carcinogenesis, (10).    Previously, we have reported that the colorectal carcinoma cell lines HT29 and PC/JW are more resistant to the  growth inhibitory effects of sodium butyrate (1mM) than the PC/AA adenoma cells (10).    The AA/C1 cells were therefore treated with sodium butyrate (1mM) in an attempt to isolate cells with increased resistance to sodium butyrate and the cell line AA/C1/SB was obtained.    AA/C1/SB cells were distinguishable from the parent AA/C1 line as they had a higher colony forming efficiency on plastic although they remained anchorage dependent and non tumorigenic.    Interestingly those cells pretreated with 1mM sodium butyrate were insensitive to the inhibitory effects of further treatments with the same concentrations and less sensitive to higher concentrations of sodium butyrate (9).

Growth in Suspension. The malignant conversion of benign tumours requires further genetic changes in the tumour cell.    To transform the adenoma cells to an anchorage independent phenotype both AA/C1 and AA/C1/SB cells were treated with a range of concentrations of the carcinogen N-methyl-N$^1$-nitro-N-nitrosoguanidine (MNNG) (0.1 to 10µg/ml).    The purpose of treating both cell lines was to determine whether the change resulting from the sodium butyrate treatment rendered the cells more susceptible to transformation by MNNG.    When tested for anchorage independence, the only cells able to growth in agarose were the AA/C1/SB cells treated with the high concentration of 10µg/ml MNNG (9).    The anchorage independent line was designated AA/C1/SB10 and the first detectable colony forming efficiency (CFE) in agarose was 0.16% at passage 65.    However, this CFE increased substantially with passage and has so far reached 17.3% at passage 82 (9).

Tumorigenicity in Athymic Nude Mice. The cell lines have been regularly injected into nude mice, and monitored over the following 6 months period for tumorigenicity.    All AA/C1 and AA/C1/SB cells, have remained non tumorigenic (tested up to passage 75). Furthermore, all animals injected with AA/C1/SB10 cells below passage 70 remained tumour free.    A proportion of mice injected with AA/C1/SB10 cells at passage 73 and higher have developed small (approximately 0.5cm$^3$) but persistent tumours at the site of injection which have not increased in size and have not developed into progressively growing tumours. However, a number of mice injected with AA/C1/SB10 cells have developed large progressively growing adenocarcinomas (>1cm$^3$). In summary, from a total of 36 mice injected with AA/C1/SB10 cells from passage 73, ten have developed small but persistent tumours and eleven have gone on to develop large progressively growing tumours at the site of inoculation. Furthermore, the number of mice which develop progressive tumors directly correlates with the passage number of the cells; those mice inoculated with the later passage numbers are more likely to develop the progressive tumour (9).

<u>Chromosome analysis of the cell lines</u>. PC/AA at early passage was diploid and at late passage (passage 50-60) became aneuploid (5,8). The karyotypes from 10 different spreads from each of the cell lines AA/C1, AA/C1/SB and AA/C1/SB10 (between passage numbers 66 and 70) showed that all 3 cell lines were aneuploid and although complex shared common abnormalities. The common abnormalities include the presence of 1-2 copies of an abnormal chromosome 1 as well as 1-2 normal copies of chromosome 1. The abnormal chromosome 1 was originally thought to be a pericentric inversion of chromosome 1 with partial chromosome loss (9). However, c-banding indicated loss of the centromeric heterochromatin of the abnormal chromosome 1 and improved G-banding indicated that the marker chromosome may consist of a translocation involving chromosomes 18 and 1. This was confirmed later by *in situ* hybridization using a biotin-labelled probe for the centromeric region of chromosome 18 (in collaboration with Joy Delhanty, University College, London). Other notable abnormalities include up to 6 copies of chromosomes 7, 9 and 13 and monosomy of chromosome 18 (9). The karyotypes of the late passage tumorigenic AA/C1/SB10 cells indicate a progressive loss of the remaining normal chromosome 18 so that the majority of cells have no normal chromosome 18 (Williams, Hague & Paraskeva - unpublished results).

<u>Summary of Transformation Experiment</u>. The isolation, through multiple steps, of the tumorigenic AA/C1/SB10 cells from the PC/AA adenoma cell line represents the first example of the malignant progression of human colonic adenoma cells *in vitro*. We have just completed a study of the genetic changes which occur during the conversion of the PC/AA adenoma to a carcinoma and have found, quite remarkably, an increase in cellular levels of p53 protein, acquisition of homozygosity of the mutant *K-ras* gene (the parent adenoma cell line PC/AA is heterozygous for *K-ras* gene mutation), a rearrangement at chromosome 1p35 and loss of both normal copies of chromosome 18 (Williams A.C., Marshall C.J., Harper S., Hague A. and Paraskeva C. - manuscript in preparation). This study provides the first reported experimental evidence for the adenoma to

carcinoma sequence and cytogenetic and molecular evidence shows that this *in vitro* progression has some relevance to *in vivo* carcinogenesis. These studies emphasize the remarkable stability of human cells in that it has taken multiple events to convert an already premalignant cell line into a tumorigenic one (9).

## Resistance to Transforming Growth Factor ß and Tumour Progression

Transforming growth factor ß although originally described as a positive growth stimulator can also act as a growth inhibitor depending on the target cell type (11). Although the growth of many normal epithelial cells is inhibited by TGFß their transformed counterparts are often resistant to its inhibitory effects. The resistance of these transformed cell lines to TGFß supports the idea that escape from negative growth control might be an important step during carcinogenesis (11). Although previous studies have indicated that, in general, colorectal cancers are resistant to TGFß there had been no studies with either normal or premalignant human colonic epithelium to rule out the possibility that human colonic epithelium is intrinsically resistant to TGFß.

We have found that three adenoma derived cell lines, AA/C1, RG/C2 and RR/C1, are all significantly inhibited by transforming growth factor ß at concentrations as low as 0.05-0.5ng/ml whereas 5 different colorectal cancer cell lines are resistant to concentrations of TGFß up to 10ng/ml (Fig 2 taken from Manning, Williams, Game & Paraskeva, Oncogene 1991, In Press). Furthermore, the tumorigenic transformed derivatives of AA/C1, designated AA/C1/SB10 (see also above) and AA/C1/SB10M are significantly more resistant to TGFß than the parent adenoma cells up to 10ng/ml TGFß (Fig 2). These studies show that not only are adenoma cell lines significantly inhibited by low concentrations of TGFß (0.5ng/ml) but the conversion of one of these adenoma cell lines *in vitro* to a tumorigenic phenotype is accompanied by a reduced response to the inhibitory effects of TGFß (10ng/ml). The fact that both AA/C1 and RG/C2 were derived from relatively large adenomas (5,6) and that they are both 3T3 feeder dependent, clonogenic and immortal indicates that these cell lines, although anchorage dependent and non-tumorigenic, represent relatively late stage adenomas (ie adenomas with a relatively high malignant potential (6)). Of further interest, both AA/C1 and RR/C1 contain *ras* gene mutations (13 and Williams, Marshall and Paraskeva - unpublished results) which suggests that the presence of *ras* gene mutations do not confer complete resistance to TGFß. These studies indicate that late stage adenomas are still responsive to the growth inhibitory effects of TGFß and that loss of this responsiveness to TGFß occurs at a relatively late stage in colorectal carcinogenesis.

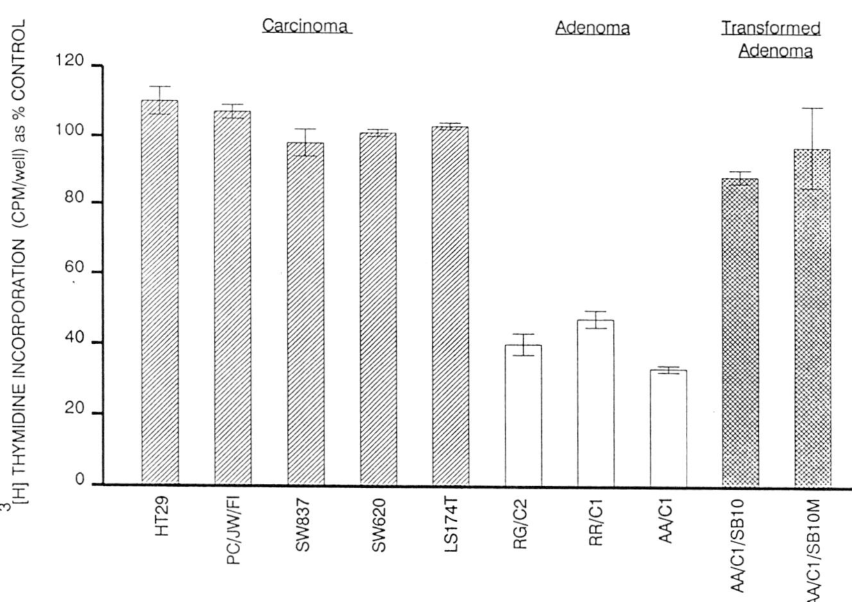



## Figure 2

The effect of 24 hours treatment with 10ng/ml TGFß on DNA synthesis of five colorectal carcinoma cell lines, three adenoma cell lines and two tumorigenic transformed derivatives (AA/C1/SB10 and AA/C1/SB10M) of the adenoma cell line AA/C1; showing the adenoma cells to be significantly more sensitive to the growth inhibitory effects of TGFß than the carcinoma or transformed adenoma cells (taken from Manning et al., Oncogene, 1991, In Press). Similar results were obtained using TGFß at 0.05 - 0.5 ng/ml.

## Carcinogenesis, Cellular Senescence and Chromosome 1

Normal human cells in culture have a limited life-span beyond which the cells cease proliferation and undergo a process termed cellular senescence that results in cell death. Many human cancer derived cell lines have escaped cellular senescence, grow in culture indefinitely and are referred to as immortal. The escape from cellular senescence seems to be an important and central step in carcinogenesis. Recently Barrett and colleagues (14) reported that human chromosome 1q may participate in the control of cellular senescence and that it contains a growth arrest or senescence gene(s). We have also reported that abnormalities involving chromosome 1 may be involved in tumour progression and in the *in vitro* immortalisation of human colorectal adenoma cell lines. These abnormalities can either be deletions on the short arm of chromosome 1(p) or formation of an isochromosome 1(q) resulting in 3 or 4 copies of the long arm of chromosome 1 in each cell (8,12). Molecular analysis has also shown important changes on chromosome 1 in several different cancers including colorectal cancers (3,15). Normal human cells are notoriously stable and they very rarely spontaneously become immortal *in vitro* indicating that several events which may include both the activation of oncogenes and loss of tumour suppressor genes may be necessary before cells escape senescence (14). Consistent with this view is our report that acquisition of *in vitro* immortality is a relatively late event in human colorectal carcinogenesis and that generally only large colorectal adenomas with a high malignant potential (which may have already accumulated 3-5 genetic changes (3)) give rise to immortal cell lines whereas cell cultures derived from small adenoma generally senesce (6,12). The limited life-span of normal human cells under present cell culture conditions does not appear to allow sufficient genetic events to accumulate *in vitro* for the cells to become immortal spontaneously.


## Importance of the Microenvironment in Hereditary Cancer and its Possible Significance to *in vitro* Transformation Systems

We have previously raised the possibility that differences in the *in vivo* microenvironment may result in there being different events involved in the development of sporadic versus hereditary tumours (16). When considering the development of adenomas and carcinomas in FAP patients it is important to remember that every cell in the colon is heterozygous at the FAP locus. Because each cell is heterozygous this has led to the belief that simply by chance there is an increased risk of the development of an adenoma because of the high number of "initiated" or altered target cells, thus making it inevitable that at least one or more of these "initiated" cells will acquire the remaining hit(s) necessary for tumour formation. This would be the case whether or not a further genetic change or tumour promotion is necessary for the development of the benign tumour. However, another possibly important factor is that in hereditary patients each cell, as well as being heterozygous at the FAP locus, is surrounded by cells heterozygous at the same locus. In this situation there are no surrounding normal cells, neither epithelial nor stromal, to restrain or suppress the growth of the FAP cells. In sporadic patients rare somatic mutations giving rise to heterozygosity at the FAP locus will result in altered cells which are surrounded by normal cells. In this situation the influence of the surrounding normal cells may make it less likely for the sporadic heterozygous cell to progress to an adenoma. In sporadic patients the action of a tumour promoter and/or another genetic event may be necessary to allow clonal expansion of the altered cell. This would imply that the local environment within the colon of an FAP patient is more amenable to the growth of the heterozygous cells than the local environment surrounding a heterozygous sporadic cell in a normal colon. Under these conditions it is possible that in the FAP patients the development of the adenomas may not require either a further genetic change or tumour promotion (because they do not require tumour promoters for clonal expansion) whereas in sporadic patients one or more of these other events is necessary (16).

The possible importance of the *in vivo* microenvironment in both hereditary and sporadic cancers has to be considered in the design of *in vitro* transformation assays and carcinogenesis studies in general. In particular *in vitro* systems need to be devised which allow the clonal expansion of rare altered cells and to test for potential tumour promoters. Although a great deal is known about the genetic changes implicated in colorectal carcinogenesis (3,4) very little is known about the possible role of epigenetic changes and tumour promoters and further research in this area is clearly necessary.

This work was supported by grants from the British Cancer Research Campaign and Medical Research Council.

## REFERENCES

1.    W. F. Bodmer, C. J. Bailey, *et al.* <u>Nature</u> (Lond) 328, 614 (1987).

2. M. Leppart, M. Dobbs, *et al*, Science 238, 1411 (1987).

3. E. R. Fearon and B. Vogelstein. Cell 61, 759 (1990).

4. K. W. Kinzler, M.C. Nilbert *et al.* Science 251, 1366 (1991).

5. C. Paraskeva, B. G. Buckle, *et al.* Int. J. Cancer 34, 49 (1984).

6. C. Paraskeva, S. Finerty, *et al.* Cancer Res. 49, 1282 (1989).

7. T. Muto, H.J.R. Bussey, *et al* Cancer 36, 2251 (1975).

8. C. Paraskeva, A. Harvey, *et al.* Int. J. Cancer 43, 743 (1989).

9. A.C. Williams, S. J. Harper, *et al.* Cancer Res. 50, 4724 (1990).

10. R. D. Berry and C. Paraskeva. Carcinogenesis, 9, 447 (1988).

11. A. B. Roberts and M. B. Sporn. Advances in Cancer Res. 51, 107 (1988).

12. C. Paraskeva, Int. J. Cancer 46, 753 (1990).

13. C. J. Farr, C. J. Marshall *et al.* Oncogene 3, 673 (1988).

14. O. Sugarawa, M. Oshimuro, *et al.* Science 247, 707 (1990)

15. I. Leister, A. Weith, *et al.* Cancer Res.. 50, 7232 (1990).

16. C. Paraskeva and A. C. Williams. Br. J. Cancer 61, 828 (1990).


From: *Neoplastic Transformation in Human Cell Culture,*
Eds.: J. S. Rhim and A. Dritschilo ©1991 The Humana Press Inc., Totowa, NJ

# A HUMAN RENAL EPITHELIAL MULTISTEP MODEL OF IN VITRO CARCINOGENESIS


A. Haugen[1], L. Maehle[1], D. Ryberg[1], I. L. Hansteen[2]

[1]Department of Toxicology, National Institute of Occupational Health, P.O.Box 8149 Dep, 0033 Oslo 1, Norway, [2]Department of Occupational Medicine, Telemark Hospital, 3900 Porsgrunn, Norway.


Experimental *in vitro* models to transform human cells should provide clues to the mechanisms of development of human tumors and could identify agents that might cause human cancer. Studies of neoplastic transformation in epithelial cells are critical to an understanding of human cancer since more than 80% of human cancers are of epithelial origin. Human cells are highly resistant to changes in the mechanisms that limit their *in vitro* life span (1,2). Thus, there are few reports describing carcinogen-induced neoplastic transformation of epithelial cells (3,4). *In vitro* models of multistep transformation provide the opportunity to study cells at different stages of the transformation process. Studies strongly suggest that neoplastic transformation, both *in vivo* and *in vitro*, is a multistep process involving events of initiation, promotion and progression (5). Cellular immortality is considered to be one of the first phenotypic changes in this process and can be induced in primary cells by chemical carcinogens or by oncogene transfection. The conversion to the malignant stage is the second critical step. At least some of these stages may involve dominantly-acting genes. There is also evidence that loss or inactivation of several tumor suppressor genes is required for the the initation or progression of certain tumors.

The kidney is a target organ for chemical carcinogenesis. We have recently developed an *in vitro* multistep model for the study of human epithelial carcinogenesis of renal cells (6,7). Relatively little is known about the etiology and kidney cancer. Certain occupational

exposures and cigarette smoking may be implicated in the
disease (8). Kidney cancer is usually sporadic, but may
also occur in a hereditary form (9). The relevance of
cellular *ras* gene activation to human renal cell
carcinoma (RCC) is not well understood. However,
abnormalities in the *ras* gene have been identified in
human RCC (10).

          The environmental and occupational hazards of
metal exposure are of great concern. Epidemiological
studies of workers in industries with nickel exposure and
experimental studies have demonstrated that certain
nickel compounds are potent carcinogens (11). However,
little is known about the mechanisms of carcinogenicity
of nickel compounds.

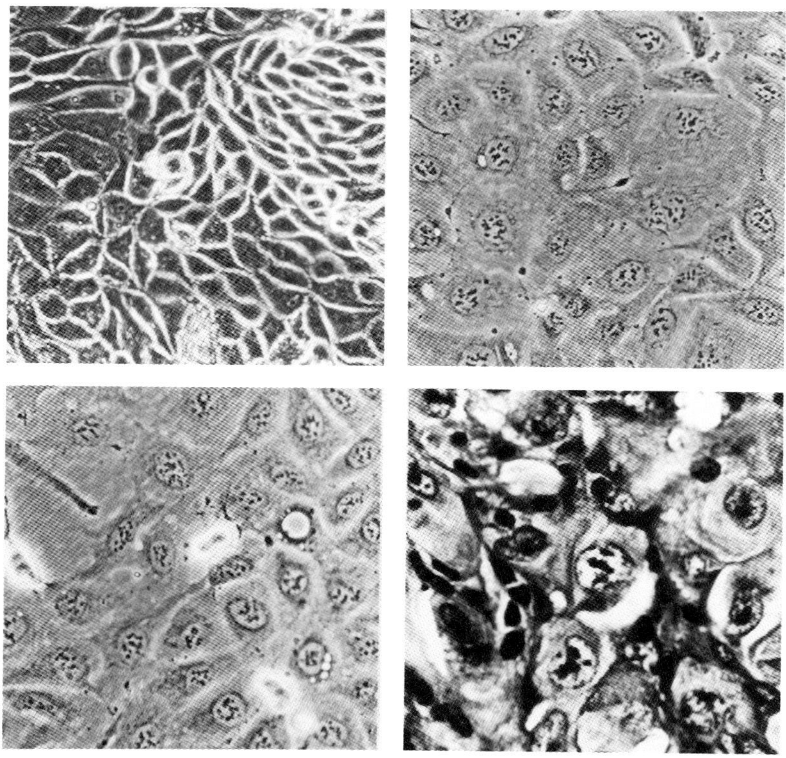

Fig 1 Phase-contrast photomicrographs showing morphology
of (a) NHKE cell; (b) IHKE cells; (c) THKE cells; (d)
Histology of the tumor, hematoxylin and eosin.

Primary cultures of normal human kidney epithelial (NHKE) cells were propagated by the explant outgrowth culture procedure. After 2 weeks epithelial cells had grown out 0.5-1.0 cm around the kidney cortex explant. NHKE cells have polygonal morphology forming domes in confluent cultures. The cells contains the epithelial markers keratin and desmosomes as revealed by electron microscopy and immunofluorescence. NHKE cells were treated with nickel(II) as previously described (6). The initial responses of immortalized human kidney (IHKE) cells to nickel(II) are altered  morphology and immortalization (IHKE cells) after a latent period of 70 to 100 days, but the cells did not undergo malignant transformation. The IHKE cells have reduced serum requirement, increased saturation density and cloning efficiency, and anchorage-independent phenotype. Untreated cells were unable to grow in soft agar. Chromosome preparations revealed a marked variation in chromosome number (range 70-86). Abnormalities of the chromosomes 1,7,9,11,13,14 and 20, increased numer of chromosome 17 and loss of normal chromosomes 20 and 22 were observed. Common for the IHKE cells were many marker chromosomes (6).

Subsequent transfection of IHKE cells with v-Ha-*ras* (pZip-*ras*) (Fig 1) induces the acquisition of neoplastic transformation (tumorigenicity in athymic nude mice).

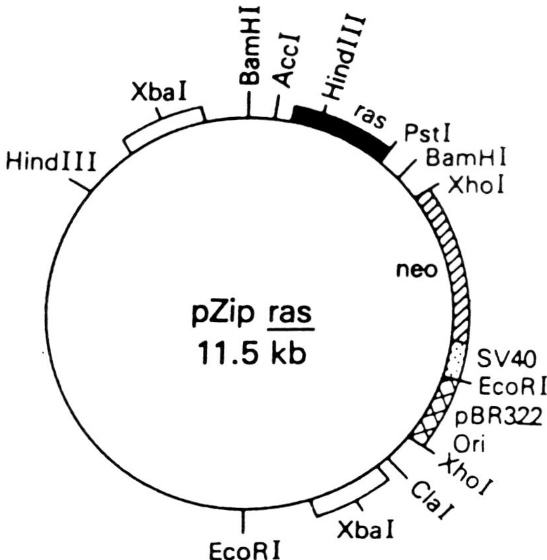


Fig 2 Diagram of the recombinant plasmid

Cells infected into athymic nude mice grew progressively to reach a diameter of more than 1 cm within 13-28 weeks (Table 1). The tumors contained large, irregular cells compatible with experimental renal tumors (fig 1d). IHKE cells and cells transfected with pZipNeoSV(x) did not produce tumors in nude mice. Southern and northern blot analysis of tumor cell lines (THKE) cells showed integration and expression of the v-Ha-*ras* gene in the cells. The 1.4 kd band was absent in the IHKE cells. No transcript homologous to the v-Ha-*ras* sequence was detected in the IHKE cells transfected with pZipNeoSV(X) (Fig 3).

### TABLE 1 – TUMOR FORMATION IN NUDE MICE

| Cell strain or clone | Tumor formation |
| --- | --- |
| IHKZE-C1/pZip*ras* | 4/4 |
| IHKZE-C2/pZip*ras* | 4/5 |
| IHKE/pZipNeoSV(X) | 0/5 |
| IHKE/untransfected | 0/15 |

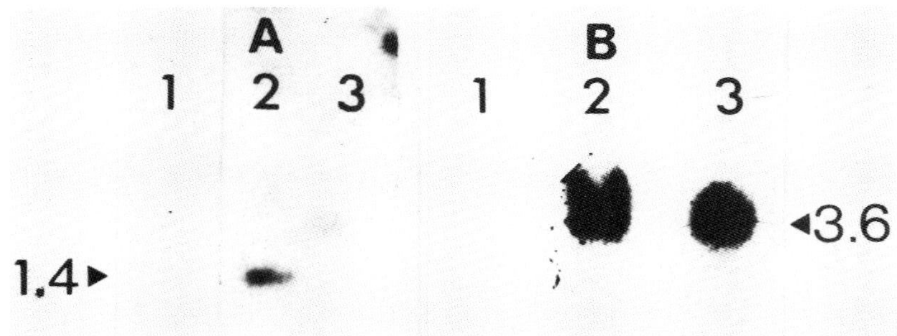


Fig 3 Southern and northern blot analysis (a) DNA from IHKE cells (lane 1); THKE (lane 2); pZipNeoSV(X) transfected IHKE(lane 3).(b) *Ras* transcript in RNA from IHKE cells (lane 1); IHKE transfected with pZip-*ras*, (THKZE)(lane 2); THKE (lane 3).

Chromosomal analysis of the cells revealed modal chromosome number 3n in IHKZE cells and both 4n and 5n in tumor cell lines established *in vitro* from the tumors (THKE cells). The following marker chromosomes were found in both cell lines: MXp(pter- q23), M2p(pter-q21), M6p(pter- q16) and i10q. Rearrangement involving chromosome 3 was found in 2 THKE cell lines. Additional abnormalities were loss of chromosomes 4,8,15,19,20 and 22, and gain of chromosomes 13,17,M1q(p21-qter),M7p(pter-q21),M(20:22)ter rea(20q-22q) (7).

Studies have shown that complete transformation of primary cells requires the collaboration of an immortalization and a transforming agent (3,4). We have shown that *in vitro* treatment with Ni(II) leads to immortalization of NHKE cells after a latency period of 70-100 days. Furthermore, integration of v-Ha-*ras* oncogene is suffic-ient for tumorigenic conversion of the Ni-immortalized cells. A wide variety of chromosomal aberrations were generated by nickel treatment. The cells did not form tumor indicating that the cells are incompletely transformed. It appears likely that a combination of genetic alterations may contribute to the conversion of a normal cell to the malignant state. In an attempt to explore targets of mutations by nickel(II) we examined whether mutations in p53 gene has occurred. The cells were found to contain a mutation in codon 6 (unpublished results). Mutant p53 with alterations in certain conserved areas of the gene have been shown to co-operate with the Harvey *ras* oncogene to transform rat fibroblasts (12).

In conclusion, nickel treatment of NHKE cells results in immortality, but not tumorigenicity. These immortal cells were further converted into malignancy by transfecting the cells with v-Ha-*ras* oncogene consistent with a multistep process leading to a malignant phenotype.

**REFERENCES**


1.    J. A. DiPaolo, <u>J. Natl. Cancer Inst.</u> 70,3 (1983).
2.    C.C. Harris <u>Cancer Res.</u> 47,1 (1987).
3.    J.S. Rhim, G. Jay *et al.* <u>Science</u> 227,1250 (1985).
4.    J.S. Rhim, J. Fujita *et al.* <u>Science</u> 232,338 (1986).
5.    E. Farber and R. Cameron <u>Cancer Res.</u> 31,125 (1980).
6.    G. Tveito, I. L. Hansteen *et al.* <u>Cancer Res.</u> 49, 1829 (1989).
7.    A. Haugen, D. Ryberg, *et al.* <u>Int. J. Cancer</u> 45,572 (1990).

8.    J. K. McLaughlin and L. M. Schuman.  In: A. M.
      Lilienfeld (ed.), Rev. Cancer Epidemiol. Vol. 2,
      170-210, Elsevier/North-Holland, New York (1983.
9.    B. Zbar, H. Branch and M. Linehan <u>Nature</u> 327, 721
      (1987).
10.   J. L. Bos. <u>Mutat. Res.</u> 195, 255 (1988).
11.   R. Doll, J. D. Mathews and L. G. Morgan. <u>Br. J.Med.</u>
      34, 102 (1977).
12.   P. Hinds, C. Finlay and A. J. Levine. <u>J. Virol.</u>
      63,739 (1989).

From: *Neoplastic Transformation in Human Cell Culture,*
Eds.: J. S. Rhim and A. Dritschilo ©1991 The Humana Press Inc., Totowa, NJ

# IMMORTALIZATION AND ONCOGENE TRANSFORMATION OF HUMAN ESOPHAGEAL EPITHELIAL CELLS


Gary D. Stoner[1], Bret A. Light[2], and Curtis C. Harris[2]

[1]Department of Pathology, Medical College of Ohio, Toledo, OH. 43614, [2]Laboratory of Human Carcinogenesis, National Cancer Institute, Bethesda, MD. 20205


## INTRODUCTION

Carcinoma of the esophagus is a disease that shows very striking geographic variations in incidence (1). The highest incidence rates are along the eastern coast of Africa, northern coast of France, southern coast of the Caspian Sea, and in several countries in Asia which comprise the Asian esophageal carcinoma belt. In most countries, the disease is more prevalent in males than in females. In addition, esophageal cancer occurs consistently among the poor in most areas of the world, where the diet is often restricted and nutritional imbalance is common.

Etiological factors associated with the development of esophageal cancer include the smoking and chewing of tobacco (2), consumption of alcoholic beverages (3), and of salt-cured, salt-pickled and moldy foods, especially those contaminated with members of the _Fusarium_ species which produce several toxins (4), and _Geotrichum_ _candidum_ which promotes the formation of nitrosamines (5). Other dietary factors implicated in the etiology of

esophageal cancer are trace elements, vitamins,
tannins, and hot beverages and foods (6).

Histologically, approximately 50-70% of
human esophageal cancers are either poorly or
well differentiated squamous cell carcinomas
(7).  Another 5-10% are adenocarcinomas that
originate either from the esophageal mucus
glands or in regions of the esophagus where
there is preexistent esophageal damage (e.g.,
esophagitis).  The remainder are undifferentiated tumors.

The conversion of normal human esophageal
cells to cancer cells is associated with a
variety of genotypic and phenotypic changes.
Cytogenetic studies with human esophageal
carcinoma cell lines revealed frequent
structural abnormalities (usually deletions) in
chromosomes 1, 3, 9 and 11 (8).  There was
evidence of gene amplification in the form of
homogeneously staining regions and double-
minute chromosomes in both primary and
metastatic tumors (9).  Molecular studies
revealed the amplification of the epidermal
growth factor receptor gene (10), and coamplification of the <u>hst</u>-1 and <u>int</u>-2 genes in
esophageal carcinomas (11).  Elevated levels of
the EGF receptor are associated with the
malignant potential of esophageal tumors (12).
Coamplification of the <u>hst</u>-1 and <u>int</u>-2 genes
has prognostic significance in terms of the
survival of esophageal cancer patients (13).
There is no evidence for point mutations in
codons 12, 13 or 61 in the H-, K- or N-<u>ras</u>
genes in human esophageal cancers (14),
although our laboratory has demonstrated H-<u>ras</u>
activation in codon 12 of N-nitrosobenzyl-
methylamine-induced rat esophageal tumors (15).
The conversion of normal human esophagus to
esophageal carcinoma is also associated with
changes in the profile of keratin proteins (16-
17), and the elaboration of tumor associated

antigens such as human chorionic gonadotrophin, human placental lactogen, alpha-fetoprotein, carcinoembryonic antigen and nonspecific cross-reacting antigen (18).

Normal human cells rarely undergo spontaneous transformation _in vitro_, and they are difficult to transform with carcinogenic agents (19). In our experience, normal human esophageal cells are no exception to this rule (20). In recent years, an approach to the development of human cell systems for studies of _in vitro_ transformation has involved: (a) immortalizing the cells with viral genes introduced by one or more transfection procedures (21), and (b) treatment of the immortalized cells with either chemical carcinogens or transfected oncogenes to achieve transformation to the tumorigenic endpoint (22, 23). This approach was used in the present study to develop an _in vitro_ system for investigations of the neoplastic transformation of normal human esophageal (NHE) epithelial cells. NHE cells were immortalized by transfection with Simian virus-40 (SV40) early region genes, and the immortalized cells were transfected with plasmids containing either an activated K-_ras_ gene or the _hst_-1 gene. Immortalized cells transfected with the _hst_-1 gene but not the K-_ras_ gene acquired the ability to produce tumors in athymic, nude mice. This cell transformation system will be useful for investigating the molecular events associated with the conversion of normal human esophageal epithelial cells to tumorigenic cells.

## MATERIALS AND METHODS

### A. Cell Culture

Normal human esophageal epithelial cells (NHE) were derived from outgrowths of autopsy tissue from noncancerous individuals (20). The outgrowths were subcultured into T-flasks coated with a mixture of fibronectin-collagen-bovine serum albumin as described (20). NHE cells were cultured in esophageal growth medium (EGM) consisting of MCDB 153 basal medium (24) supplemented with 5 ng/ml epidermal growth factor, 1.4 $\mu$M hydrocortisone, 0.1 mM ethanolamine, 0.1 mM phosphoethanolamine, 5 $\mu$g/ml insulin, 40 $\mu$g/ml bovine pituitary extract, 250 $\mu$g/ml bovine serum albumin, and 0.5 $\mu$g/ml epinephrine. The $Ca^{2+}$ concentration was 0.1 mM. Antibiotics (100 units/ml penicillin G, 100 $\mu$g/ml kanamycin, 50 $\mu$g/ml gentamicin) were added as needed. Cultures were monitored for <u>Mycoplasma</u> contamination by culture on anexic agar and by DNA fluorochrome staining of an indicator culture (25). No contamination was detected.

### B. Transfection

Subcultures of NHE cells were transfected with the plasmid, pRSV-T, containing the SV40 early region genes and the Rous sarcoma virus long terminal repeat as described (20). After the appearance of transformed foci, the cells were subcultured and underwent approximately 50-60 population doublings before entering "crisis". After 6-8 months in crisis, a single colony of surviving cells was transferred into a T-flask and subcultured. The subcultured cells eventually developed into a cell line designated HET-1A. HET-1A cells are hypodiploid; sensitive to serum- and $Ca^{2+}$- induced terminal differentiation; contain tonofilaments, immunoactive keratins and SV40T antigen genes; have a doubling time of 26-28 hours; and are nontumorigenic in athymic, nude mice (20). DNA fingerprinting confirmed that HET-1A cells are derived from esophageal epithelium from a single individual (20). To date, HET-1A cells have undergone more than 400 population doublings.

SV40T-antigen-immortalized HET-1A cells were transfected with an activated K-_ras_ gene or the _hst_-1 gene to determine if these oncogenes would convert the cells to the tumorigenic phenotype. Plasmid DNA, pZipNeoSV(X), containing the _hst_ or K-_ras_ oncogenes as well as a neomycin resistance (Neo)gene was coprecipitated with strontium phosphate onto HET-1A cells. Oncogene transfected cultures were allowed to grow to confluency in 100-mm dishes and were then subcultured into T-75 flasks. HET-1A cells that incorporated and expressed pZipNeoSV(X) were selected for by the addition of G418 (100 μg/ml) to the medium for a period of 14 days. This procedure resulted in the development of Neo, K-_ras_ and _hst_-1 transfected HET-1A cell lines that were designated 1A Neo, 1A K-_ras_ and 1A-_hst_-1.

To date, 1A-Neo, 1A-K-_ras_, and 1A-_hst_-1 cell lines have been characterized with respect to morphology (light microscopy), presence of keratin proteins (immunoperoxidase analysis), colony forming efficiency and growth rate (clonal growth assays), and tumorigenic potential (in irradiated, athymic nude mice) according to procedures described before (20). In addition, the presence of the Neo gene, and of the K-_ras_ and _hst_-1 oncogenes in the cell lines was determined by Southern blot analyses. Five μg of DNA from each of cell lines HE-457 (a precrisis line from which the HET-1A cells were derived), HET-1A, 1A-Neo, 1A-K-_ras_ and 1A-_hst_-1 was cut with restriction enzymes and

transferred to nylon membranes.  The membranes
were hybridized with the following radiolabeled
probes: (a) Bam HI-Hind III 1.13 Kb fragment
from pBRNeo for the Neo gene; (b) AatI-Eco
RII 0.3 Kb fragment from pZipNeoSV-v-K-_ras_ for
the K-_ras_ gene; and (c) AvaII-AvaII 0.3 Kb
fragment of pZipNeoSV-_hst_-1 for the _hst_-1 gene.
Finally, the presence of the SV40T-antigen
genes in these cell lines was confirmed by
Southern blot analyses (20).

Table 1 summarizes the properties of HET-
1A, 1A-Neo, 1A-K-_ras_ and 1A-_hst_-1 cell lines.
Analysis of the data indicates that: (a) all
cell lines have morphological and functional
characteristics of epithelial cells; (b) the
profile of SV40T-antigen, Neo, K-_ras_ and _hst_-1
genes in the cell lines is as expected; (c) the
Neo, K-_ras_ and _hst_-1 genes did not influence
the growth rate or colony forming efficiency of
HET-1A cells; and (d) only HET-1A cells
transfected with the _hst_-1 oncogene acquired
the ability to produce tumors following
injection into athymic, nude mice.  The tumors
(1-1.5 cm in diameter) persisted for several
months in the host, but did not acquire the
ability to metastasize.  By histopathology, the
tumors were found to be poorly differentiated
squamous cell lesions with a moderate degree of
invasiveness.  Karyotypic analyses of cell
lines derived from 2 of the 5 tumors showed
that the tumors were composed of human cells
containing marker chromosomes similar to those
observed in HET-1A cells (20).

In summary, an epithelial cell culture
system has now been developed for studies of
the neoplastic transformation of human
esophageal epithelial cells.  NHE cells were
immortalized by transfection with SV40T-antigen
early region genes.  The immortalized cells
acquired tumorigenic potential in nude mice

after transfection with the <u>hst</u>-1 gene but not the K-<u>ras</u> gene.  These results are in agreement with studies of human esophageal squamous cell carcinomas in which the <u>hst</u>-1 gene is amplified and the K-<u>ras</u> gene is not mutationally activated.

Table 1. Properties of HET-1A, 1A-Neo, 1A-K-<u>ras</u> and 1A-<u>hst</u>-1 cell lines.

| Properties | HET-1A | 1A-Neo | 1A-K-<u>ras</u> | 1A-<u>hst</u>-1 |
|---|---|---|---|---|
| Morphology | Epi[a] | Epi | Epi | Epi |
| Keratins | + | + | + | + |
| SV40T-anti-gen gene | + | + | + | + |
| Neo gene | − | + | + | + |
| K-<u>ras</u> gene | − | − | + | − |
| <u>hst</u>-1 gene | − | − | − | + |
| Growth rate (PDT)[b] | 24-26 hrs. | 24-26 hrs. | 24-26 hrs. | 24-26 hrs . |
| CFE[c] | 25-35% | 25-35% | 25-35% | 25-35% |
| Tumori-genicity[d] | 0/20 | 0/10 | 0/10 | 5/10 |

a Epi = epitheloid
b PDT = population doubling time
c CFE = colony forming efficiency
d Data indicate no. of mice with tumor/no. of mice injected with 5 x $10^6$ cells.

REFERENCES

1.  D.M. Parkin, J. Stjernsward, <u>et al.</u> <u>Bull. WHO</u>, 62, 163 (1984).
2.  A.J. Tuyns. In: C.J. Pfeiffer (ed.), Cancer of the Esophagus, p. 3, CRC Press, Inc., Boca Raton, Florida (1982).
3.  A.J. Tuyns, G. Pe'quignot, <u>et al.</u> <u>Bull. Cancer</u>, 65, 69 (1978).
4.  C-C. Hsia, B-L. Tzian, <u>et al.</u> <u>Carcinogenesis</u> 4, 1101 (1983).
5.  M.H. Li, C. Ji, <u>et al.</u> <u>Nutr. Cancer</u>, 8, 63 (1986).
6.  M. Frank-Stromberg. <u>Cancer Nursing</u>, 12, 53 (1989).
7.  S.L. Robbins, R.S. Cotran, <u>et al.</u> In: Pathologic Basis of Disease, p. 804, W.B. Saunders, Philadelphia, 1984.
8.  J. Whang-Peng, S.P. Banks-Schlegel, <u>et al.</u> 45, 101 (1990).
9.  E. Rodriguez, P.H. Rao, <u>et al.</u> <u>Cancer Res.</u>, 40, 6410 (1990).
10. M.C. Hollstein, A.M. Smits, <u>et al.</u> <u>Cancer Res.</u>, 48, 5119 (1988).
11. M. Tsutsumi, H. Sakamoto, <u>et al.</u> <u>Jpn. J. Cancer Res. (Gann)</u> 79, 428 (1988).
12. S. Ozawa, U. Masakazu, <u>et al.</u> <u>Cancer</u> 63, 2169 (1989).
13. Y. Kitagawa, M. Ueda, <u>et al.</u> <u>Cancer Res.</u>, 51, 1504 (1991).
14. T. Victor, R. DuTiot, <u>et al.</u> <u>Cancer Res.</u>, 50, 4911 (1990).
15. Y. Wang, M. You, <u>et al.</u> <u>Cancer Res.</u>, 50, 1591 (1990).
16. S.P. Banks-Schlegel,and C.C. Harris. <u>Cancer Res.</u> 44, 1153 (1984).
17. M.P. Grace, K.H. Kim, <u>et al.</u> <u>Cancer Res.</u>, 45, 841 (1985).
18. C.L. Burg-Kurland, D.M. Purnell, <u>et al.</u> <u>Cancer Res.</u>, 46, 2936 (1986).
19. J.J. McCormick, V.M. Mayer. <u>Mutat. Res.</u>, 199, 273 (1988).

20. G.D. Stoner, M.E. Kaighn, <u>et al.</u> <u>Cancer Res.</u>, 51, 365 (1991).
21. J.S. Rhim, G. Jay, <u>et al.</u> <u>Science</u> 227:1250 (1985).
22. J.S. Rhim, J. Fujita <u>et al.</u> <u>Science</u> 232:338 (1986).
23. C.A. Reznikoff, L.J. Loretz, <u>et al.</u> <u>Carcinogenesis</u>, 9, 1427 (1988).
24. S.T. Boyce, and R.G. Ham  In: M. Webber and L. Sekely (eds.) In Vitro Models for Cancer Research, p. 245, CRC Press, Boca Raton, Florida (1985).
25. R. DelGuidice, and H.E. Hopps. In: G.J. McGarrity, D.G. Murphy, and W.W. Nichols (eds.), Mycoplasma Infection of Cell Cultures, p.57, Plenum Publishers, New York (1987).

# A NON-TUMORIGENIC HUMAN LIVER EPITHELIAL CELL CULTURE MODEL FOR CHEMICAL AND BIOLOGICAL CARCINOGENESIS INVESTIGATIONS

John F. Lechner[1,2], Duane T. Smoot[1], Andrea M. A. Pfeifer[3], Katharine H. Cole[1], Ainsley Weston[1], John D. Groopman[4], Peter G. Shields[1], Takayoshi Tokiwa[1] and Curtis C. Harris[1,5]

[1]Laboratory of Human Carcinogenesis, Division of Cancer Etiology, NCI, NIH, Bethesda, MD 20892; [2]Current address: Inhalation Toxicology Research Institute, P.O. Box 5890, Albuquerque, NM 87158; [3]Nestec Ltd. Research Ctr., Lausanne, Switzerland; [4]The Johns Hopkins University School of Hygiene & Public Health, Baltimore, MD 21205; [5]From whom reprints should be requested: Building 37, Room 2C01, Bethesda, MD 20892, Tel: (301) 496-2048, FAX: (301) 496-0497.

## ABSTRACT

A new medium has been formulated that will support *in vitro* replication of normal human liver epithelial cells for 4 passages (12 population doublings). The replicating cells uniformly contain keratin 18, but keratin 19 is not detectable. In addition, albumin remains discernable in many of the cells throughout their culture life-span. The SV40 large T-antigen gene has been introduced into the genome of cells from six cultures that were initiated from both adult and neonatal donors. The life spans of two of these are indefinite whereas, the others have extended population doubling potentials. The transformed cells have near-normal karyotypes and, initially, they express cytokeratin 18, albumin, and cytochromes. With continued passaging, however, they became positive also for cytokeratin 19 and loose expression of most hepato-specific proteins. However, when incubated as roller cultures, the cells re-acquire the ability to metabolize benzo[a]pyrene, aflatoxin $B_1$, and dimethylnitrosamine to electrophilic derivatives that form carcinogen-DNA adducts. Further, when co-cultured with fibroblasts or on extracted basement membrane material, the cells synthesize albumin and acute phase proteins.

Therefore, by using appropriate culture conditions, the "immortalized" human liver epithelial cells may serve as a useful model for chemical and biological carcinogenesis studies.

## INTRODUCTION

Traditionally, cultures of hepatocytes are initiated at high cell density in media containing 10-20% serum and a few factors such as insulin, glucagon and epidermal growth factor (1-4). These cells remain functional as assessed by measuring hepatocyte functions, *e.g.*, carcinogen metabolism and cell-mediated mutagenesis for 2-7 days. In addition, they carry out extensive repair DNA when exposed to genotoxic agents (4-12). However, cytokinetic events are rare in these cultures. One noticeable departure from this norm was the work of Kaighn and Prince (13), who established clonally-derived cultures of human hepatocytes from fetal, infant and adult donors. An unappreciated features of their cultures was that, although the replicating cells expressed hepatocyte-specific markers, they did not exhibit the typical hepatocyte morphology. Instead, the cells more closely resembled fibroblasts. In retrospect, however, these observations support the hypothesis that there exists a population of cells that is either less differentiated or can undergo "retrograde differentiation" (14) and that these cells are capable of undergoing several divisions *in vitro*. If the "retrograde differentiation" hypothesis is correct then, potentially, the most efficacious approach to establishing replicative cultures of adult human hepatocytes would be to first, develop methods to culture the "retrograde-differentiated liver epithelial cells" and subsequently devise conditions that promote their re-differentiation into hepatocytes.

## RESULTS AND DISCUSSION

Factors and medium additives, *e.g.*, insulin; glucagon; EGF; somatotropin; transferrin; fatty acids; lipoproteins; pyruvate and DMSO have been shown to increase the rate of hepatocyte DNA synthesis *in vitro* (2,3,15-21). In addition, numerous supplements, *e.g.*, cholera toxin, triiodothyronine, bovine pituitary extract, carcinoma cell conditioned medium, and phosphoethanolamine have been shown to enhance the growth of various types of normal human epithelial cells (22). Our medium formulation (LCM; liver cell medium (23)) was designed

Table 1:   LIVER CELL MEDIUM (LCM)

<u>Nutrients</u>:
    PFMR-4 modified to contain:

| | |
|---|---|
| | 0.4mM calcium; |
| | 0.3mM ornithine; |
| | 0.0mM arginine. |

<u>Hormones and Factors</u>:

| | |
|---|---|
| Insulin | 10.4mg/ml |
| Epidermal growth factor | 5.0ng/ml |
| Transferrin | 10.0$\mu$g/ml |
| Cholera toxin | 25.0ng/ml |
| Hydrocortisone | 0.2$\mu$M |
| Triiodothyronine | 10.0nM |
| Retinoic acid | 10.0nM |

<u>Other Additives</u>:

| | |
|---|---|
| Phosphoethanolamine | 0.5$\mu$M |
| Ex-Cyte V[a] | 312.0$\mu$g/ml |
| Bovine pituitary extract[b] | 7.5$\mu$g/ml |
| Chemically-denatured serum[c] | 10.0% |
| Hep-G2 conditioned medium[d] | 35.0% |

[a]Miles Diagnostics, Pentex Products.
[b]Prepared as described in (49).
[c]Prepared as described in (36).
[d]Prepared by incubating 80% confluent Hep-G2 human hepato-blastoma cells in LCM (without the conditioned medium) for 3 days. The conditioned medium is filter sterilized before use.

---

to incorporate much of this literature.  The basal nutrients are a version of Ham's F12 (24), referred to as PFMR-4 (25) except that the PFMR-4 formula has been modified to be: without arginine; the $[Ca^{2+}]$ reduced to 0.4mM; having 0.3mM ornithine; and arbitrarily supplemented with the additives shown in Table 1.

Normal human hepatocytes are obtained by collagenase/dispase perfusion (9) of the lower lobe of livers of non-cancerous "immediate autopsy" donors (26).  The cells are inoculated at a moderate cell density of 6,700 cells/cm$^2$ into flasks that had been precoated with Vitrogen® collagen (23). The cells are incubated over night in Waymouth's medium (27) containing 10% serum.  The next day they are rinsed and the medium is replaced LCM.  Within a few days, sporadic mitotic cells are be seen throughout the cultures.  The cells (Figure

1) will undergo as many as four successive (1:4 split ratio) subculturing or an estimated 12 population doublings, with a cell doubling time of 3 days, before division ceases. 3$^{rd}$ passage cells are uniformly positive for keratin 18 but negative for keratin 19, a keratin species not found in hepatocytes but present in ductal cells (28,29). In addition, 30-50% of the same passage cells express human albumin.

The SV40 large T-antigen gene has been introduced into the genome of cells from six cultures that were initiated from both adult and neonatal donors. Cells from the first, second and third donors were transfected with a DNA construct containing the SV40 T-antigen gene linked to the Rous sarcoma virus LTR (30). The forth and fifth donor's cells were transformed by the zip vector infection technique (31), and the sixth donor's cells by lipofection (32) of the above SV40 T-antigen gene plasmid construct. Foci of cells with morphologies varying from epithelial-like to fibroblastic-like were discernible using all of these protocols 6-8 weeks later. The transformed cultures are denoted THLE-#, for "transformed human liver epithelial-#). The THLE-0 culture was lost during third passage due to an incubator accident. We attempted to isolate and subculture individual clones of THLE-1 cells. However, these efforts were unsuccessful; the cells were exceptionally sensitive to cell dissociating enzymes and they consistently sloughed from the culture dish

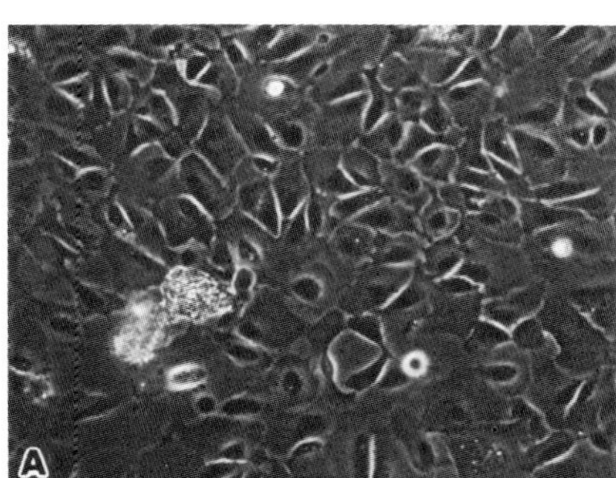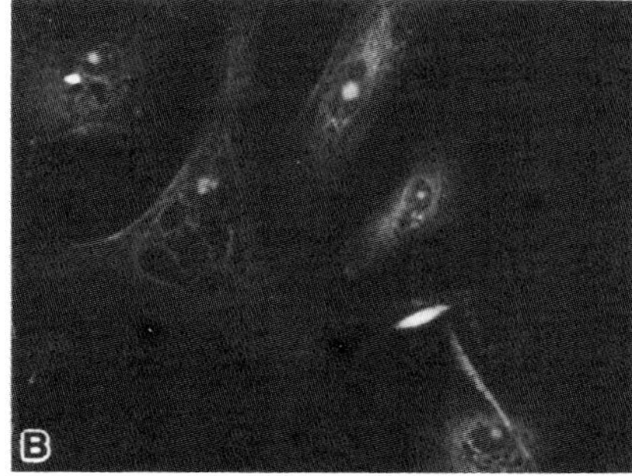

<u>Figure 1</u>   Photomicrographs of human liver epithelial cells. 1a, second passage culture; note mitotic figure (arrow). 1b, immunostaining for keratin 18 of third passage cells.

surface within two days after having been sub-cultured. Therefore, the remaining colonies were pooled as a mass culture. THLE-1 cells initially underwent 4 sub-culturings where upon mitotic figures became non-discernable. Ornithine was then replaced with arginine and the cells recommenced replicating. In arginine-containing LCM, the cells continued to grow until they entered irreversible senescence at the $11^{th}$-$12^{th}$ passage (1:4 split ratio).

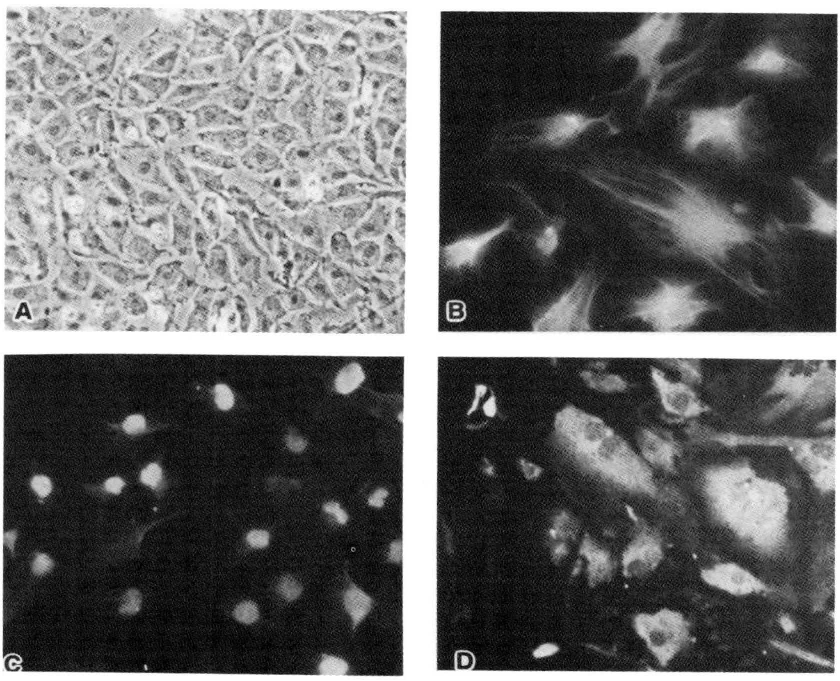

<u>Figure 2</u>  Photomicrographs of SV40 T-antigen gene immortalized human liver epithelial cells THLE-2. la, fifth passage cells; lb, immunostaining for keratin 18; lc, immunostaining for SV40 T-antigen gene; ld, immunostaining for human albumin.

THLE-1 cells would not form colonies even when incubated in arginine-containing LCM; thus, their clonal growth rate could not be measured. However, 5th passage moderately dense cultures exhibited a mean generation time of 36 hrs. When THLE-1 cells were examined at the 3rd passage, roughly 30% of the cells expressed the SV-40 T-antigen gene and virtually 100% of the cells expressed the SV40 T-antigen in their nuclei two passages later. Passage 3 cells were uniformly positive for keratin 18 and negative for keratin 19, suggesting that the cells arose from hepatocytes or from cells of the hepatocyte lineage. However, even though the cells were 100% positive for keratin 18 at the 10th passage, 30% of the cells also exhibited keratin 19. Transferrin, fibrinogen and albumin expression was ascertained using 10th passage cells. None of the cells showed evidence of transferrin or fibrinogen. On the other hand, 20% of the cells were positive for albumin. These albumin expressing cells were always found in clusters of 8-12 cells and analogous to what has been reported for rat liver epithelial cells (33), the number of albumin positive cells increased to 30-40% if the cells were incubated for 48 hrs in medium supplemented with 10% serum.

THLE-1 cells undergo senescence after 40-45 population doublings. Thus, the majority of our efforts have been focused on THLE-2 (Figure 2) and THLE-3 cells, which exhibit indefinite population doubling potentials (THLE-4 and THLE 5 cells are recent additions to our collection and have not been in culture long enough to evaluate their culture life-span potentials). The karyotypes of THLE-2 and THLE-3 cells are near diploid. In addition, and in similarity to THLE-1 cells, both THLE-2 and THLE-3 cells were initially keratin 18 positive and keratin 19 negative but with passage express both keratins. In contrast to THLE-1 cells, both THLE-2 and THLE-3 cells will form colonies; their colony forming efficiencies are 35% and 20%, respectively and their corresponding clonal growth rates are 1.3 and 0.9 population doublings/day. However, like THLE-1 cells, numerous attempts to dissociate and subculture individual clones of either THLE-2 or THLE-3 cells (using trypsin or dispase or collagenase or simple scraping) have been unsuccessful.

The clonal growth requirements of THLE-2 and THLE-3 cells have been evaluated using single medium supplement elimination experiments. The data using early passage THLE-2 cells is shown in Figure 3; except for the effects of serum and TGF-$\beta_1$, results with +20th passage THLE-2 and THLE-3 cells were similar. Note that significant growth did not occur if the medium was devoid of arginine of if serum or TGF-$\beta_1$ were added to the medium (neither serum nor TGF-$\beta_1$ inhibited growth of +20 passage THLE-2 or THLE-3 cells). Also, the data in Figure 3 show that some of the additives in LCM are actually detrimental for optimal growth (comparable experiments remain to be conducted using normal human liver epithelial cells). In contrast, clonal growth was minimal to absence if the medium was not supplemented with THLE-2 conditioned medium (see dose-response, Figure 4) or chemically-denatured serum (34-36) (see dose-response, Figure 5). On the other hand, THLE-3 cell conditioned medium was markedly less effective in promoting clonal growth. Thus for culturing the transformed liver epithelial cells, the medium was modified such that arginine was present, cholera toxin, retinoic acid and ex-cyte were eliminated and Hep-G2 cell conditioned medium was replace with medium conditioned by THLE- cells.

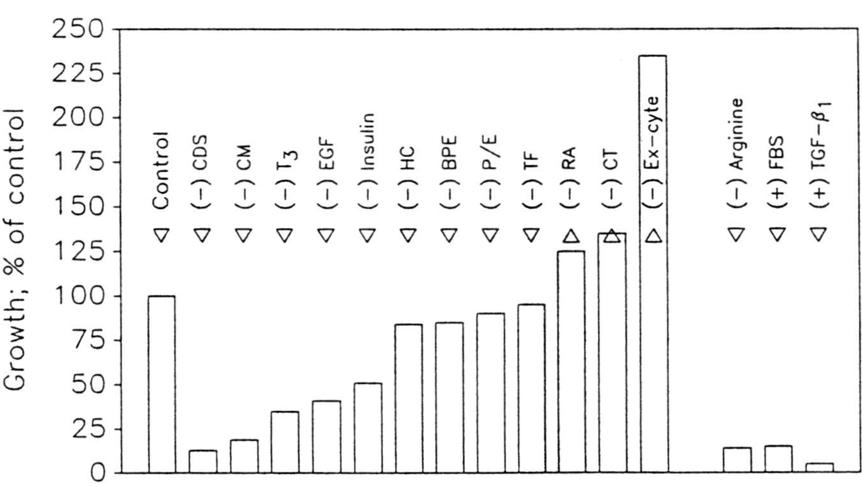



**Figure 3**  Effect of medium supplement elimination on clonal growth rate of THLE-2 cells.

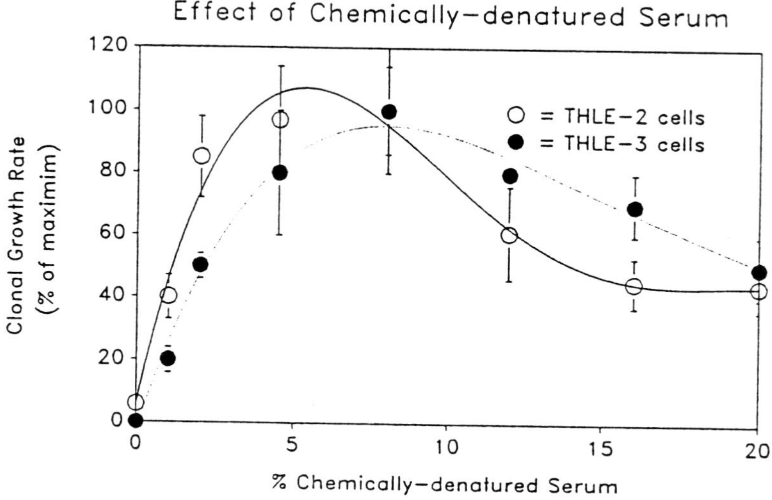


**Figure 4**  Clonal growth dose-response for THLE-2 cells for THLE-2 cell conditioned medium.

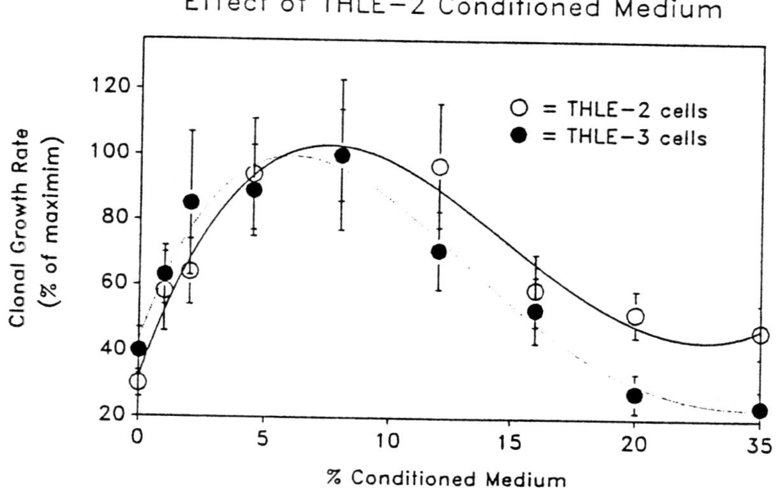


**Figure 5**  Clonal growth dose-response for THLE-2 cells for chemically-denatured serum (36).

The second assumption of our hepatocyte culture strategy is that it should be possible to devise techniques and media that promote the cells to express differentiated hepatocellular characteristics. High concentrations of amino acids, hyperosmolality, TGF-$\beta_1$, bioresponse modifying peptides, DMSO, sodium butyrate, collagen matrices, basement membranes and co-culturing with rat liver oval cells are known culture conditions that promote the expression of liver-specific proteins (2,37-46). Thus, prior to initiating our *in vitro* differentiation experiments, there was considerable information in the literature to guide our efforts. The first technique evaluated was the collagen/fibroblast mesenchyme "tissue equivalent" matrix technique described by Bell and associates (47). No expression of albumin could be detected when either THLE-2 or THLE-3 cells were incubated on these matrices. However, elaboration of ferritin by THLE-2 cells was increased from 10 $\mu$g/ml/$10^6$ cells/24hrs when the cells were incubated on plastic surfaces to 17.2 $\mu$g/ml/$10^6$ cells/24hrs when attached to these matrices. On the other hand, preparation of these matrices is complex and a comparable increases in ferritin elaboration was noted by incorporating DMSO into the medium. We have also evaluated "transwell membrane" technology using Costar® transwell membrane chambers. Ferritin elaboration by cultures incubated on these membranes is double that expressed when the cells are incubated on cell culture plastic surfaces. However, when human foreskin fibroblasts are present on the under surface of the membrane, ferritin levels in the medium increase to 66 $\mu$g/ml/$10^6$ cells/24hrs. Finally, both THLE-2 and THLE-3 cells become positive for human albumin, as assessed by immuno-specific histochemical staining when incubated on commercial basement membrane extract (Matrigel®).

In order for the immortalized cells to truly efficacious for chemical carcinogenesis studies, they should also be capable of metabolizing pro-carcinogenic compounds to electrophilic forms that adduct to cellular DNA. Again, initial investigations (Table 2) have revealed that DNA-carcinogen adducts can be detected in these cells if incubated under appropriate culture conditions. Specifically, Aflatoxin $B_1$ and benzo[a]pyrene adducts are low to absent if the cells are incubated as monolayers. However, as roller cultures, both of these pro-carcinogens form significant levels of adducts. Also, although DNA adducts are formed when monolayer cultures are incubated with

Table 2:  EFFECT OF CULTURE CONDITION ON DNA-ADDUCT FORMATION
IN HUMAN LIVER EPITHELIAL CELLS (preliminary results)

<u>AFLATOXIN B$_1$</u>
THLE-2 cells
    Flask                                    0.0   fmole / $\mu$g DNA
    Flask + Arochlor                         0.0   fmole / $\mu$g DNA

    Roller bottle                            0.39  fmole / $\mu$g DNA
    Roller bottle + Arochlor                 0.35  fmole / $\mu$g DNA

THLE-3 cells
    Flask                                    0.0   fmole / $\mu$g DNA
    Flask + Arochlor                         0.0   fmole / $\mu$g DNA

    Roller bottle                            0.38  fmole / $\mu$g DNA
    Roller bottle + Arochlor                 0.27  fmole / $\mu$g DNA

<u>DIMETHYLNITROSAMINE</u>
THLE-2 cells
    Flask                                   40.0   fmole / $\mu$g DNA
    Roller bottle                          105.7   fmole / $\mu$g DNA

THLE-3 cells
    Flask                                   --------------------
    Roller bottle                           17.4   fmole / $\mu$g DNA

<u>BENZO[A]PYRENE</u>
THLE-2 cells
    Flask                                    0.0   fmole / $\mu$g DNA
    Flask + Arochlor                         0.0   fmole / $\mu$g DNA

    Roller bottle                            1.5   fmole / $\mu$g DNA
    Roller bottle + Arochlor                 7.0   fmole / $\mu$g DNA

THLE-3 cells
    Flask                                    6.7   fmole / $\mu$g DNA
    Flask + Arochlor                         --------------------

    Roller bottle                            6.62  fmole / $\mu$g DNA
    Roller bottle + Arochlor                 9.5   fmole / $\mu$g DNA
    Roller bottle + benzflavone              0.0   fmole / $\mu$g DNA

dimethylnitrosamine, the amount of adduct markedly increases when the cells are cultured in roller bottles. This observation reflects the earlier observations of Kaighn and Prince (13), who showed that roller-culture conditions caused higher expressions of liver-specific proteins by cultures of normal human liver epithelial cells; we will extent these studies and also assess the effects of roller-culture conditions of expression of hepato-specific proteins as well.

The p450 enzymes involved in the metabolism of aflatoxin $B_1$, dimethylnitrosamine and benzo[a]pyrene await to be determined. Preliminary Northern blotting has shown only the presence of the mRNA for the IA1 cytochrome. However, the relative intensity of the message is increased in cells exposed to benzo[a]pyrene and arochlor relative to only benzo[a]pyrene. On the other hand, the adduct data (Table 2) suggests that cytochromes in addition to p450IA1 maybe functioning in these cells. Specifically, arochlor does not affect adduct formation by aflatoxin $B_1$. In addition, a role for p450IA2 is suggested since benzflavone abolishes benzo[a]pyrene adduct formation (48). However, further experimentation is required to validate these interpretations of the data in Table 2.

In conclusion, we have devised (at least minimal) culture conditions for replicative cultures of normal human liver epithelial cells. In addition, some of these cultures have been transformed to apparently immortal forms that are non-tumorigenic. Finally, by adjusting culture conditions, these immortal human liver epithelial cells can be induced to express some hepato-specific proteins and metabolize pro-carcinogens to electrophilic forms that adduct with cellular DNA.

REFERENCES


1. M.A. Sells, J. Chernoff, A. Cerda, *et al*. <u>In Vitro Cell Dev. Biol</u>. 21, 216 (1985).

2. N.C. Luetteke, G. Michalopoulos. In: The Isolated Hepatocyte: Use in Toxicology and Xenobiotic Biotransformation, E.J. Rauckman, G.M. Padilla, eds. (Academic Press, New York, 1987), pp. 93-118.

3. D. Acosta, D. Anuforo, D.B. Mitchell, K.S. Santone, K.F. Nelson, <u>Lab. Animal</u>, 31 (1985).

4. S.C. Strom, D.K. Monteith, K. Manoharan, A. Novotny. In: The Isolated Hepatocyte: Use in Toxicology and Xenobiotic Biotransformation, E.J. Rauckman, G.M. Padilla, eds. (Academic Press, New York, 1987), pp. 265-280.

5. N.L. Bucher. In: The Isolated Hepatocyte: Use in Toxicology and Xenobiotic Biotransformation, E.J. Rauckman, G.M. Padilla, eds. (Academic Press, New York, 1987), pp. 1-19.

6. K.E. Cole, T.W. Jones, M.M. Lipsky, B.F. Trump, I.C. Hsu, <u>Carcinogenesis</u> 10, 139 (1989).

7. H. Autrup, C.C. Harris, S.M. Wu, *et al*. <u>Chem. Biol. Interact</u>. 50, 15 (1984).

8. D. Ratanasavanh, P. Beaune, G. Baffet, *et al*. <u>J. Histochem. Cytochem</u>. 34, 527 (1986).

9. I.C. Hsu, M.M. Lipsky, K.E. Cole, C.H. Su, B.F. Trump, <u>In Vitro</u> 21, 154 (1985).

10. K.E. Cole, I.C. Hsu, B.F. Trump, <u>Cancer Res</u>. 46, 1290 (1986).

11. I.C. Hsu, C.C. Harris, M.M. Lipsky, S. Snyder, B.F. Trump, <u>Mutat. Res</u>. 177, 1 (1987).

12. K.E. Cole, T.W. Jones, M.M. Lipsky, B.F. Trump, I.C. Hsu, <u>Carcinogenesis</u> 9, 711 (1988).

13. M.E. Kaighn, A.M. Prince, <u>Proc. Natl. Acad. Sci. USA</u> 68, 2396 (1971).

14. N. Fausto, J. E. Mead, <u>N. Y. Acad. Sci.</u> 593, 231 (1990).

15. H.L. Leffert, K.S. Koch, P.J. Lad, H. Skelly, B. de Hemptinne. In: Hepatology: A Textbook of Liver Diseases, D. Zakim, T.D. Boyer, eds. (W.B. Saunders Co., Philadelphia, 1982), pp. 64-75.

16. F. Ballet, M.E. Bouma, S.R. Wang, N. Amit, J. Marais, R. Infante, <u>Hepatology</u> 4, 849 (1984).

17. J.L. Cruise, G. Michalopoulos, <u>J. Cell Physiol</u>. 125, 45 (1985).

18. N. Fausto, J.E. Mead, <u>Lab. Invest</u>. 60, 4 (1989).

19. M. Chessebeuf, P. Padieu, <u>In Vitro</u> 20, 780 (1984).

20. M. Salas-Prato, J.F. Tanguay, Y. Lefebvre, *et al*. <u>In Vitro Cell Dev. Biol</u>. 24, 230 (1988).

21. I. Isom, I. Georgoff, M. Salditt-Georgieff, J.E. Darnell,Jr., <u>J. Cell Biol</u>. 105, 2877 (1987).

22. D. Barnes, G. Sato, <u>Anal. Biochem</u>. 102, 255 (1980).

23. J.F. Lechner, K.E. Cole, R.R. Reddel, L. Anderson, C.C. Harris, <u>Cancer Detect. Prev</u>. 14, 239 (1989).

24. R. G. Ham, <u>Proc. Nat. Acad. Sci. USA</u> 53, 288 (1965).

25. J.F. Lechner, M.S. Babcock, M.M. Marnell, K.S. Narayan, M.E. Kaighn. In: Methods in Cell Biology, C.C. Harris, B.F. Trump, G.D. Stoner, eds. (Academic Press, Inc., New York, 1980), pp. 195-225.

26. B.F. Trump, C.C. Harris, <u>Hum. Pathol</u>. 10, 245 (1979).

27. C. Waymouth, <u>J. Nat. Cancer. Inst.</u> 22 1003 (1959).

28. W.W. Franke, D. Mayer, E. Schmid, H. Denk, E. Borenfreund, <u>Exp. Cell Res</u>. 134, 345 (1981).

29.  L. Germain, M.J. Blouin, N. Marceau, <u>Cancer Res</u>. 48, 4909 (1988).

30.  R.R. Reddel, Y. Ke, B.I. Gerwin, *et al.* <u>Cancer Res</u>. 48, 1904 (1988).

31.  A. Pfeifer, G.E. Mark, L. Malan-Shibley, S.L. Graziano, P. Amstad, C.C. Harris, <u>Proc. Natl. Acad. Sci. USA</u> 86, 10075 (1989).

32.  P. L. Felgner, T. R. Gadek, *et al.* <u>Proc. Nat. Acad. Sci. USA</u> 84 7413 (1987).

33.  J.B. McMahon, W.L. Richards, A.A. del Campo, M.K. Song, S.S. Thorgeirsson, <u>Cancer Res</u>. 46, 4665 (1986).

34.  E.J. van Zoelen, T.M. van Oostwaard, S.W. de Laat, <u>J. Biol. Chem</u>. 261, 5003 (1986).

35.  E.J. van Zoelen, T.M. van Oostwaard, P.T. van der Saag, S.W. de Laat, <u>J. Cell Physiol</u>. 123, 151 (1985).

36.  M.A. LaVeck, A.N.A. Somers, L.L. Moore, B.I. Gerwin, J.F. Lechner, <u>In Vitro</u> 24, 1077 (1988).

37.  R.C. Jambou, J.N. Snouwaert, G.A. Bishop, J.R. Stebbins, J.A. Frelinger, D.M. Fowlkes, <u>Proc. Natl. Acad. Sci. USA</u> 85, 9426 (1988).

38.  M.R. Hill, R.D. Stith, R.E. McCallum, <u>J. Immunol</u>. 137, 858 (1986).

39.  H. Baumann, R.E. Hill, D.N. Sauder, G.P. Jahreis, <u>J. Cell Biol</u>. 102, 370 (1986).

40.  P.E. Schwarze, A.E. Solheim, P.O. Seglen, <u>In Vitro</u> 18, 43 (1982).

41.  R. Enat, D.M. Jefferson, N. Ruiz-Opazo, Z. Gatmaitan, L.A. Leinwand, L.M. Reid, <u>Proc. Natl. Acad. Sci. USA</u> 81, 1411 (1984).

42.  B. Clement, C. Guguen-Guillouzo, J.P. Campion, D. Glaise, M. Bourel, A. Guillouzo, <u>Hepatology</u> 4, 373 (1984).

43. J.C. Dunn, M.L. Yarmush, H.G. Koebe, R.G. Tompkins, <u>FASEB J</u>. 3, 174 (1989).

44. T. Tokiwa, M. Miyagiwa, Y. Kusaka, A. Muraoka, J. Sato, <u>Cell Biol. Int. Rep</u>. 12, 131 (1988).

45. T. Nakagawa, Y. Nakao, T. Matsui, *et al*. <u>Br. J. Cancer</u> 51, 357 (1985).

46. E.G. Bade, B. Nitzgen, <u>In Vitro. Cell Dev. Biol</u>. 21, 245 (1985).

47. E. Bell, H.P. Ehrlich, D.J. Buttle, T. Nakatsuji, <u>Science</u> 211, 1052 (1981).

48. M. E. McManus, W. M. Burgess, *et al*. <u>Cancer Res.</u> 50, 3367 (1990).

49. J.F. Lechner, M.A. LaVeck, <u>J. Tissue Culture Meth</u>. 9, 43 (1985).

From: *Neoplastic Transformation in Human Cell Culture,*
Eds.: J. S. Rhim and A. Dritschilo ©1991 The Humana Press Inc., Totowa, NJ

# ESTABLISHMENT AND CHARACTERIZATION OF

# SV40 T-ANTIGEN IMMORTALIZED HUMAN LIVER CELLS

Masayoshi **Namba**, Yoshio **Kano**,
Li-yan **Bai**, Koichiro **Mihara**,
and Masahiro **Miyazaki**

Department of Cell Biology
Institute for Cellular and Molecular Biology
Okayama University Medical School
2-5-1 Shikata, Okayama 700, Japan

SUMMARY: Human liver cells derived from an
embryo were transfected with SV40 early region
(T) DNA and two cell lines, OUMS-21 and OUMS-22,
were established. The cells of these lines were
SV40 T-antigen positive, epithelial-like,
immunoreactive against an anti-keratin 18
monoclonal antibody and produced serum albumin
in the culture medium. Karyotypic analysis
showed OUMS-21 to be diploid (42-47) with a
modal number of 44, whereas OUMS-22 was
hypotetrapoid (66-104) with a modal number of
83. No marker chromsomes were found in these
cell lines. Both lines were sensitive to
cytotoxicity of aflatoxin B1, Trp-P-1(3-amino-
1,4-dimethyl-5H-pyrido[4,3-b]indole), and
benzo[a]pyrene. These results indicate that
these cells have enzymes to activate these
carcinogens to proximate ones. The cells showed
0.2 to 1.2% cloning efficiency in soft agar, but
they were not tumorigenic when transplanted into
nude mice. Upon treatment with Harvey murine
sarcoma virus, the cells acquired
tumorigenicity in nude mice.

## INTRODUCTION

Since most human cancers develop from epithelial cells, in vitro studies utilizing human epithelial cells are ideal for analyzing the progressive multistep process of carcinogenesis of human cells. Along this line, studies on neoplastic transformation have been carried out using several types of human epithelial cells derived from the skin, cervix, breast, prostate, kidney, urinary tract, esophagus, colon, bronchus and trachea (1-12). In these studies, mostly SV40 virus DNAs and some papilloma virus DNAs were used to immortalize normal cells, which were further transformed neoplastically by ras oncogenes or chemicals. Without these oncogenic DNA viruses, immortalization of normal human epithelial cells would very rarely occur (13- 16). Recent reports also show a certain relationship between papilloma viruses and cervical cancers.

To our knowledge, there have been no reports concerning the transformation of human liver cells. Hepatocellular carcinoma is one of the most common human cancers in Africa, Southeast Asia, China, Korea and Japan. Although a strong correlation exists between chronic infection with hepatitis viruses and the development of hepatoma, the actual mechanism of the carcinogenesis of liver cells remains unknown.

To investigate the developmental mechanisms of human liver cancer, a model system for studies of the in vitro neoplastic transformation of human liver cells must be established. Since normal human liver cells have no ability to grow in culture at present, even when various sophisticated culture media are used, our strategy was first to immortalize human liver cells by introducing transforming viral genes into the cells. To achieve this, we introduced SV40T DNA into normal human liver cells in the primary culture and established immortalized cell lines. In this paper, we

describe the immortalization process, some
cellular characteristics of these cells, and
neoplastic transforamtion of the cells with
Harvey murine sarcoma virus.

## MATERIALS AND METHODS

<u>Cells and Cultures</u>: Liver tissue from an 18-
week-old embryo was minced with two crossed
scalpels and digested with 0.05% type I
collagenase. Cells obtained by the digestion
were washed with phosphate buffered saline(PBS,
pH 7.2) and seeded onto collagen-coated dishes.

<u>Transfection and Isolation of Transformed Cell
Lines</u>: Confluent cultures (about 4 x $10^6$
cells /10 cm dish) were transfected with 40 µg
supercoiled pSV3neo DNA (SV40 T) by calcium
phosphate/DNA coprecipitation on day 2 after the
initiation of the culture. After incubation for
four hours, the cells were washed with serum-
free culture medium and maintained in a culture
medium consisting of RPMI-1640 supplemented with
10% fetal calf serum, 0.2% lactalbumin
hydrolysate, 10 µM dexamethasone and 10 µg/ml
insulin. The next day the cells were
subcultured and two weeks later 100 µg/ml G418
was added to the cultures for four days to
select transformed cells.

<u>Determinations of Cell Growth and Cloning
Efficiency in Soft Agar, Chromosome Analysis,
and Transplantation</u>: The methods of these
experiments have been described in detail
elsewhere (17).

<u>Immunofluorescene</u>: To detect SV40 T antigen,
cells grown on coverslips were fixed wih acetone
for 15 min at room temperature and stained with
a hamster antibody against SV40 T antigen. For
keratin studies, cells grown on coverslips were
fixed in methanol/acetone (3/1, v/v) at $-20^0$C
for 20 min and air dried. Fixed cells were
then reacted with keratin mouse monoclonal
antibodies (KL 1; Immunotech, CK5; Sigma,

RPN.1162;    Amersham),    washed    in    PBS,   and
incubated    with    fluorescein    isothiocyanate-
conjugated rabbit anti-mouse immunoglobulin.

<u>Double  Diffusion  Analysis  of  Albumin  and α-</u>
<u>Fetoprotein</u>:   The    spent    culture    medium    was
collected after 48 hr of culture.   Albumin and
α-fetoprotein  in  the  concentrated medium were
examined by a double agar-gel diffusion method
with  antibodies  against  human  albumin and α-
fetoprotein.

<u>Treatment of Cells with Chemical Carcinogens</u>:
Aflatoxin B1,   Trp-P-1  and  benzo[a]pyrene were
dissolved   in   dimethylsulfoxide  at  1  mg/ml,
diluted with PBS  at  appropriate concentrations
before use,  and added  to cultures  24 hr after
the cells were seeded into 35  mm dishes.   Then
48   hr   later   the   cells   were   dispersed   by
trypsinization, and  the  number  of  the viable
cells  was  determined  by  trypanblue exclusion
test.

RESULTS

**Transformation of  human liver  cells with SV40T
DNA:**
    Liver    cells    into    which    SV40    T    was
introduced were maintained in culture for two
weeks and then treated  with 100  μg/ml G418 for
four  days.    For G418 treatment, we determined
these conditions , because the human liver cells
were very  sensitive to the cytotoxic effects of
the drug at more than 100  μg/ml concentrations.
A longer  expression period  was allowed because
of the slow growth  rate  of  SV40  T introduced
cells.  On  day  48  after the initiation of the
culture, two epithelial-like cell lines, OUMS-21
and  OUMS-22,   were  obtained  by  cloning  two
colonies grown in different dishes.

    Since then  OUMS-21 cells  have grown without
crisis,   reaching   over 100 population doublings
to date, OUMS-22 cells, however, have grown more
slowly.   Thus  OUMS-21 cells are considered to

have been immortally transformed, while the
immortalization of OUMS-22 must be confirmed in
the future.

**Characteristics of transformed cells:**
The morphology of these two cell lines is
shown in Fig.1. The cells appear to be immature
liver cells identical to some undifferentiated
hepatoma cells in culture. OUMS-22 cells look
more epithelial-like than OUMS-21 cells, but the
cells of both cell lines hardly display few of
the morphological characteristics of mature
parenchymal liver cells. No criss-crossed or
piled up foci were seen in the culture.

Expression of keratin 18 in these cells was
demontrated by immunocytochemistry using
monoclonal antibody CK5, which reacts
specifically with a variety of simple epithelia
(e.g.intestine, liver) but does not stain
stratified squamous epithelia or non-epithelial
cells. In contrast to these findings, the cells
did not react to monoclonal antibodies against
epidermal keratinocytes (KL 1) and glandular
epithelia(RPN.1162).

OUMS-21 and -22 cells produced albumin in the
culture medium, suggesting that these cells
originated from liver parenchymal cells (Fig.2).
However, production of α-fetoprotein was not
detected in either cell line. These cells showed
little activity of tyrosine transaminase, an

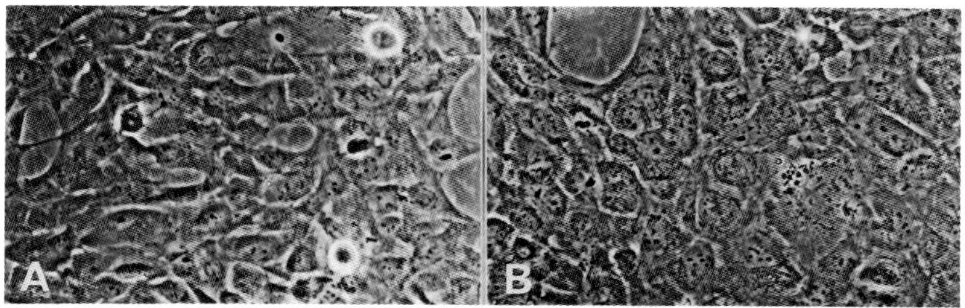

Fig.1    Phase contrast micrographs of OUMS-21 (A)
         and OUMS-22 (B)

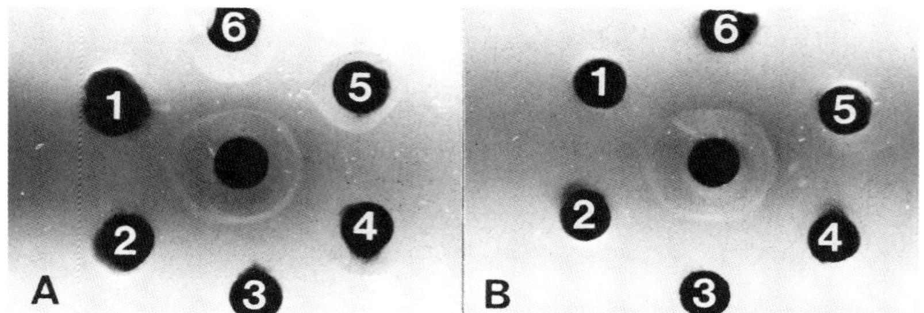

Fig.2  Albumin  production  of  OUMS-21  (A) and
OUMS-22 (B).  1: 4-,  2: 8-,  3: 16-, 4: 32-, 5:
64-,  6:  128-fold  concentrated  medium. Center
well: anti-human albumin antibody

enzyme specific to liver cells.  Furthermore,
this activity could not be induced by
treatment of the cells with dexamethasone.

The  average  population  doubling  time  of
OUMS-21 and -22 cells was about 30 hr and 40 hr,
respectively.  At  confluence,  the  saturation
density of each line was 700,000  cells/cm$^2$ and
300,000  cells/cm$^2$,  respectively.  SV40T antigen
was observed in the  nuclei  of  the transformed
cells  of  both  lines  by  immunofluorescent
staining.

As  can  be  seen  in  Fig.  3,   karyotypic

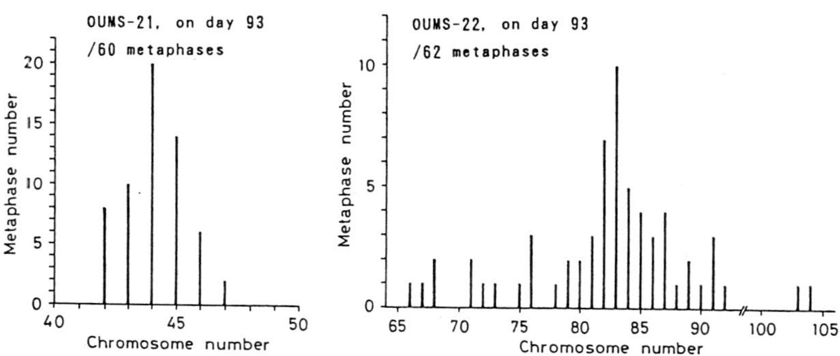

Fig.3  Distribution of chromosome numbers of
      OUMS-21 and OUMS-22

analysis showed OUMS-21 to be diploid with a modal number of 44, whereas the chromosome counts of OUMS-22 were allocated broadly from 66 to 104 with a modal number of 83. No marker chromosomes were found in these cell lines. Interestingly, these chromosomal abnormalities did not correlate with the growth characteristics of these cell lines. In fact, OUMS-21 cells with fewer abnormalities grew more rapidly than OUMS-22 cells.

Table 1. Cytotoxic Effects of Aflatoxin B1, Trp-P-1, and Benzo[a]pyrene on OUMS-21, -22 and Diploid Human Fibroblasts (IMR-90).

| Conc. | Cell number (% Control)** | | |
|---|---|---|---|
| (μg/ml) | Aflatoxin B1 | Trp-P-1 | Benzo[a]pyrene |
| **OUMS-21** | | | |
| 0 * | 100 ± 7.9 | 100 ± 0.5 | 100 ± 2.1 |
| 0.11 | 85.7 ± 2.3 | 89.4 ± 4.1 | 90.9 ± 2.9 |
| 0.33 | 73.9 ± 2.5 | 76.4 ± 0.5 | 82.5 ± 2.8 |
| 1 | 55.1 ± 3.0 | 60.1 ± 2.4 | 84.3 ± 4.3 |
| **OUMS-22** | | | |
| 0 * | 100 ± 4.1 | 100 ± 4.1 | 100 ± 4.2 |
| 0.11 | 95.5 ± 8.3 | 86.1 ± 2.9 | 95.2 ± 1.3 |
| 0.33 | 87.9 ± 3.8 | 74.5 ± 0.9 | 91.6 ± 0.6 |
| 1 | 81.2 ± 3.5 | 61.8 ± 2.5 | 87.7 ± 4.8 |
| **IMR-90** | | | |
| 0 * | 100 ± 1.9 | 100 ± 4.4 | 100 ± 1.0 |
| 0.11 | 100.7 ± 1.2 | 103.5 ± 0.8 | 99.5 ± 3.5 |
| 0.33 | 98.7 ± 1.5 | 101.5 ± 2.7 | 100.6 ± 1.6 |
| 1 | 98.6 ± 0.5 | 95.2 ± 1.6 | 101.0 ± 2.3 |

**Sensitivity of immortalized liver cells to chemical carcinogens:**

If these cultured liver cells have enzymes to metabolize the carcinogens to proximate active ones, their growth should be impaired by the metabolites. Therefore the inhibitory effects of aflatoxin B1, Trp-P-1 and benzo[a]pyrene on cell proliferation were examined. As shown in Table 1, OUMS-21 and -22 cells showed sensitivity to the killing effects of aflatoxin B1, Trp-P-1 and benzo[a]pyrene, whereas normal human fibroblasts showed no sensitivity to these carcinogens.

**Anchorage-independent growth and transplantability:**

OUMS-21 and -22 cells demonstrated about 1.2% and 0.2% cloning efficiency, respectively, in soft agar. Then $10^7$ cells of each cell line were transplanted subcutaneouly into nude mice, but no tumors were visible three months after injection. When the cells were treated with Harvey murine sarcoma virus, they acquired tumorigenicity when transplanted in nude mice.

DISCUSSION

The present liver cell lines were not tumorigenic. This implies that immortalization alone is insufficient to induce tumorigenicity. The neoplastic transformation of human cells is thought to result from multiple cellular changes. In fact, we demonstrated that normal human fiborblasts were transformed into neoplastic cells with ras oncogenes after they were immortalized by CO-60 gamma rays (18-21). However, ras oncogenes may not always be involved in liver carcinogenesis. Other chemicals and hepatitis viruses are also considered to be hepatocarcinogens. Thus the present immortalized cell lines should prove useful for investigating the multistep carcinogenesis of human liver cells with putative liver carcinogens.

Restriction fragment length polymorphism (RFLP) studies on hepatocellular carcinoma revealed tumor-specific loss of heterozygosity (LOH) on several chromosomes, including 11p, 13q,4p11-q21,16q and 17p(22).Therefore, once our present cultured liver cells are neoplastically transformed, the correlation between these chromosome aberrations and the processes of tumorigenic changes in cells will be studied in detail.

## ACKNOWLEDGEMENTS

This work was supported by a Grant-in-Aid for Cancer Research from the Ministry of Education, Science and Culture, Japan.

## REFERENCES

1. Rhim, J.S. Yoo, J.H. et al. Cancer Res. 50(Suppl), 5653s (1990).
2. DiPaolo, J.A. Woodworth, C.D. Oncogene 4, 395 (1989)
3. Band, V. Zajchowski, D. et al. Proc. Natl. Acad. Sci. USA 87, 463 (1990).
4. Chang, S.E. Keen, J. et al. Cancer Res. 42, 2040 (1982).
5. Kaighn, M.E. Reddel, R.P. et al. Cancer Res. 49, 3050 (1989)
6. Poirier, V. Tyler, S.J. et al. Int. J. Cancer 42, 887 (1988).
7. Christian, B.J. Kao, C. et al. Cancer Res. 50, 4779 (1990).
8. Reznikoff, C.A. Loretz, L.J. et al. Carcinogenesis 9, 1427 (1988).
9. Stoner, G.D. Kaighn, M.E. et al. Cancer Res. 51, 365 (1991).
10. Berry, R.D. Powell, S.C. et al. Br. J. Cancer 57, 287 (1988).
11. Pfeifer, A.M.A. Mark III, G.E. et al. Proc. Natl. Acad. Sci. USA 86, 10075 (1989)
12. Gruenert, D.C. Basbaum, C.B. et al. Proc. Natl. Acad. Aci. USA 85, 5951 (1988).
13. Stampfer, M.R. Bartley, J.C. Proc. Natl. Acad. Sci. USA 82, 2394 (1985).

14. Boukamp, P. Petrussevska, R.T. et al. J.
    Cell Biol. 106, 761 (1988)
15. Tveito, G. Hansteen, I-L. et al. Cancer Res.
    49, 1829 (1989).
16. Soule, H.D. Maloney, T.M. et al. Cancer Res.
    50, 6075 (1990).
17. Namba, M. Nishitani, K. et al. Int. J.
    Cancer 35, 275 (1985).
18. Namba, M. Nishitani, K. et al. Int. J.
    Cancer 37, 419 (1986).
19. Namba, M. Nishitani, K. et al. Mutat. Res.
    199, 415 (1988).
20. Namba, M. Nishitani, K. et al. Anticancer
    Res. 8, 947 (1988).
21. Namba, M., Nishitani, K. et al. In: K.H.
    Chadwick et al.(eds.), Cell transformation
    and radiation-induced cancer. 67-74, Adam
    Hilger, Bristol and New York (1989).
22. Slagle, B.L. Zhou, Y-Z. et al. Cancer Res.
    51, 49 (1991).

# TRANSFORMATION OF HUMAN TRACHEAL GLAND EPITHELIAL CELLS *IN VITRO*

D.P. Chopra[1], A.P. Joiakim[1], B. Retherford[1], P.A. Mathieu[1], and J.S. Rhim[2].

[1]Institute of Chemical Toxicology, Wayne State University, Detroit, MI. 48201, [2]National Cancer Institute, Bethesda, MD. 20892

Cancer of respiratory tract is among the most common neoplasms in the U.S and European countries but etiology and mechanisms of neoplastic transformation are not understood. Different types of respiratory tract lesions including squamous metaplasia, squamous cell carcinoma and adenocarcinoma have been described. Since the respiratory tract contains different epithelia i.e. mucosal epithelium and submucosal glands, it is possible that various lesions have different cell types of origin. Much effort has been devoted to the study of tracheal and bronchial mucosal cells which have been successfully cultured and neoplastically transformed (1-3). The untransformed and transformed cells in vitro however, lose their inherent property of mucus secretion. Submucosal glands in human trachea constitute the major tissue contributing to respiratory mucus and may also constitute the cell of origin of respiratory adenocarcinoma. We have propagated in serum-free medium, mucin producing epithelial cells from the human tracheal glands (4). The cell cultures however, undergo senescence after few passages precluding studies on biochemical and molecular mechanisms of growth and differentiation which require large numbers of cells. We have transformed the human tracheal gland epithelial (HTGE) cells by infection with adenovirus 12-SV40 hybrid virus (Ad12-SV40).

It is believed that protooncogenes play an important role in the regulation of cell proliferation and function (5). Since abnormalities in the expression and/or structure of protooncogenes or activity of oncogene products apparently are involved in the development and maintenance of transformed phenotypes (6,7), we have examined the expression of oncogenes in untransformed and Ad12-SV40 transformed HTGE cells. It was found that c-erbB-2 is over expressed in the transformed cells as compared to non-transformed cells. In order to establish if c-erbB-2 expression is directly associated with transformed phenotypes, we also examined the effects of c-erbB-2 antibody on growth and transformation phenotypes of the cells.

Primary HTGE cells were propagated by the explant-outgrowth procedure (4). The culture medium used was serum-free KBM (Clonetics, San Diego, CA) supplemented with insulin (5 $\mu$g/ml, Sigma, St. Louis, MO), hydrocortisone (0.5 $\mu$g/ml, Sigma), EGF (10 ng/ml, Gibco, NY), bovine pituitary extract (25 $\mu$g/ml, Sigma) and antibiotics. The cultures were maintained at 37°C in an atmosphere of 5% $CO_2$ in air. Outgrowth cultures were infected with Ad12-SV40 at a multiplicity of 1:100. Twenty-four hours later, the virus-containing medium was withdrawn, cultures rinsed with fresh complete medium and incubated. At confluent density, the cultures were routinely passaged and observed for transformed phenotypes at different passages. Primary and low passage cultures (Fig. 1) exhibited many properties of epithelial cells such as desmosomes between cells, microvilli on cell surfaces, and keratin positive markers (Fig. 2).

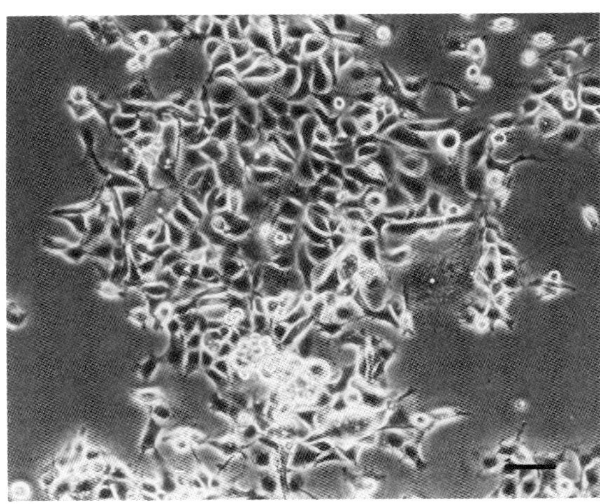

Fig. 1.  Phase contrast photomicrograph of Ad12-SV40 infected cells at 8th passage.  Bar = 20$\mu$m

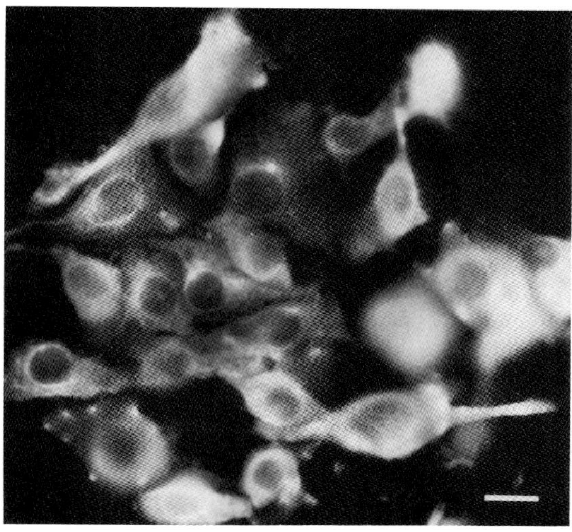

Fig. 2. Indirect immunofluorescent staining of the Ad12-SV40 infected cells (passage 7) showing the presence of cytokeratin filaments. Bar = 5$\mu$m

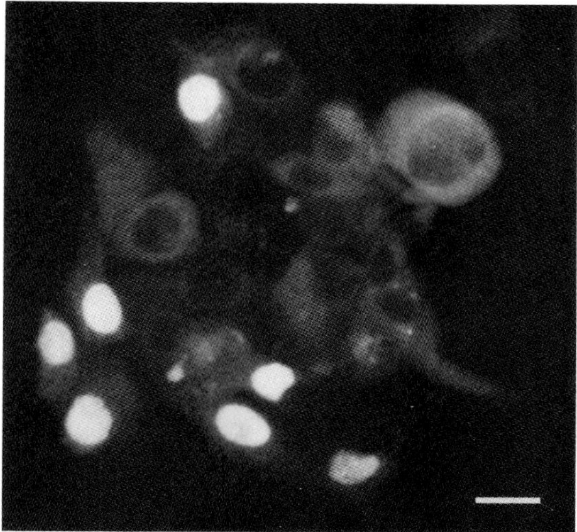

Fig. 3. Indirect immunofluorescent staining of transformed cell (passage 7) for SV40-T antigen. Bar = 5$\mu$m

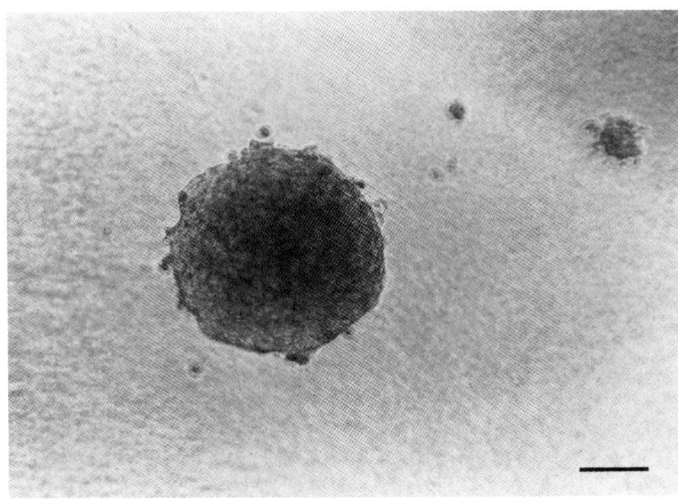

Fig. 4. Photomicrograph of colonies in semi-solid medium.
Bar = 30μm

Most cells exhibited intercellular interdigitations and their cytoplasm
contained bundles of tonofilaments, well developed rough
endoplasmic reticulum, Golgi complexes and membrane bound
secretory vesicles. Immunofluorescent staining for large T-antigen
at passage 7 was observed within nuclei of approximately 40% of
the cells (Fig. 3). The production of infectious virus, as examined
by lysis of Green Monkey kidney cells was negative at passage 23.
The population doubling time of the cells was approximately 33
hours. At passage 14, the cells exhibited focus formation and
formed colonies (Fig. 4) in semisolid medium (AIG) with a colony
forming efficiency of approximately 19-33%. The transformed cells
were not tumorigenic (passage 19) in nude mice.
   We examined the expression of protooncogenes and epidermal
growth factor receptor (EGF-R) in untransformed and transformed
cells by Northern Analysis using total RNA. Total cellular RNA (6
x10$^6$ cells) was extracted and purified by a guanidinium thiocyanate
procedure and cesium trifluro-acetate gradient centrifugation (8).
The probes used in this work were as follows:  pc-fos-3 (ATCC
#41041), a genomic DNA of c-fos protooncogene (a 7.10 kilobase
(kb) insert) cloned into the EcoR1-Sst1 site of PBR322; pCER204

(ATCC #57584), a cDNA of c-erbB-2 protooncogene (4.0 kb), cloned into the StuI site of pCD; pSVcmyc1 (ATCC #41029), a genomic DNA clone of c-myc protooncogene (4.8 kb), cloned to the BamHI-Xba1 site of pSV2 vector; and pE7 (ATCC #57346), a cDNA clone of epidermal growth factor receptor (2.4 kb) cloned into the Cla1, site of pBR322. Fifty ng of the probes were radiolabelled [$^{32}$P] = dCTP at > 3000Ci/mMol) by the random primer method using a Pharmacia LKB kit (Pharmacia LKB Biotechnology, Piscataway, NJ). Approximately $10^6$ cpm/ml of the probes were used for the hybridization.

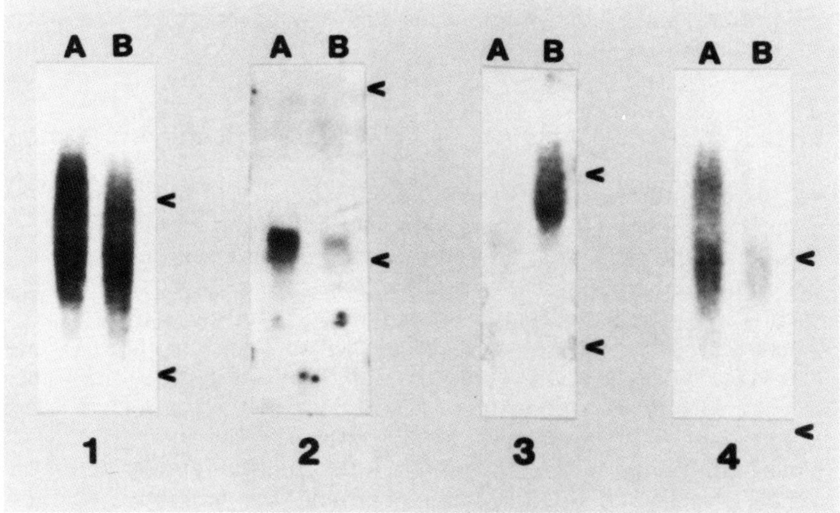

Fig. 5. Northern analysis of total cellular RNA for oncogenes and epidermal growth factor receptor transcripts. Total cellular RNAs from normal and immortalized gland cells were isolated; 25μg aliquots of RNAs were fractionated by electrophoresis on 1% agarose gels containing formaldehyde, transferred to nylon membranes. The membranes were hybridized with [$^{32}$P] cDNA probes: 1, c-fos protooncogene; 2, c-myc protooncogene; 3, c-erbB-2 protooncogene and 4, epidermal growth factor receptor. Lane A, RNA from untransformed cells and Lane B, from transformed cells. Arrows indicate the position of 28s (upper) and 18s (lower) rRNAs.

Results showed that among the genes examined (Fig. 5), c-fos was the most highly expressed oncogene in both the untransformed and transformed cells; no significant difference however, was observed in its expression between the two groups. Oncogene c-erbB-2 showed several-fold higher expression in the transformed cells. EGF-R showed somewhat higher expression in the untransformed than the transformed cells. Higher expression of c-erbB-2 in the transformed cells is intriguing as this gene has been reported to be over expressed in neoplasms of many glandular tissues including those of breast (9), salivary gland (10), ovarian (11), thyroid (12) and stomach (13, 14). The gene is also known as c-neu and encodes a 185 kD transmembrane glycoprotein with inherent tyrosine kinase activity which is believed to be a receptor for an unknown ligand.


Effects of c-erbB-2 Antibody on Growth and Transformed Phenotype

Recent studies have reported amplification of the human protooncogene c-erbB-2 in several adenocarcinomas of human tissues. Gene amplification and resulting over-expression of oncogene proteins is believe to be involved in cell transformation by chronically stimulating signal transduction pathway and over-expression of c-erbB-2 have been shown to transform NIH/3T3 cells (15, 16). Therefore we tested the ability of anti-c-erbB-2 antibody to modulate growth and AIG of HTGE cells. If the product of c-erbB-2 oncogene is functioning as a stimulator of growth and transformation phenotypes, then c-erbB-2 antibody may indirectly inhibit growth and AIG. In the experiment to examine the effects on growth, 35mm dishes containing 2 ml culture medium were plated with $5 \times 10^4$ cells per dish. Twenty-four hours later, three cultures were terminated and cell numbers determined using a hemacytometer. The remaining cultures were divided into five groups; three groups were treated with different concentrations (50, 100, 200 ng/ml) of the c-erbB-2 antibody, one group was treated with non-immune rabbit IgG (200 ng/ml), and one group served as untreated control. Culture medium was changed three times per week and fresh test factors added: Cultures were terminated at 13 days after treatment and the number of cells in each group determined (Fig. 6).

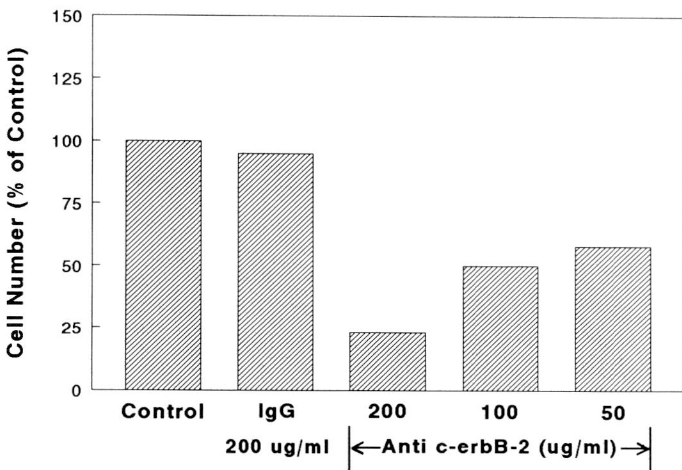


Fig 6. Inhibition by c-erbB-2 antibody of growth of transformed HTGE cells. Non-immune IgG was used as a control.

Addition of the c-erbB-2 antibody to the cultures caused a dose-dependent inhibition of growth. As compared to the untreated control, the growth inhibition was approximately 76%, 23% and 12% at 200, 100, and 50 ng/ml of c-erbB-2 antibody. The non-immune IgG had no significant effect on growth of HTGE cells.

In another set of experiments, the effect of c-erbB-2 antibody was examined on the transformed phenotype AIG. For this, cultures were treated for 13 days with different concentrations of the antibody as above and subsequently cultured in semi-solid medium for an additional 10 days and the number of colonies enumerated. Non-immune rabbit IgG (200 ng/ml) was used as a control. c-erbB-2 antibody also inhibited AIG in a concentration dependent manner (Fig. 7). The inhibition of colony forming efficiency (CFE) was 65%, 38%, 5% at 200,100, and 50 ng/ml respectively. The IgG apparently had some stimulatory effect on CFE as compared to the untreated control cultures.

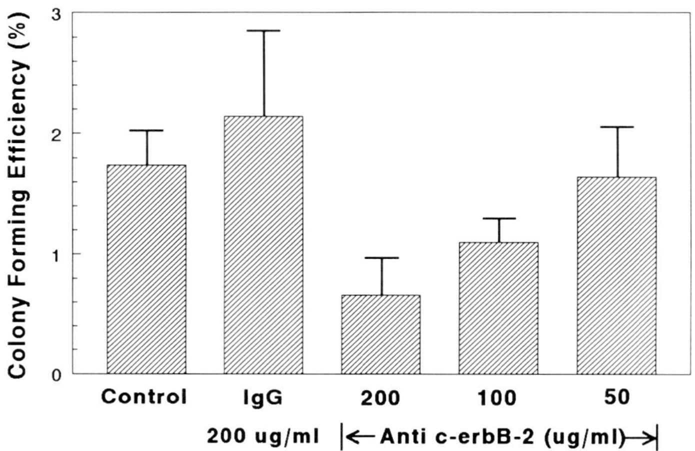



Fig. 7. Inhibition by c-erbB-2 antibody of colony forming efficiency in semi-solid medium of transformed HTGE cells. Non-immune IgG was used as a control.

In summary we have transformed HTGE cells by infection with Ad12-SV40 hybrid virus. They exhibited enhanced growth as compared to the non-transformed cells, exhibited AIG but were non-tumorigenic. The transformation involves over-expression of c-erbB-2 oncogene. The c-erbB-2 antibody specifically inhibited growth and AIG of the transformed cells. The mechanism by which c-erbB-2 antibody inhibits growth and AIG remains to be investigated.

## REFERENCES


1.      R.R. Reddel, Y. Ke, et al. <u>Cancer Res</u>. 48, 1904 (1988).

2.      R.R. Reddel, Y. Ke, et al. <u>Oncogene Res</u>. 3, 401 (1988).

3.   G.H. Yoakum, J.K. Lechner, et al. <u>Science</u> 227, 1174 (1985).

4.   D.P. Chopra, R.L. Shoemaker, et al. <u>In Vitro Cell. Develop. Biol.</u> 27, 13 (1991)

5.   E.D. Adamson. <u>Development</u> 99, 449 (1987)

6.   D.J. Slamon. <u>New Eng. J. Medicine.</u> 317, 955 (1987).

7.   D.J. Slamon, J.B. deKernion. <u>Science</u> 224, 256 (1984).

8.   H. Okayama, M. Kawaichi, et al. In: R. Wu and L. Grossman (eds.) <u>Methods of Enzymology.</u> vol 154, 3-27, Academic Press, NY, (1987).

9.   M.J. Van de Vijiver, R. van der Bersselaer, et al. <u>Mol. Cell. Biol.</u> 7, 2019 (1987).

10.   K. Semba, N. Kamata, et al. <u>Proc. Natl. Acad. Sci. USA.</u> 82, 6497 (1985)

11.   D.J. Slamon, W. Godolphin, et al. <u>Science</u> 244, 707 (1989)

12.   R. Aasland, J.R. Lillehaug. <u>Brit. J. Cancer</u> 57, 358 (1988).

13.   J. Yokota, T. Yamamoto, et al. <u>Lancet</u> i, 756 (1986)

14.   J.B. Park, J.S. Rhim, et al. <u>Cancer Res.</u> 49, 6605 (1989)

15.   P.P. DiFiore, J.H. Pierce, et al. <u>Cell</u> 51, 1063 (1987).

16.   R.M. Hudziak, J. Schlessinger, et al. <u>Proc. Natl. Acad. Sci. USA.</u> 84, 7159 (1987).

Acknowledgement

   This research was supported by USPHS grants RO1-HL41979 and RO1-HL33142 from the National Heart, Lung and Blood Institute.

From: *Neoplastic Transformation in Human Cell Culture,*
Eds.: J. S. Rhim and A. Dritschilo ©1991 The Humana Press Inc., Totowa, NJ

# STABLE EXPRESSION OF SV40 LARGE T-ANTIGEN GENE IN PRIMARY HUMAN SCHWANN CELLS

J.L. Rutkowski[1], J.S. Rhim[2], K.W.C. Peden[3], and G.I. Tennekoon[1]

[1]Depts. of Pediatrics and Neurology, Univ. of Michigan, Ann Arbor, MI; [2]National Cancer Inst., Bethesda, MD; and [3]National Inst. of Allergy and Infectious Disease, Bethesda, MD.

Schwann cells, which arise from the neuroepithelium, are glial cells of the vertebrate peripheral nervous system. During development, they grow along nerve axons and eventually ensheathe or myelinate them. In the genetic disease neurofibromatosis, transformed Schwann cells form usually benign but disfiguring tumors that emerge from peripheral or cranial nerves. To investigate the events leading to cell transformation, we have developed a tissue culture system for propagating human Schwann cells.

A population of mitotically active Schwann cells was isolated from a human nerve biopsy, and the large T-antigen gene from simian virus 40 (SV40) was introduced either by viral infection or by transfection of plasmid DNA enclosed in liposomes. Stable cell lines were obtained with the vectors listed below. Cell lines were generated and continuously subcultured for at least 50 population doublings without crisis before studies were initiated. Data characterizing the properties of these cell lines are presented.

*Viruses*
    -wild-type SV40 (SV40wt)
    -A58 temperature-sensitive strain of SV40 (tsA58)
    -adenovirus 12/SV40 hybrid (AD/SV)
*Plasmids*
    -Rous sarcoma virus promoter/SV40 T antigen (RSV-T)
    -SV40 promoter/T antigen (SV-T)
    -wild-type metallothionein promoter/T antigen (MTwt-T)
    -synthetic promoter with 4 metal regulatory elements
        from the MT promoter/T antigen (MT4-T)


## RESULTS

### Morphological Phenotype and T-antigen Expression

Cell lines established with T antigen driven by the
metallothionein promoter or its derivative were maintained
in the presence of zinc to induce transcription.  T antigen was
detected in the nucleus by indirect immunofluorescent
staining, but when zinc was removed from the medium, T-
antigen expression decreased to low (MTwt-T) or
undetectable (MT4-T) basal levels.  These cell lines, with or
without zinc, appeared morphologically similar to the
parental strain.  All of the cell lines generated with the T-
antigen gene driven by the viral promoters (SV-T, RSV-T,
SV40wt, tsA58, AD/SV) expressed the oncoprotein at very
high levels and the cells acquired morphological features of a
transformed phenotype, i.e., smaller cells with less cytoplasm
that grew in dense, fusiform layers.  Although T-antigen
levels decreased in the tsA58 line when the temperature was
increased from 32 to 39°C, the cells did not regain a normal
morphology.


### Growth in Culture

Cells were seeded at a density of $10^5$ cells/35mm dish, then
released with trypsin and counted after 1, 2, 4, 7, or 10 days.

The doubling time (determined during log phase growth) of the parental strain was 91 hr.  In the MT4-T cell line, removing zinc from the medium slowed the doubling time from 29 to 77 hr and from 17 to 31 hr in the MTwt-T line. Cell lines in which T antigen was driven by viral promoters grew very rapidly (doubling time < 20 hr).

The number of cells per dish approached saturation by day 10 and only the MT4-T line (in the absence of zinc) retained normal contact inhibition.  All of the other cell lines lost contact inhibition and achieved saturation densities from 5-9 times that of the parental strain.

## Serum-dependent Growth

Cells were seeded at a density of $10^5$ cells/35mm dish in medium containing 10%, 2%, 1% , or 0% fetal bovine serum (FBS) and counted 7 days later.  None of the cell lines survived without serum, but the AD/SV and RSV-T cell lines grew well in low-serum media.  The SV-T, tsA58, and SV40wt cell lines grew slowly in 1 or 2% serum.  The parental strain and both MT cell lines survived in low-serum media but could not grow without 10% FBS.

## Growth in Soft Agar

Single cells ($6\times10^3$)were seeded in medium containing 3% agar and 20% FBS over a layer of 5% agarose.  The top agar was covered with 1 ml of medium containing 20% FBS and the number of single cells and colonies per dish were counted after 21 days.  KHOS/NP (a transformed osteosarcoma cell line used as a positive control) formed colonies typically 200 μm in diameter with an efficiency of 60%.  The SV-T, SV40wt, and  AD/SV cell lines all formed smaller colonies in soft agar (25-100 μm) with efficiencies ranging from 22-38%. The parental strain and both MT cell lines remained as single cells.

# SUMMARY AND CONCLUSIONS

<u>CELL LINES</u>

| PROPERTIES | MT4 | MTwt | SV-T | RSV-T | SV40wt | tsA58 | AD/SV |
|---|---|---|---|---|---|---|---|
| Life span | + | + | + | + | + | + | + |
| Transformed morphology | -- | -/+ | + | + | + | + | + |
| Growth rate | -- | + | ++ | ++ | ++ | + | ++ |
| Saturation density | -- | + | + | + | ++ | + | ++ |
| Growth in low serum | -- | -- | + | ++ | + | + | ++ |
| Growth in soft agar | -- | -- | + | nd | ++ | nd | ++ |

+   significantly different from parental cells          - - no change
++  greater than a two-fold difference                    nd  not determined

As shown in the table above, all of the cell lines had an extended life span in culture relative to the parental cell strain, which began to senesce at about 20 population doublings.  However, only the MT4-T line retained all of the properties of the parental strain and this cell line should provide a useful system to study transformation *in vitro*. Cell lines expressing high levels of T antigen divided rapidly, lost contact inhibition, and aquired serum- and anchorage-independence.

Thus, Schwann cells appear to transform more readily in culture than other human epithelial cells, since high levels of T antigen alone were sufficient to induce a transformed phenotype.  Epidermal keratinocytes and bronchial epithelial cells are not transformed by T antigen expressed by viral promoters, and only the AD/SV hybrid virus is able to extend their life span in culture (1).  A second event, such as treatment with a chemical carcinogen or infection with a retrovirus, is required for their neoplastic transformation.

# REFERENCE

1.  J. Rhim. <u>Anticancer Res.</u> 9, 1345 (1989).

From: *Neoplastic Transformation in Human Cell Culture*,
Eds.: J. S. Rhim and A. Dritschilo ©1991 The Humana Press Inc., Totowa, NJ

# MALIGNANT TRANSFORMATION OF HUMAN FIBROBLASTS *IN VITRO*


J. Justin McCormick and Veronica M. Maher

Carcinogenesis Laboratory - Fee Hall,
Michigan State University,
East Lansing, MI 48824-1316


## ABSTRACT


Although carcinogens cause human tumors, normal human
fibroblasts in culture have not been successfully transformed
to malignancy by exposure to carcinogens.  It is now
recognized that malignant transformation involves multiple
changes within a cell and, therefore, successive clonal
selection of cells containing such changes must occur.  One
explanation for the failure to induce *in vitro* malignant
transformation of human cells could be inability to recognize
cells that have undergone intermediate changes so as to
expand the population, expose the cells a second time, cause
further changes, etc.  Therefore, we transfected finite life
span diploid human fibroblasts with oncogenes known to be
active in cells derived from human fibrosarcomas or effective
in transforming animal fibroblasts to determine the
phenotypes they produced.  Transfection of a *sis* gene, or an
H-, or N-*ras* oncogene caused the cells to acquire many
characteristics of malignant cells, but not to acquire an
infinite life span or become malignant.  We recently
succeeded in developing  an infinite life span human
fibroblasts cell strain, designated MSU-1.1, which has a
stable, near-diploid karyotype, composed of 45 chromosomes
including two marker chromosomes.  We have shown that these
cells can be transformed to malignancy by transfection of the
H-, K-, or N-*ras* oncogene.  All of the malignant H-, K-, or
N-*ras* transfected derivatives examined have exhibited the
stable karyotype of the original MSU-1.1 cells.  We have also

found rare spontaneous clonal variants of MSU-1.1 that are malig- nantly transformed and have shown that carcinogen treatment can cause the MSU-1.1 cells to become transformed into malignant cells.

## *IN VITRO* TRANSFORMATION OF FINITE LIFE SPAN HUMAN FIBROBLASTS BY TRANSFECTION OF ONCOGENES

Exposure to chemical carcinogens or radiation is considered to cause most human cancer, but human fibroblasts in culture have not been successfully transformed to malignancy by such agents. Malignant transformation is a multi-step process, and there is growing evidence that at least five changes are required and that these are clonally acquired. A normal cell that by chance acquires one of these changes must undergo clonal expansion so that among the progeny cells, a cell with the first change can acquire a second change, and so on until by sequential clonal expansions, a malignant cell arises. One explanation for the failure to induce such transformation of human cells in culture could be inability to recognize the phenotypes of cells that have undergone intermediate changes, so that these cells can be isolated, expanded, and exposed a second time to cause further changes, etc. To identify possible intermediates, we transfected diploid human fibroblasts with oncogenes known to be active in cell lines derived from fibrosarcomas or effective in transforming animal fibroblasts, such as H-*ras*, or N-*ras*, or a *sis* oncogene and determined the phenotypes produced. The *sis* oncogene codes for a protein structurally and immunologically related to the B chain of platelet-derived growth factor (PDGF(B)) (1,2). Oncogenes from DNA tumor viruses such as simian virus 40 (SV40) or the papilloma viruses were not utilized in these studies since they do not have a homolog in the DNA of human cells. The plasmids we constructed or used for these experiments also contained a gene coding for a selectable marker so the transfectants could be identified and selected by drug resistance and examined for one or the other characteristics of tumor-derived cells, such as morphological alteration, focus formation, ability to form colonies in soft agar, growth-factor independence, and tumorigenicity.

Using this approach, we and our colleagues (3) found that diploid human fibroblasts transfected with the v-*sis* oncogene grew to 6- to 10-fold higher saturation densities than control cells transfected with the vector plasmid alone, formed large, well-defined foci, exhibited growth factor independence, growing well in the absence of serum, and formed colonies in soft agar at a high frequency. But they retained their normal fibroblastic morphology, exhibited a finite life span in culture, and were not tumorigenic.

Similar studies were carried out using the T24 H-*ras* oncogene derived from the human EJ bladder carcinoma cell line (4) or human N-*ras* oncogenes (5) inserted into vectors designed to give various levels of expression of the oncogene. The *ras* oncogenes that were flanked by suitable enhancer and promoter sequences caused the cells to acquire many characteristics of malignant cells, i.e., morphological transformation, anchorage independence, focus-formation, etc., but they did not acquire an infinite life span and did not form tumors in athymic mice.

Since the human fibrosarcoma-derived cell line HT1080 expresses both a mutated N-*ras* gene (6) and the B chain of PDGF (7), we attempted to develop strains expressing both oncogenes. Our efforts to introduce the v-*sis* oncogenes into the *ras*-transformed cell strains described above and a *ras* oncogene into the *sis*-transformed cells were thwarted by the finite life span of these human diploid fibroblasts. Even though the first oncogene transfection experiments were carried out with early-passage cells, the drug-resistant transfectant cell strains isolated and expanded to serve as recipients for the second oncogene represent individual clones. The progeny cells from such clones can be expanded through 20 to 24 additional population doublings, yielding from $1 \times 10^6$ to $16 \times 10^6$ cells, but the cells in the transfectant clones from the second transfection can only undergo a few population doublings before they senesce. This early senescence is not unexpected since Holliday et al. (8) showed that the life span of cells in culture is reduced by 10 to 15 population doublings if they are cloned, a phenomenon that is sometimes referred to as a "bottleneck effect".

TRANSFORMATION OF INFINITE LIFE SPAN HUMAN FIBROBLASTS BY TRANSFECTION OF ONCOGENES

Since these *ras* transfectants were approaching the end of their life span at the time they were injected into **athymic mice, we reasoned that** they may simply not have possessed sufficient replicative capacity to form tumors. Therefore, we and our colleagues set out to generate an infinite life span human fibroblast cell strain that would be otherwise normal. The most common method of generating infinite life span human cell lines is to infect them with SV40 (9) or transfect them with plasmids, such as pSV3, that contain the early region of SV40, including the region coding for large T-antigen (10). However, human fibroblasts that express T-antigen exhibit changes in morphology, become aneuploid, and exhibit anchorage independence, and since these are also the characteristics of tumor-derived cells, such altered cells have limited usefulness in studies designed to gain insight into the step-wise changes required for a normal cell to become a malignant cell.

In our attempt to generate an infinite life span human fibroblast cell strain that had undergone only minimal changes, we were guided by the work of Weinberg and his colleagues (11) who showed that transfection of rat embryo fibroblasts with a v-*myc* oncogene increased the frequency at which the cells developed into infinite life span cell strains. We transfected early passage, foreskin-derived normal human fibroblasts, designated LG1, with a plasmid carrying the *neo* gene and a v-*myc* gene. The transfectants were selected for Geneticin resistance, and clonally-derived cell strains were isolated and propagated for many generations. Eventually all cell strains senesced, but among the senescing progeny of one cell strain, clones of viable cells could be seen. These eventually gave rise to an infinite life span cell strain that we designated MSU-1.1 (12). These cells have a normal fibroblastic morphology, do not form foci, but produce a low frequency of small colonies in soft agarose, and display a near-diploid karyotype of 45 chromosomes including two distinctive marker chromosomes, and do not form tumors in athymic mice. The karyotype has remained stable, still showing the identical pattern more than 200 generations since its origin. The MSU-1.1 cells were analyzed using a battery of "paternity tests" and were shown to be derived from the parental cell strain that had been used for transfection. They were also shown to express the v-*myc* gene (12).

The infinite life span MSU-1.1 cells were then used as the recipient cells for transfection with plasmids containing an H-*ras* (13), N-*ras* (14), or K-*ras* oncogene (15). Because the recipient MSU-1.1 cells express the *neo* gene, the transfectants were identified by their ability to form foci of morphologically transformed cells on a background monolayer of fibroblastic cells. Cells isolated from the foci were analyzed and found to express the *ras* protein of the transfected gene. The transformed cells exhibited the same altered characteristics found in the *ras*-transformed finite life span diploid fibroblasts described above, but in addition they made progressively-growing, invasive sarcomas when injected into athymic mice. Cells isolated from the tumors had a human karyotype, contained the two distinctive marker chromosomes of MSU-1.1 cells, and were Geneticin resistant as expected.

Our interpretation of these experiments was that a suitable expression level of a *ras* oncogene in this infinite life span human fibroblast cell strain was sufficient to bring about malignant transformation. To be sure that the MSU-1.1 cells were not unique, we transfected two other infinite life span human fibroblast cell strains (KMST-6 and GM637) with the plasmid carrying the H-*ras* oncogene in the same vector construct (13). The KMST-6 cell strain, which arose following repeated radiation treatment (16), and the GM637 strain, which arose following SV40 infection and subsequent immortalization, are highly aneuploid, morphologi-cally-transformed, and capable of forming foci and colonies in soft agar, but they do not form tumors in athymic mice. Following transfection with a plasmid carrying the H-*ras* oncogene and a *neo* gene, the transfectants were selected for resistance to Geneticin. When the transfectants were expanded into large populations and injected into athymic mice, they formed progressively-growing, invasive sarcomas. Since KMST-6 and GM637 cells do not constitutively express *myc*, the results suggested that it was the infinite life span phenotype of the MSU-1.1 cells, rather than their expression of *myc*, that complemented the expression of the H-*ras* oncogene and allowed malignant transformation.

The results of these studies demonstrate that human fibroblasts are not refractory to transformation, as was previously thought. They suggest that for such cells to become malignantly transformed in the human body, they must undergo repeated clonal selection to yield cells that express the appropriately activated proto-oncogenes. The use of transfection techniques to transform these cells in culture was especially helpful since it made it possible for us to directly identify a specific transformed phenotype with the expression of a specific dominantly-acting oncogene.

## NUMBER OF CHANGES REQUIRED TO DEVELOP AN INFINITE LIFE SPAN CELL STRAIN

One of the major interests of workers in the field of carcinogenesis is to determine the number and kinds of independent changes required for normal cells to acquire specific transformed properties. Studies using human cells in culture can be useful for answering such questions. But if results obtained in culture are to be applied to the problem of the mechanisms that operate to cause human cancer, it is necessary to demonstrate that the process in culture recapitulates what occurs in humans. From our studies and that of many other investigators it seems clear that acquiring an infinite (or very greatly extended) life span in culture is a prerequisite if a cell is to acquire sequentially all the changes needed to become malignant. Whether this is the case for cells in the human body is not known for certain. What is known is that cells derived from malignant human tumors frequently give rise to infinite life span cell lines when placed in culture, but cells from normal tissues never do so.

In the course of the above studies with the MSU-1.1 cell strain, we examined stocks of cells from the original *myc*-transfectant that had been frozen during the time that the cells were senescing to determine when the cells with the two unique marker chromosomes first appeared. We found that in a stock frozen early there was a pure population of diploid cells. These cells were designated MSU-1.0. An intermediate passage taken from the freezer was found to contain two populations, one diploid like MSU-1.0, the other identical to MSU-1.1. Both the MSU-1.0 and MSU-1.1 cell strains have undergone more than 200 population doublings since their siblings senesced, without any change in chromosome complement. Both express the v-*myc* protein and have the same integration site for the transfected v-*myc* and *neo* genes. Since the chance of human cells acquiring an infinite life span in culture is very rare, the data suggest that MSU-1.1 cells are derived from MSU-1.0 cells. Table 1 compares the growth characteristics of the MSU-1.1 and MSU-1.0 cells with the parental LG1 cells and two of the MSU-1.1 malignantly-transformed cell strains. What is clear is the diploid, infinite life span MSU-1.0 cells exhibit growth character-

**Table 1.  Growth Characteristics of Various Cell Strains in the MSU-1 Lineage**

| Cell Strain | Colonies in Agarose per $10^3$ Cells Plated (diameter $\geq$ 40 $\mu$m) | (diameter $\geq$ 120 $\mu$m) | Growth Factor Indepen- dence | Malig- nancy |
|---|---|---|---|---|
| LG1 | 0.5 | 0.01 | – | – |
| MSU-1.0 | 0.5 | 0.01 | – | – |
| MSU-1.1 | 10 | 0.01 | + | – |
| MSU-1.1 H-*ras* | 250 | 68 | +++ | High Grade |
| MSU-1.1 N-*ras* | 270 | 70 | +++ | High Grade |

istics identical to those of the parental finite life span
LG1 cells.  This is an important finding because it clearly
shows that the only selective advantage these infinite life
span cells have is that they can continue to replicate when
the rest of the cell population senesces.

While we have not yet succeeded in formally proving that
unregulated expression of the transfected *myc* gene played a
causal role in generating the infinite life span cells, we
consider this highly likely.  Evidence for this hypothesis
includes the apparent causal role of *myc* in causing infinite
life span rat fibroblasts (17), our finding that we have been
able to generate additional infinite life span human
fibroblast strains after transfection of the *myc* gene (J. J.
McCormick, unpublished studies), and a report by Kinsella et
al. (18) that infection with a *myc*-containing virus produced
an infinite life span human fibroblast strain.  If we
postulate that *myc* expression played a causal role, at least
one additional change was required to generate the infinite
life span MSU-1.0 cell strain since it arose from the progeny
of a single Geneticin-resistant cell, and we showed that all
of the progeny of the clonally-derived population expressed
the same level of *myc* protein, yet the vast majority of the
population went into crisis and senseced.  In fusion
experiments between infinite life span and finite life span
cells, the hybrid cells formed have a finite life span.  This
suggests that an infinite life span results when cells lose
a gene(s) for mortality.  Since it is unlikely that such
genes are sex-linked, escape from senescence may well require
the loss of ability to make functional gene product from both
copies of a gene.  If each of these assumptions is correct,

MSU-1.0 cells would differ from their parental finite life span cells not only because they constitutively express the *myc* gene, but also because they have undergone two other genetic changes.

## NUMBER OF CHANGES REQUIRED TO CONVERT AN INFINITE LIFE SPAN CELL TO MALIGNANCY

As indicated above, the majority of our studies to date have been carried out with the MSU-1.1 cell strain because it was isolated first. Preliminary studies show that the MSU-1.0 cells cannot be malignantly transformed by transfection of various *ras* oncogenes, indicating that the MSU-1.1 cells have acquired at least one additional transformed property. Table 1 shows that MSU-1.1 cells differ from MSU-1.0 cells in that they can grow at a modest rate without exogenous growth factors and make colonies in agarose at a low, but detectable frequency. We have found that, unlike LG1 cells and MSU-1.0 cells, MSU-1.1 cells synthesize a low level of PDGF(B), which may be responsible for these characteristics. However, MSU-1.1 cells also carry two unique marker chromosomes that apparently arose independently, and one of these involves a partial trisomy of chromosome 1, which requires a third event. Just which of these changes in the MSU-1.1 cells is necessary if cells are to be malignantly transformed is under study. In addition, at least two changes were required to convert the H-*ras* or N-*ras* gene into a transforming oncogene. First, the proto-oncogene had to acquire a mutation in a specific codon, and second that oncogene had to be overexpressed so that the total level of *ras* gene product present in the cells could be three to seven-fold higher than normal. (The H-*ras* or N-*ras* oncogene in a low expression vector is ineffective in transforming MSU-1.1 cells to malignancy, J. J. McCormick, unpublished studies.)

As shown in Table 1, we have succeeded in deriving by sequential clonal selection, a series of cell strains of a single lineage that exhibit increasing anchorage independent growth and decreasing dependence on exogenous growth factors. Fully malignant cells form colonies in agarose with a diameter $\geq$ 40 $\mu$m at a frequency of 25% or greater and grow well without exogenous growth factors. These techniques can be used to select rare spontaneous variant cells that exhibit

these same properties.  The clonal isolation and expansion
of cells that express such properties is critical because the
chance of a cell acquiring an additional genetic change in
a specific gene is low.  Only when one has expanded a clone
of cells that express some phenotype into a large population
($\geq 10^6$ cells) can one find rare variants that have acquired
an additional transformation-related genetic change.  Human
cells in culture are genetically stable and ordinarily do not
exhibit abnormally high mutation frequencies.

Our best estimate from the present studies is that at
least six genetic changes are required to convert normal
human fibroblasts into malignant cells.  Some of these
changes involve dominant-acting oncogenes, such as *myc* and
*ras*.  Other changes have not yet been identified with a
specific gene.  Some may involve other dominant-acting genes;
others may involve recessive suppressor genes.  It is clear
from the studies we have completed that at many steps in the
pathway, alternative genes may be activated, indicating that
a simple linear model is inadequate.

## ROLE OF GENETIC INSTABILITY IN MALIGNANT TRANSFORMATION

All of the malignant H-, K-, or N-*ras*-transfected
derivatives of MSU-1.1 cells that we have examined have
exhibited the stable karyotype of the original MSU-1.1 cells.
They form characteristic malignant tumors in athymic mice and
have proven positive in experimental studies of metastasis
(13-15).  The cells derived from these tumors have the same
stable karyotype as the precursor transfectant cells that
were injected into athymic mice.

We have also found rare clonal variants of MSU-1.1 cells
that spontaneously transformed into malignant cells, and we
have shown that malignant variants of MSU-1.1 cells can be
induced by carcinogen treatment.  Exposure to carcinogen
caused a dose-dependent increase in foci formation, and cells
from such foci grew to a higher density in medium containing
1% serum than did the MSU-1.1 cells from which they were
derived.  A substantial fraction of these focus-derived
strains proved to be malignant. Unlike the H-, K-, or N-*ras*-
transfected malignant MSU-1.1 cell strains or the cells
derived from the tumors they produced, each of the
carcinogen-induced, focus-derived malignant cells or the
spontaneously transformed cells exhibited unique chromosomal

changes, in addition to the marker chromosomes of the MSU-1.1 strain. These changes in karyotype are stable. Taken together, the data indicate that activated *ras* oncogenes, even when expressed at high levels, do not cause genetic instability in transfectant cell strains. They further suggest that spontaneous and/or carcinogen-induced oncogene activation (or tumor suppressor gene inactivation) commonly takes place as a result of major chromosome alterations.

## ACKNOWLEDGEMENTS

We wish to express our indebtedness to our colleagues, Drs. John E. Dillberger, Dennis G. Fry, Peter J. Hurlin, Calvert Louden, Thomas L. Morgan, Daniel M. Wilson, and Dajun Yang, and Ms. Suzanne  Kohler for their valuable contributions to the research summarized here. The excellent technical assistance of Stephen Dietrich, Lonnie D. Milam, Elvet Potter, Clay Spencer, and Clarissa Stropp is gratefully acknowledged. The research was supported by DOE Grant DE-60524, DHHS Grant CA21289 from the NCI, and DHHS Contract ES65152 from the NIEHS.

## REFERENCES

1.  R. F. Doolittle, M. W. Hunkapiller, L. E. Hood, S. G. Devare, S. G., K. C. Robbins, S. A. Aaronson, and H. N. Antoniades. <u>Science</u> 221, 275-276 (1983).
2.  K. C. Robbins, H. N. Antoniades, S. G. Devare, M. W. Hunkapiller, and S. A. Aaronson. Nature London 305, 605-608 (1983).
3.  D. G. Fry, L. D. Milam, V. M. Maher, and J. J. McCormick. <u>J. Cellul. Physiol</u>., 128, 313-321 (1986).
4.  P. J. Hurlin, D. G. Fry, V. M. Maher, and J. J. McCormick. <u>Cancer Res</u>., 47, 5752-5757 (1987).
5.  D. M. Wilson, D. G. Fry, V. M. Maher, and J. J. McCormick. <u>Carcinogenesis</u> 10, 635-640 (1990).
6.  R. Brown, C. J. Marshall, S. G. Pennie, and A. Hall. <u>EMBO J</u>. 3, 1321-1326 (1984).
7.  P. Pantazis, P. G. Pellicci, R. Dalla-Favera, and H. N. Antoniades. <u>Proc. Nat. Acad. Sci. USA</u> 82, 2404-2408 (1985).
8.  R. Holliday, L. I. Huschtscha, G. M. Tarrant, and T. B. L. Kirkwood. <u>Science</u>, 198, 366-372 (1977).
9.  G. H. Sack, Jr. <u>In Vitro</u> 17, 1-19 (1981).

10. S. E. Chang, <u>Biochim. Biophys. Acta</u> 823, 161-164 (1986).
11. H. Land, L. F. Parada, and R. A. Weinberg. <u>Nature London</u> 304, 596-602 (1983).
12. T. L. Morgan, D. Yang, D. G. Fry, P. J. Hurlin, S. K. Kohler, V. M. Maher, and J. J. McCormick. <u>Exp. Cell. Res</u>. in press (1991).
13. P. J. Hurlin, V. M. Maher, and J. J. McCormick (1989) <u>Proc. Nat. Acad. Sci. USA</u> 86, 187-191 (1989).
14. D. M. Wilson, D. Yang, J. E. Dillberger, S. E. Dietrich, V. M. Maher, and J. J. McCormick. <u>Cancer Res</u>. 50, 5587-5593 (1990).
15. D. G. Fry, L. D. Milam, J. E. Dillberger, V. M. Maher, and J. J. McCormick. <u>Oncogene</u> 5, 1415-1418 (1990).
16. M. Namba, K. Nishitani, F. Hyodoh, F. Fukushima, and T. Kimoto. <u>Int. J. Cancer</u> 35, 275-280 (1985).
17. M. Schwab and M. Bishop, <u>Proc Nat. Acad. Sci. USA</u>. 85, 9585-9589 (1988).
18. A. R. Kinsella, L. Fiszer-Maliszewska, E. L. D. Mitchell, Y. Guo, M. Fox, and D. Scott. <u>Carcinogenesis</u> 11, 1803-1809 (1990).

From: *Neoplastic Transformation in Human Cell Culture,*
Eds.: J. S. Rhim and A. Dritschilo ©1991 The Humana Press Inc., Totowa, NJ

MITOGEN-INDEPENDENCE AND AUTOCRINE GROWTH FACTOR

SECRETION DISPLAYED BY HUMAN MESOTHELIOMA CELLS

AND ONCOGENE-TRANSFECTED MESOTHELIAL CELLS.


James G. Rheinwald[1], Ross Tubo[1],
Beatrice Zenzie, Therese O'Connell[1],
and Anita Terpstra

Dana-Farber Cancer Institute, Harvard
Medical School, Boston, MA 02115
[1]Present address:  Department of
Research and Development, BioSurface
Technology, Inc., 64 Sidney Street,
Cambridge, MA 02139


## ABSTRACT


The mesothelium is the simple squamous
epithelium that lines the pleural, pericardial
and peritoneal cavities and covers the outer
surfaces of the organs contained within these
cavities.  We have identified the growth factor
and nutritional requirements of normal human
mesothelial cells for clonal and serial
proliferation in culture.  An optimal medium is
M199/MCDB105 (1:1 v/v) + 10ng/ml EGF or bFGF +
0.4 $\mu$g/ml HC + $\geq$5% bovine serum.  Several
mesothelioma cell lines we have examined grow
optimally in the absence of EGF or FGF and they
secrete a mitogen ("transformed mesothelial
growth factor" (TMGF)) which can satisfy the
EGF/FGF requirement of normal mesothelial cells.
When a mutationally activated H-<u>ras</u> gene or the
SV40 large T gene is introduced <u>via</u> calcium
phosphate- or defective retrovirus-mediated
transfection into normal mesothelial cells, the

resulting cells are able to grow independent of
added EGF.  The SVLT transfectants are also HC-
independent, exhibit a reduced requirement for
serum, and become replicatively immortal, but
they are not tumorigenic in nude mice.  Ras
transfectants apparently differ in growth
characteristics from normal cells only by their
EGF/FGF independence.  Ras or SVLT transfectants
secrete a mitogen with the same biological
activity as the TMGF secreted by mesothelioma
cells.  TMGF appears to be a novel heparin-
binding growth factor that remains to be
characterized.

## Properties of Normal Human Mesothelial Cells in Serial Culture

Patients with metastatic cancer in one of
the body cavities often accumulate liters of
"ascites" fluid (in the peritoneum) or
"effusion" fluid (in the pleura or pericardium).
It has long been known that normal human
mesothelial cells slough off into this fluid
(for example, see 1-4).  Our studies of the
mesothelial cell began with our discovery that
attempts at growing ovarian carcinoma cells from
ascites fluid almost invariably resulted in the
selective growth of normal mesothelial cells in
the culture medium we were using (5).  We soon
identified an optimal culture medium for human
mesothelial cells, consisting of a 1:1 mixture
(v/v) of M199 and either MCDB202 or MCDB105,
supplemented with 5-10 ng/ml EGF or bFGF, 0.4
$\mu$g/ml HC, and $\geq$ 5% bovine serum (6,7).  In this
medium, normal human mesothelial cells grow from
very low density platings and can be serially
propagated with a population doubling time of $\leq$
24 hours until senescence after 40-50 population
doublings.  The growth factor requirements of
human mesothelial cells, their sensitivities to
growth inhibitors, their expression of
differentiation proteins, and their histogenic
potential in culture and in vivo are very
different from those of keratinocytes (i.e.,

stratified squamous epithelial cells),
fibroblasts, and large vessel endothelial cells
(Table 1).  Thus, attempts to classify them as
either an epithelial or connective tissue cell
are misguided; the mesothelial cell is a unique
cell type.

Mesothelial cells adopt a distinctive
morphology in culture.  They do not form closely
adherent colonies as typical epithelial cell
types do.  In their optimal growth medium they

Table 1.  The mesothelial cell (Meso)
exhibits assorted characteristics of endothelial
cells (Endo), fibroblasts (Fibro), and
keratinocytes (K'cyte) and other true epithelial
cell types (Eps).

|  | Meso | Endo | Fibro | K'cyte, other Eps |
|---|---|---|---|---|
| Keratins | + | - | - | + |
| Vimentin | + | + | + | (-) |
| PAI-1 | ++ | ++ | + | (-) |
| connective tissue formation | + | - | + | - |
| simple squamous epithelium formation | + | + | - | - |
| terminal differentiation | - | - | - | + |
| EGF mitogenic | + | - | + | + |
| KGF mitogenic | - | - | - | + |
| TGF-b inhibitory | - | - | - | + |

grow in a dispersed fashion with a stubby, somewhat fibroblastoid morphology.  Mesothelial cells are not as long and spindly as humanfibroblasts, however; they form a broad, ruffled plasma membrane along one side and migrate laterally (6).  Under optimal growth conditions, they mimic fibroblasts by continuing to divide after reaching a confluent monolayer, ultimately forming a multilayer of elongated cells at saturation densities of up to $2 \times 10^5$ cells/cm$^2$.  If EGF is withdrawn from preconfluent cultures, however, mesothelial cells flatten, slow their growth to a doubling time $\geq$ 80 hours, and form an epithelioid monolayer at a saturation density of ~$3 \times 10^4$ cells/cm$^2$, resembling their normal _in vivo_ histology (6).


### Growth Regulation and Reversible Dedifferentiation of Cultured Human Mesothelial Cells

In _vivo_, mesothelial cells normally form a non-dividing, simple squamous epithelium. Within several days of being placed in primary culture in their optimal growth medium, the cells assume their characteristic _in vitro_ morphology, described above.  This morphologic conversion from that of the quiescent, _in vivo_ state to that of the rapidly growing _in vitro_ state is accompanied by a decrease in keratin synthesis and content, an increase in vimentin synthesis and content (6), and the synthesis and secretion of large amounts of fibronectin (8). Keratin synthesis and content returns to high levels whenever EGF is removed from the medium, growth slows, and the cells again assume a flattened, epithelioid morphology.

The remarkable capacity of normal mesothelial cells to reversibly dedifferentiate or "transdifferentiate" to a fibroblastoid phenotype explains the striking histologic heterogeneity of mesotheliomas, many of which contain both epithelioid and fibroblastoid regions (see 9-11). Because of their histopathologic appearance, mesotheliomas were once regarded as fibrosarcomas. However, mesothelioma cells in tumors merely exhibit the phenotypic range exhibited by normal mesothelial cells in culture. This helps to explain why some, but not all, of the fibroblastoid cells within mesotheliomas are stained by anti-keratin antibodies (12). It seems that during malignant transformation mesothelial cells lose their dependence upon external mitogens, convert from a quiescent to a growing state and, therefore, also begin to express a fibroblast-like differentiation program.

### Mesothelioma-Derived Cell Lines and Oncogene-Transfected Mesothelial Cells: Mitogen-Independence and Growth Factor Secretion

Many cell lines derived from human malignant mesothelioma exhibit mitogen-independent growth in culture (Terpstra and Rheinwald, unpublished). We found that the mesothelioma line JMN1B (a subline which we isolated from the JMN line of Behbehani et al., 13)) grows optimally in culture without EGF or FGF and secretes a mitogen which can satisfy the EGF/FGF requirement of normal human mesothelial cells. We have named this mitogenic activity "transformed mesothelial growth factor" (TMGF). These interesting characteristics of JMN1B cells prompted us to analyze the phenotypic changes that might result from the introduction of a single, specific oncogene into normal diploid mesothelial cells.

When a mutationally activated H-_ras_ gene (14) or the gene encoding the SV40 large T antigen (SVLT) (Cicila and Rheinwald, unpublished) is introduced into normal mesothelial cells, the resulting tranfectants exhibit morphologic alterations, disorganized growth patterns, and mitogen-independent growth.

The <u>ras</u> transfectants are independent of EGF for
rapid growth, but they are not immortal nor do
they form tumors in athymic <u>nude</u> mice.  The <u>SVLT</u>
transfectants are EGF- and HC-independent and
also exhibit a reduced requirement for serum.
Some SVLT transfectants escape senescence and
become replicatively immortal, but they are not
tumorigenic in <u>nude</u> mice.  Medium conditioned by
either <u>ras</u>- or SVLT-transfected cells contains a
mitogen with the same biological activity as the
TGMF secreted by the JMN1B line.


## Toward the Identification of TMGF

Normal mesothelial cells in culture are
induced to express a number of lymphokines,
including G-CSF, GM-CSF, M-CSF, and IL-1b, when
they are exposed to inflammatory mediators such
as bacterial endotoxin (lipopolysaccharide, LPS)
or tumor necrosis factor (TNF) (15).  EGF and
TNF act synergistically to induce maximal levels
of lymphokine transcripts.  Interestingly, the
EGF-independent mesothelioma line JMN1B and <u>ras</u>
oncogene-transfected cells exhibit autonomous
expression of G-CSF, GM-CSF, M-CSF, IL-1b, and
IL-6 mRNA (15,16).  Our experiments have
demonstrated that neither G-CSF, M-CSF, GM-CSF,
nor IL-6 are mitogenic to mesothelial cells and
that IL-1b is only a very weak mesothelial
mitogen; thus TMGF is different from any of
these factors.

We are currently in the process of
characterizing TMGF.  Antibody neutralization
and receptor blocking experiments show that TMGF
is not EGF or TGF-$\alpha$, nor any other factor that
acts via the EGF receptor.  Pure acidic and
basic FGF have become commercially available
since our earlier analyses of mesothelial cell
mitogenic requirements (6,14,17), and we have
found that these factors can satisfy the "EGF
requirement" of normal mesothelial cells.
However, PDGF, TGF-b, IGF-1, and insulin cannot.
TMGF shares some properties with basic FGF, in

that both bind to heparin-Sepharose, both induce neurite extension of PC-12 cells, and the mitogenic activities of both are inhibited by heparin. However, radioimmunoassay using an antiserum specific for basic FGF has revealed that TMGF is not basic FGF, consistent with our finding that TMGF is non-mitogenic to large vessel endothelial cells. Recent experiments indicate that TMGF is different from other heparin-binding factors related to FGF, such as K-FGF and KGF, and from the heparin-binding, EGF-like factor amphiregulin. We are currently attempting to purify sufficient material to characterize TMGF precisely.

Normal human mesothelial cells in culture represent an important experimental system for studying epithelial cell biology and oncogenesis. The growth factor requirements and differentiation characteristics of this interesting and unique cell type in culture have been characterized in detail. Their amenability to genetic manipulation will facilitate molecular studies of the aberrations in cell regulation exhibited by mesothelioma.

## ACKNOWLEDGEMENTS

These investigations were supported by grants to J.G.R. from the National Cancer Institute, the National Institute on Aging, and the National Foundation for Cancer Research, and by an American Cancer Society Faculty Research Award to J.G.R.

## REFERENCES

1. R. S. Cunningham. *Am. J. Phys.* 59, 1 (1922).
2. C. W. Castor, B. Naylor. *Lab Invest.* 20, 437 (1969).
3. G. Singh, A. Dekker, et al. *Acta Cytol.* 22, 487 (1978).

4.   W. Domagala, L. G. Koss. <u>Virchows Arch. B. Cell Path.</u> 30, 231 (1979).

5.   Y-J. Wu, L. M. Parker, et al. <u>Cell</u> 31, 693 (1982).

6.   N. D. Connell, J. G. Rheinwald. <u>Cell</u> 34, 245 (1983).

7.   J. G. Rheinwald. In: R. Baserga (ed.), Cell Growth and Division: A Practical Approach. 81-94, IRL press, Oxford, (1989).

8.   J. G. Rheinwald, J. L. Jorgensen, et al. <u>J. Cell Biol.</u> 104, 263 (1987).

9.   P. Klemperer, C. B. Rabin. <u>Arch. Pathol.</u> 11, 385 (1931).

10.  A. P. Stout, M. R. Murray. <u>Arch. Pathol.</u> 34, 951 (1942).

11.  J. M. Corson, G. S. Pinkus. <u>Am. J. Pathol.</u> 108, 80 (1982).

12.  R. Schlegel, S. Banks-Schlegel, et al. 1980. <u>Am. J. Pathol.</u> 101, 41 (1980).

13.  A. M. Behbehani, W. J. Hunter, et al. <u>Hum. Pathol.</u> 13, 862 (1982).

14.  R. A. Tubo, J. G. Rheinwald. <u>Oncogene Res.</u> 1, 407 (1987).

15.  G. D. Demetri, B. W. Zenzie, et al. <u>Blood.</u> 74, 940 (1989).

16.  G. D. Demetri, T. J. Ernst, et al. <u>J. Clin. Invest.</u> 86, 1261 (1990).

17.  P. J. LaRocca, J. G. Rheinwald. <u>In Vitro</u> 21, 67 (1985).

From:  *Neoplastic Transformation in Human Cell Culture,*
Eds.: J. S. Rhim and A. Dritschilo  ©1991 The Humana Press Inc., Totowa, NJ

STRUCTURE AND GROWTH REGULATION IN NORMAL, TRANSFORMED AND

MALIGNANT HUMAN ENDOMETRIAL CELL CULTURES.

D.G. Kaufman, C.A. Rinehart and C.D. Albright

University of North Carolina at Chapel Hill,

Chapel Hill, NC 27599-7525, USA

## INTRODUCTION

Malignant transformation may have unique aspects for the different cell types from the many  different tissues of the body.  There are unique features of regulation of growth in different cells and tissues and for fetal or neonatal cells as compared to adult cells.  For these reasons it is necessary to look at the unique aspects of malignant transformation in a wide spectrum of human cells in order to discover major common themes that characterize the transformation process.  Our goal in the studies that are reported here, is to characterize this process as it occurs in cells of one tissue, the endometrium.

Cancers of the  endometrium affect many women each year, but relatively little is known about malignancies of this tissue.  To learn more about the biology of normal endometrial tissue and different forms of endometrial cancer, we studied human endometrial cells in culture.  We studied normal biology with cultures of the principal cell types from normal human endometrium.  We compared these to cell cultures of malignant tumors of this tissue.  We also studied normal endometrial stromal cells that had been treated with chemical carcinogens or tumor promoters, or that had been transfected with oncogenes.

## CELL CULTURES FROM NORMAL ADULT ENDOMETRIUM

Endometrium is derived from embryonic mesoderm. It is largely composed of two cell types: epithelial cells and endometrial stromal cells. Endometrial stromal cells are the most numerous cells in the tissue, and they surround glands and blood vessels. Endometrial stromal cells differ from the fibroblasts which form the stroma of most tissues. Endometrial stromal cells contain steroid hormone receptors, and respond to changes in the hormonal environment by undergoing morphological and biochemical changes during the menstrual cycle (1). Stromal cells differentiate to become decidual cells at placental sites of implantation during pregnancy. Endometrial epithelial cells line the endometrial cavity and form the endometrial glands. They also have hormone receptors, and respond to changes in hormone levels with changes in cell proliferation rates and in differentiation.

Under standard culture conditions (e.g., DMEM, 10% FBS), two types of cells grow in primary cultures of human endometrium (2). Comparisons of histochemical and immunohistochemical staining patterns of cultured cells and frozen sections of endometrium identified epithelial and stromal cells (3). Stromal cells can be subcultured readily and have been seen to undergo reversible morphologic changes that resemble the differentiation of these cells in vivo. When cultured in standard media with serum, epithelial cells could not be subcultured, and were soon overgrown by stromal cells. New methods of serum-free culture on basement membrane material were recently developed for culture of epithelial cells (4). Epithelial cells and gland fragments are grown in primary culture on Matrigel, which contains laminin, type IV collagen, heparan sulfate proteoglycan, and entactin. Gland fragments attach and flatten to form cell monolayers that grow as colonies. Outgrowth of the colonies is vigorous for several weeks.

Under these conditions, growth of the endometrial epithelial cells is not restricted to the monolayer.

Gland like organoids form above the monolayer colonies after several weeks in culture. Morphogenesis of gland-like structures begins as small tubules, and proceeds to formation of large gland-like structures (4). Microscopy of these structures in cross section reveals radially-oriented cells encircling a central lumen. Individual cells are highly polarized, with abundant microvilli and tight junctions at the apical surface. Nuclei typically are positioned basolaterally, and a basal lamina is apparent. They resemble endometrial glands found in vivo (4).

TREATMENT WITH CHEMICAL CARCINOGENS AND TUMOR PROMOTERS

Efforts were made to transform human endometrial stromal cells with the chemical carcinogen N-methyl-N'-nitro-N-nitrosoguanidine (MNNG) and with tumor promoters. Human endometrial stromal cells treated repetitively with MNNG developed progressive alterations including morphologic changes, increased growth rates and saturation densities, and the capacity for anchorage-independent growth. Compared to control cells, carcinogen-treated cells displayed atypical morphology characterized by irregularities in cell and nuclear size and shape, increased nuclear:cytoplasmic ratios, and cellular crowding (5). Alterations in levels of expression of several oncogenes, including Ha-ras, c-myc and fos, were seen in MNNG-treated endometrial stromal cells. These cells, however, did not form tumors when transplanted into nude mice.

If MNNG-treated stromal cells were treated for long intervals with low doses of tumor promoters TPA (6) or diethylstilbestrol (DES) (7), further alterations were produced in cells as if they had received further treatments with MNNG. These results suggest that TPA and DES may act as tumor promoters in human cells. In contrast to MNNG-treated cells, normal cells treated with TPA appeared to differentiate and had reduced growth capacity. These results suggest that tumor promoters may have dichotomous effects on cells: enhancing growth if the cells had undergone an initiating event, and inhibiting normal cells.

TRANSFORMATION WITH TEMPERATURE SENSITIVE SV40 T ANTIGEN

Our inability to achieve malignant transformation
of normal adult human endometrial cells by treatments with
chemical carcinogens and/or tumor promoters in vitro was
like the results reported for other human cell cultures
from several other labs [reviewed in (8)]. This result
may be due to the limitations on cellular lifespan of
normal adult human cells in vitro. We then sought to
extend the lifespan of the stromal cells by transfecting
into them a viral gene known to extend lifespan.

Normal adult human stromal cells were transfected
with a plasmid that bears an origin-defective construct of
the SV40 mutant A209 (tsSV40) with a temperature-sensitive
large T antigen (9). The use of origie-defective (ori-)
SV40 constructs produces a higher rate of transformation,
and increases the frequency of production of immortalized
populations. Endometrial stromal cells were transfected
either prior to their plating in primary culture or in low
(PDL < 6) passage. Colonies of morphologically altered
cells began to appear 4 to 6 weeks after transfection.
Transfected cells were smaller than their normal stromal
cell parents; they continued to grow past confluence,
eventually forming large multilayered colonies. The growth
pattern of cells transfected with tsSV40, however, retains
a large degree of order and exhibited little criss-
crossed growth pattern. The untransfected stromal cells
proliferate faster at the nonpermissive temperature (39°C)
than at the permissive temperature (33°C). Cells transfected with ori- tsA209 SV40 cease proliferation upon
shift to the nonpermissive temperature, if they have been
propagated past their normal lifespan of 20 population
doublings (9). Pre- and post-crisis clones have been
isolated. These cells demonstrate temperature-dependent
alterations in cell proliferation and inter- and intracellular structure.

## LARGE T ANTIGEN EFFECTS ON ACTIN ORGANIZATION

Actin in endometrial stromal cells is rigidly organized into an elaborate system of stress fibers which span the cytoplasm and often overlap. In stromal cell strains, temperature had no effect on actin organization in the range of 33°C to 39°C. In tsSV40 transfected stromal cells, the stress fibers are disrupted and disorganized. Apparently unpolymerized actin is concentrated near the plasma membrane. Inactivation of the large T antigen by shift to the restrictive temperature results in reassembly and reorganization of the stress fibers (10).

## IMMORTALIZATION

All the tsSV40 transfected adult diploid endometrial stromal cells eventually entered a senescence "crisis". Several clones have escaped from this period of crisis. Characterization has been most extensive for two of these. The two unrelated cell lines both appear to be capable of unlimited growth. Both lines continue to require functional large T antigen for growth. Cytogenetic analysis indicates a continuing increase in chromosome number during the post crisis period of growth. M4 cell line is hypertetraploid, and B10T1 cell line is hypotetraploid.

The histories of these two cell lines, named M4 and T1, are described in Table 1. Cell line M4 was isolated by cloning ring from one of the colonies which appeared following transfection. In early passage M4 had a 2n DNA content. M4 entered crisis at population doubling (PD) 58. After about 8 weeks many colonies appeared simultaneously, and the culture resumed proliferation. Cell line B10 was cloned following transfection of a different specimen. B10 had a 4n DNA content as soon as cell numbers were sufficient to allow analysis by flow cytometry. This clone entered crisis at PD 28. After 12 weeks two colonies appeared in the culture dish, and were subcultured separately. One of these, B10T1 has been maintained in culture and characterized. It has now achieved PD 125.

To determine if the cells retained their dependence
upon the large T antigen, their growth potential was
ascertained at nonpermissive temperature.   Both M4 and T1

TABLE 1. Description of Post-Crisis Cell Lines

| Precrisis Line | DNA Content | Crisis at PD | Postcrisis Line | Current PD |
|---|---|---|---|---|
| M4 | 2n | 58 | M4 | 230 |
| B10 | 4n | 28 | B10T1 | 125 |

experienced 1-2 population doublings and then ceased
proliferation following shift to $39^{\circ}$C. Two recent studies
with human fibroblasts immortalized with controllable SV40
genes indicate a continued, post-crisis dependence upon
large T antigen for growth (11,12).   The transfected
endometrial stromal cells continue to be viable for at
least 2 weeks at the nonpermissive temperature.


PROPERTIES OF CELL CULTURES OF ENDOMETRIAL CANCERS

Cell cultures of human endometrial carcinomas and
sarcomas have also been studied to understand properties
of natural tumor cells and to compare these properties to
those of normal cells and cells induced by treatments of
normal cells in vitro.   Studies are evaluating alterations
in growth factor production,  cell structure and cell-to-
cell interaction in carcinoma cell lines and comparing
these characteristics with differentiation in vivo of
tumors from which these cell lines were derived.   For
example, cultures of endometrial carcinoma cells on Matrigel substrates did not develop normally-formed, gland-
structures like normal endometrial epithelial cells (13).

There is strong evidence that alterations in the coordination of cell-to-cell interactions occurs during carcinogenesis (14-16). However, the role of such interactions in endometrial carcinogenesis are not well understood. There is empirical evidence that fewer stromal cells are found between the glands in higher-risk atypical hyperplasia as compared to lower-risk adenomatous hyperplasia. Furthermore, stromal cells are virtually absent between glands in most endometrial adenocarcinomas (1). These alterations in the relationship between cell types suggests that altered intercellular communication may be an important feature of endometrial carcinogenesis.

To learn more about this aspect of the biology of endometrial carcinomas we studied effects of intercellular autocrine-paracrine communication between normal human endometrial epithelial cells (HEPC), normal stromal cells (HESC) and endometrial carcinoma cells (RL95-2). After three days in culture, HEPC and HESC were treated with serum free medium conditioned (CMt) by culture of RL95-2 cells for 24 hr. By the seventh day, HESC exhibited fewer colonies per culture and had a lower mitotic index. The growth of HEPC was also inhibited by CMt. Preliminary analysis of RL95-2 CMt by SDS-gel electrophoresis has identified several candidate proteins which may play a role in the interactions observed between the normal endometrial stromal cells and carcinoma cells. Studies to characterize these proteins and their biological effects are in progress. Production of proteins by endometrial carcinomas that inhibit the growth of stromal cells could explain the paucity of stromal cells observed between the malignant glands of endometrial carcinomas.

We also examined effects of TGF-$\beta_1$ on the growth of 8 endometrial carcinoma cell lines derived from cancers of different histologic tlpe and differentiation (17). Adding exogenous TGF-$\beta_1$ to media in which these tumor cells were grown, caused inhibition of growth of 5 of 8 cell lines including the 4 that are most differentiated (Table 2). The 3 lines that were least well differentiated were not inhibited by addition of exogenous TGF-$\beta_1$ and

these cell lines were found to produce greatly
increased quantities of messenger RNA for TGF-$\beta_1$ compared
to the other tumors. From these observations it is tempting to speculate that poorly differentiated endometrial
carcinomas produce TGF-$\beta_1$ and lose their responsiveness to
TGF-$\beta_1$. Therefore these poorly differentiated carcinoma
cells may have a growth advantage over normal epithelial
cells or better differentiated carcinoma cells because
their growth is not inhibited by TGF-$\beta_1$ secreted by non-
epithelial cells. Also, in evolving tumors, poorly differentiated cells that express TGF-$\beta_1$ and may secrete it,
might inhibit the growth of the normal cells or better
differentiated carcinoma cells. In this way more advanced
cancer cells could be selected for growth and come to
supplant normal epithelium and better-differentiated tumor
cells in forming solid, non-glandular tumors.

TABLE 2. TGF-$\beta_1$ in Human Endometrial Carcinoma Cell Lines:
  Differentiation, TGF-$\beta_1$ Expression, and Effect on Growth

| Name of Cell Line | Differentiation of Original Tumor | Relative TGF-$\beta$ | Effect of TGF-$\beta$ on Cell Growth |
|---|---|---|---|
| HEC-1-A | Moderate Diff. | 1.4 | Inhibits |
| HEC-1-B | Moderate Diff. | 0.8 | Inhibits |
| SPEC2 | Moderate Diff. | 1.4 | Inhibits |
| RL95-2 | Moderate Diff. | 1.7 | Inhibits |
| KLE | Poor Diff. | 1.8 | Inhibits |
| EA1 | Poor Diff. | 13.2 | None |
| SPEC1 | Poor Diff. | 40.0 | None |
| AN3CA | Metastatic | 59.2 | None |

These findings with endometrial carcinoma cell lines suggest that some features of endometrial cancers as they occur in vivo may be reproduced in culture. Recognition of interactions between cancer cells and normal cells and how these interactions differ from those that normally occur in this tissue may help us understand why cancers of the endometrium look and behave the way they do. It may allow us to begin to grasp underlying principles of endometrial cancer, or other kinds of cancer, as diseases of tissues.

## REFERENCES


1.   G. Dallenbach-Helleg. Histopathology of the endometrium. Springer-Verlag, New York, (1975), pp. 22-82.
2.   B.H. Dorman, V.A. Varma, J.M. Siegfried, S.A. Melin, T.A. Adamec, C.R. Norton and D.G. Kaufman. In Vitro, 18, 919 (1982).
3.   J.M. Siegfried, K.G. Nelson, J.L. Martin and D.G. Kaufman. In Vitro, 20, 25 (1984).
4.   C.A. Rinehart, B.D. Lyn-Cook, and D.G. Kaufman. In Vitro Cell. Dev. Biol., 24, 1037 (1988).
5.   B.H. Dorman, J.M. Siegfried, and D.G. Kaufman. Cancer Res., 43, 3348 (1983).
6.   J.M. Siegfried and D.G.Kaufman. Internatl. J. Cancer 32, 423 (1983).
7.   J.M. Siegfried, K.G. Nelson, J.L. Martin, and D.G. Kaufman. Carcinogenesis, 5, 641 (1984).
8.   J.J. McCormick and V.M. Maher. Mutation Res., 199, 273 (1988).
9.   C.A. Rinehart, J.S. Haskill, J.S. Morris, T.D. Butler and D.G. Kaufman. J. Virol., 65, 1458 (1991).
10.  C.A. Carter, C.A. Rinehart, C.R. Bagnell, and D.G. Kaufman. Pathobiology 59, 36 (1991).
11.  W.E Wright, O.M. Pereira-Smith, and J.W. Shay. Mol. Cell. Biol., 9, 3088 (1989).
12.  R.L. Radna, Y. Caton, K.K. Jha, P. Kaplan, G. Li, F. Tragnos, and H.L. Ozer. Mol. Cell. Biol., 9, 3093-3096, (1989).
13.  J.A. Boyd, C.A. Rinehart, L.A. Walton, G.P. Siegal and D.G. Kaufman. In Vitro Cell Dev. Biol., 26, 701 (1990).

14.   C.D. Albright, R.T. Jones, P.H. Grimley and J.H.
      Resau. Toxicol. Pathol., 18, 324 (1990).
15.   J.E. Trosko, C.C. Chang, B.V. Madhukar and J.E.
      Klaunig. Pathobiology, 58, 265 (1990).
16.   H. Yamasaki. Carcinogenesis, 11, 1051 (1990).
17.   J.A. Boyd and D.G. Kaufman. Cancer Res., 50, 3394
      (1990).

Acknowledgements:   This work was supported by NIH grant
      CA31733, and American Cancer Society grant IN-15-30.

# CONSTRUCTION OF A UNIDIRECTIONAL cDNA LIBRARY FROM A RADIORESISTANT LARYNGEAL SQUAMOUS CELL CARCINOMA CELL LINE IN AN EPSTEIN BARR VIRUS SHUTTLE VECTOR

Zahra Salehi[1], Susan Ramos[1], Gary Pearson[2], Mira Jung[1], Anatoly Dritschilo[1], and Francis G. Kern[3], Departments of Radiation Medicine[1], Microbiology[2], and Biochemistry and Molecular Biology[3], Georgetown University Medical Center, Washington, D.C. 20007

## INTRODUCTION

The identification and cloning of genes in the absence of knowledge of their corresponding proteins presents a challenge that may be overcome using expression vectors that complement a given phenotype.  This approach involves the transfection of the cDNA of cells expressing a selectable phenotype into cells which lack this phenotype.  The methodology requires a very high transfection efficiency, low background of spontaneous acquisition of the phenotype and is ultimately limited to identification of dominant genes.  In this study we have sought to test the utility of an extrachromosomal-based host-vector system to identify the gene which confers the radiation sensitive phenotype to immortalized ataxia telangiectasia (AT) fibroblasts (1,2,3,4).  We have adopted a protocol which allows for extrachromosomal maintenance of plasmids in host cells to effectively retrieve genes after transfection.  This protocol is based on the phenomenon that in human or primate cell lines expressing the Epstein Barr Virus Nuclear Antigen 1 (EBNA1), plasmids that contain the Epstein Barr virus (EBV) origin of replication (Ori P) sequences will not integrate into the genome of host cells and will be maintained episomally (5,6,7).

## MATERIALS AND METHODS AND RESULTS

**<u>Establishment of clones that produce EBNA-1</u>**.  The
host cell line used for the transfection of the cDNA
library in this study is an SV40 immortalized fibroblast
cell line, AT5BISV40 which was established by Murnane
<u>etal</u>. (12).  The AT5BISV40 cell line was transfected with
the plasmid p266CH2 (Figure 1).  This plasmid contains a
cryptic promoter directing the expression of EBNA-1.  It
also contains Ori P sequences and a transcription unit
under the control of the cytomegalovirus immediate early
gene promoter that confers resistance to the antibiotic
hygromycin.  Since the plasmid encodes EBNA-1 and contains
Ori P sequences, the plasmid p266CH2 can potentially
replicate episomally in transfected human cells.
Transfection of plasmid DNA into the AT cells was
performed according to the method of Chen and Okayama
(13).  After transfection, cells were trypsinized and
$2x10^5$, cells were plated in 100mm dishes.  Cells were
selected for resistance to hygromycin.  Initial
experiments demonstrated that the highest frequency of
transfection ($5.6x10^{-3}$) was achieved when 40 $\mu$g of plasmid
DNA was used.  A dozen clones which were resistant to
hygromycin were selected but only 3 clones were
successfully maintained in culture.

To determine whether the clones expressed EBNA-1
protein, immunofluorescence antibody staining (IFA) was
performed.  For IFA, cells were fixed in 50% acetone and
methanol and reacted with EBV positive and negative human
sera.  The fixed cells were subsequently incubated with
fluorescine labeled antibody against human immunoglobulin
gamma (IgG).  The results of IFA (data not shown)
demonstrated that only one clone expressed high levels of
EBNA-1 protein.  This clone was designated AT5BISV40/Cl.2.
The levels of EBNA-1 protein in the AT5BISV40 cells was
also analyzed by Western blot analysis.  Cell lysates of
the AT5BISV40 cells were electrophoresed on 8-16%
Trisglycine gels at 150 volts.  The gels were transferred
to nitrocellulose at 150 amps of constant current for 3
hours.  The nitrocellulose membrane was initially reacted
with EBV positive human sera and next with antihuman IgG-
($\gamma$-chain specific) alkaline phosphatase.  The
immunocomplex on the nitrocellulose membrane was
visualized by a subsequent reaction with BCIP and NTP.
The result of the Western blot analysis (Figure 2)

confirmed the initial findings of IFA and demonstrated
that while untransfected AT5BISV40 cells do not express
the EBNA-1 protein, AT5BISV40/Cl.2 expresses high levels
of this protein of the appropriate size.

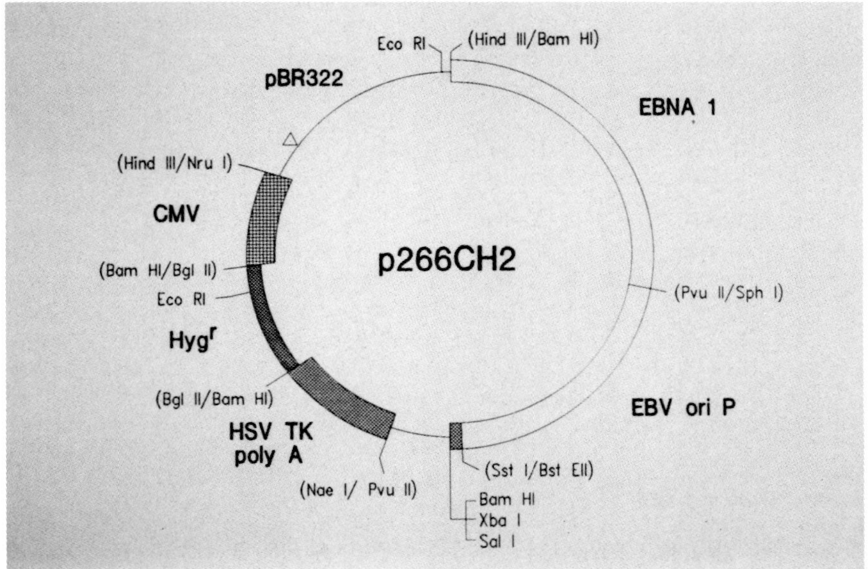


**Legend to Figure 1.** The plasmid p266CH2 is a mammalian
expression vector that encodes for EBNA-1, contains EBV
Ori P sequences, and confers resistance to the antibiotic
hygromycin.

Next we sought to determine whether the EBNA-1
expression vector, p266CH2 was maintained episomally in
transfected AT5BISV40 cells. Extrachromosomal DNA was
isolated from the total genomic DNA by using the method of
Hirt extraction (14). To determine whether the p266CH2
plasmid was integrated into the genome of AT5BISV40 cell
lines, total genomic DNA was isolated. The genomic DNA of
the AT5BISV40 cell lines were further digested with the
restriction endonucleases BamHI (which linearizes the
p266CH2 plasmid) and BglII (which does not cut the p266CH2
plasmid). The digested genomic DNAs were further
subjected to Southern blot analysis (15) and hybridized
with $\alpha^{32}$P-labeled p266CH2 plasmid. The results of the
Southern analysis (data not shown) indicated that the
plasmid p266CH2 had integrated into the genome of
AT5BISV40 cell lines. This observation suggests that the

cells harboring p266CH2 contain a deletion or mutation of
the Ori P sequences.

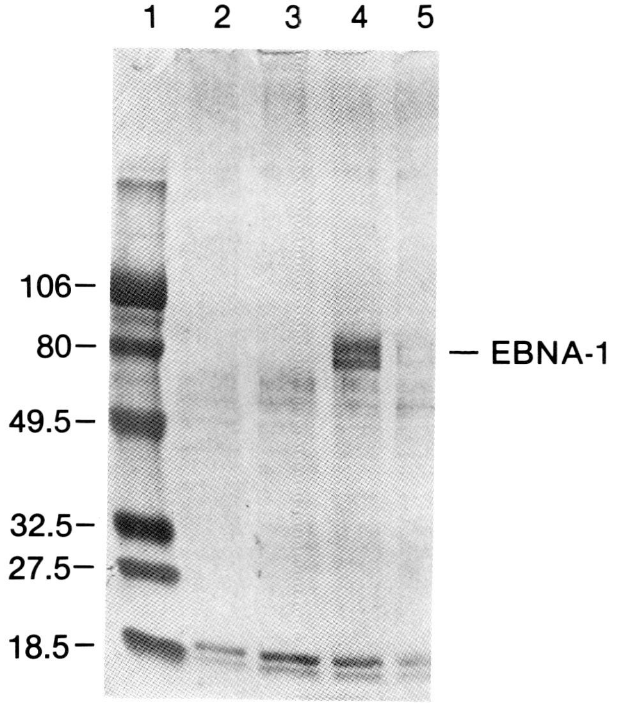



**Legend to Figure 2.** Western-blot analysis of
untransfected AT5BISV40 cells and EBNA-1 transfected
AT5BISV40 clones. Cell lysates of AT cell lines were
electrophoresed on 8-16% Trisglycine gels and transferred
to nitrocellulose filters. The nitrocellulose membranes
were initially incubated first with EBV positive human
sera and next with anti-human IgG ($\gamma$-chain specific)
conjugated to alkaline phosphatase. Lane 1: molecular
weight markers; lane 2: lysate from untransfected
AT5BISV40; lane 3: AT5BISV40/Cl.1; lane 4: AT5BISV40/Cl.2;
and lane 5: AT5BISV40/Cl.3.

Finally, to determine whether the ATSBISV40/Cl.2
cell line expressing high levels of EBNA-1 had maintained

the radiosensitive phenotype, X-ray clonogenic survival
assays were performed. The results of these assays (data
not shown) demonstrated that the degree of sensitivity of
AT5BISV40/Cl.2 as determined from the terminal slope of
radiation survival curve ($D_0$) was identical to the
parental AT5BISV40 and had a value of 0.75 Gy.

**Construction of cDNA libraries**. The cell line
chosen for the identification of the wild type allele of
the AT defect was the cell line SQ20B, which was derived
from a squamous cell carcinoma of the larynx (16). This
cell line is about 3-fold more resistant to radiation than
AT5BISV40 cell line ($D_0$=2.4 Gy vs. 0.75 Gy). Total
cellular RNA of SQ20B cells was prepared according to the
method described by Chirgwin etal. (17). PolyA+ mRNA was
subsequently selected on Clonetech oligo dT-cellulose
columns. cDNA was synthesized by a modification of the
method of Gubler and Hoffman (18). The first strand of
cDNA was synthesized using the Superscript reverse
transcriptase (BRL). The primer used for the synthesis of
the first strand of cDNA encoded for the following
sequence: $5'$CTCAGTCGACGGCCTATCGGCCGT$_{15}3'$. This sequence
hybridizes to mRNA at the 3'polyA-tail and generates the
recognition sequence for the restriction endonuclease SfiI
at the 3'end of the cDNA following synthesis of the second
strand. The 8-base pair recognition site of SfiI rarely
occurs within cDNA sequences. The double-stranded cDNA
was subsequently blunt-ended with T4 polymerase and
ligated to NotI linkers. NotI, similar to SfiI, has an 8-
base pair guanine and cytosine rich recognition site which
rarely occurs within cDNA sequences. Next, the cDNA was
sequentially digested first with SfiI and then with NotI
restriction endonucleases. To eliminate small fragments
of linkers and to select cDNA inserts with larger
molecular weight, the cDNA was size-fractionated on a BRL,
sephacryl S-500 HR column.

The protocol described above permits unidirectional
cloning of the cDNA into the plasmid pCNCNot (Figure 3)
which contains a NotI/SfiI cloning site downstream of the
cytomegalovirus promoter. The mammalian expression
vector, pCNCNot also contains for EBV Ori P sequences and
confers resistance to the antibiotic geneticin (G418).
The cDNA and pCNCNot ligation mix was used to transform E.
coli Electromax DH10B™ (BRL) by electroporation. After
electroporation bacteria were plated on nitrocellulose

filters that were placed on LB agar plates supplemented
with 400 $\mu$g/ml ampicillin and 10 $\mu$g/ml kanamycin.  About
430,000 colonies were collected and the plasmid DNA of the
clones corresponding to the cDNA library of the SQ20B cell
line was isolated on cesium chloride density gradients.

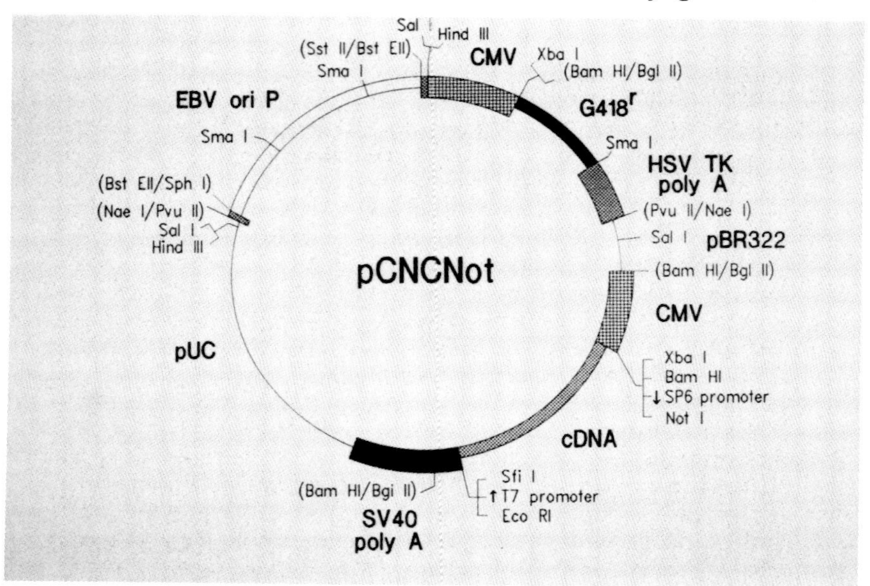


**Legend to Figure 3.**  The plasmid pCNCNot is a eukaryotic
expression vector that contains EBV-Ori P sequences and
two transcription units both under the control of the
cytomegalovirus immediate early gene promoter.  The first
confers resistance to G418 and the second contains NotI
and SfiI cloning sites which are spanned by SP6 and T7
promoters.

The cDNA library in pCNCNot was effectively linearized by
the restriction endonucleases NotI and SfiI and sequential
digestions with SfiI and NotI restriction endonucleases
excised the cDNA inserts from the pCNCNot plasmid (Figure
4).  The cDNA fragments of the SQ20B cell line ranged
between 400 base pairs to 4Kb.  The average size of the
inserts was greater than 1.5Kb.

To isolate the defect of AT cell line, about 40 $\mu$g
of SQ20B cDNA library was used to transfect 1x10$^7$
AT5BISV40/Cl.2 cells.  After transfection, 2x10$^5$ cells

were plated in 175 cm² tissue culture flasks and the cells
were selected with hygromycin and G418.  The efficiency of
transfection was very high and was about 1.2%.  About
48,000 colonies were selected with both hygromycin and
G418 and pooled.  The results of the Southern analysis on
the Hirt supernatant DNA from (Figure 5) AT5BISV40/Cl.2
cells that have been transfected with the SQ20B cDNA
library, demonstrated that the plasmids are maintained
extrachromosomally in these cells.  The AT5BISV40/Cl.2
colonies are currently being selected with X-irradiation.
We are trying to isolate individual clones from
AT5BISV40/Cl.2 cells which have converted from the
radiosensitive phenotype of ataxia cells to a wild type
level of radiation sensitivity.

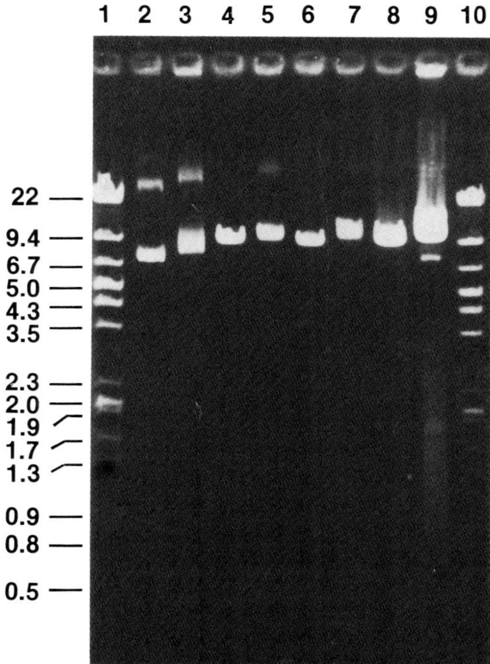

**Legend to Figure 4.**  Restriction endonuclease analysis of
a SQ20B cDNA library in the plasmid pCNCNot.  The DNA
samples were electrophoresed on 1% agarose gels at 25

volts overnight.  Lane 1: contains λ DNA restriction
fragments as molecular weight markers; lane 2: 500 ng
pCNCNot undigested plasmid DNA; lane 3: 500 ng undigested
SQ20B cDNA library uncut; lane 4: pCNCNot digested with
SfiI; lane 5: SQ20B cDNA library digested with SfiI; lane
6: PCNCNot digested with NotI; Lane 7: pCNCNot digested
with NotI; lane 8: SQ20B cDNA library digested with NotI.
Lane 8 and Lane 9 contain pCNCNot and SQ20B cDNA library
sequentially digested with SfiI and NotI, respectively.

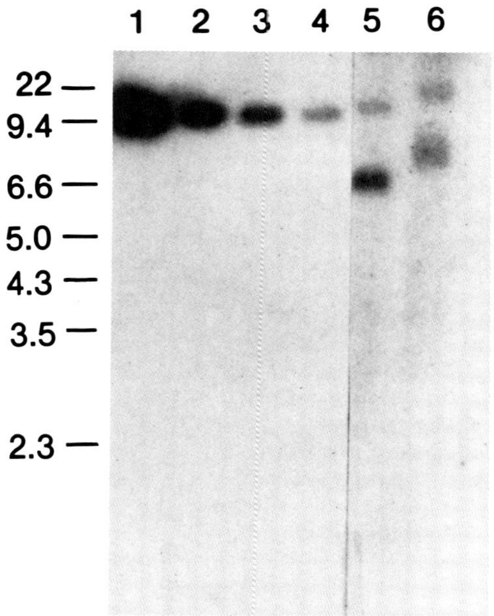

**Legend to Figure 5.**  Detection of the presence of
extrachromosomal DNA in AT5BISV40/Cl.2 cell lines
transfected with either the plasmid pCNCNot alone or with
a SQ20B cDNA library in pCNCNot by Southern blot analysis
of Hirt supernatants.  The Hirt supernatants of pooled
G418 resistant colonies from pCNCNot and SQ20B cDNA
library transfected cells were digested with the restriction endonuclease NotI and electrophoresed on 1% agarose
gels at 25 volts overnight.

The gels were transferred to nitrocellulose and hybridized

with $1 \times 10^6$ cpm/ml of nick translated $\alpha^{32}$P-labeled pCNCNot
DNA.  Lanes 1,2,3, and 4 correspond to 400, 100, 25, and
12.5 pg of the plasmid p266CH2 linearized with NotI,
respectively.  Lane 5: Hirt supernants of AT5BISV40/Cl.2
transfected with the pCNCNot vector only.  Lane 6: Hirt
supernant from cells transfected with a library containing
cDNA inserts from the SQ20B cell line.

In this study we have attempted to identify and
isolate the gene which confers the radiation sensitive
phenotype to SV40 immortalized AT fibroblasts (AT5BISV40).
We have successfully established derivatives of the ataxia
cell lines that express EBNA-1 protein and can thus
maintain stable episomal replication of plasmids that
contain EBV Ori P sequences.  We have been able to
demonstrate that a cDNA library from a radioresistant
laryngeal squamous carcinoma cell line cloned into the EBV
Ori P containing mammalian expression vector pCNCNot is
transfected with a high efficiency and maintained
episomally in an EBNA-1 producing AT5BISV40/Cl.2 cell
line.

The cloning of cDNA at NotI and SfiI sites of the
plasmid PCNCNot also allows for size fractionation of cDNA
libraries since the recognition sites for NotI and SfiI
restriction endonuclease rarely occur within cDNA
sequences.  The NotI/SfiI cloning site of the plasmid
PCNCNot also encodes for the sequences of T7 and SP6
promoters.  Thus, a cDNA library constructed in this
plasmid can also be used to transcribe sense and antisense
RNA for subsequent use in subtractive hybridizations.

## REFERENCES


1.  Taylor AMR, Harnden DG, Arlett CF, etal. (1975) **Nature** 258:427-429.
2.  Cox R, Hosking GP, Wilson J (1978) **Archives of Diseases of Children** 53:386-390.
3.  Weichselbaum RR, Nove J, Little JB (1980) **Cancer Res.** 40:920-925.
4.  Arlett CF, Harcourt SA (1980) **Cancer Research** 40:926-932.
5.  Yates J, Warren N, Sugden B (1985) **Nature** 313:812-815.
6.  Yates J, Warren N, Reisman D, etal. (1984) **PNAS** 3806-3810.
7.  Lupton S, Levine AJ (1985) **Mol. Cell Biol.** 5:2533-2542.
8.  Sugden B, Marsh K, Yates J (1985) **Mol. Cell. Biol.** 5:410-413.
9.  Margolskee RF, Kavathas P, Berg P (1988) **Mol. Cell Biol.** 8:2837-2847.
10. Kahn RA, Kern FG, Clark J, etal. (1991) **JBC** 266:2606-2614.
11. Deiss LP, Kimchi A (1991) **Science** 251:117-120.
12. Murnane JP, Fuller LF, Painter RB (1985) **Experimental Cell Res.** 158:119-126.
13. Chen C, Okayama H (1987) **Mol. Cell. Biol.** 7:2745-2752.
14. Hirt B (1967) **J. Mol. Biol.** 26:265-369.
15. Southern E (1975) **J. Mol. Biol.** 98:503.
16. Weichselbaum RR, Dahlberg W, Beckett M, etal. (1986) **PNAS** 83:2684-2688.
17. Chirgwin JW, Przybyla AE, MacDonald RJ, etal. (1979) **Biochemistry** 18:5294.
18. Gubler U, Hoffman BJ (1983) **Gene** 25:263-269.
19. I would like to thank Eugenia Tuturea and Tin Cao for expert technical assistance. This work was supported by DHHS grants to FGK (CA50376) and AD (CA45408) from the National Cancer Institute.



From: *Neoplastic Transformation in Human Cell Culture,*
Eds.: J. S. Rhim and A. Dritschilo ©1991 The Humana Press Inc., Totowa, NJ

# Contributors

**Allen-Hoffmann, B. Lynn** • *Department of Pathology, University of Wisconsin, Madison, Wisconsin*

**Band, Vimla** • *Division of Radiation and Cancer Biology, New England Medical Center, Boston, Massachusetts*

**Barrett, J. Carl** • *Laboratory of Pulmonary Pathobiology, National Institute of Environmental Health Sciences, Research Triangle Park, North Carolina*

**Braun, Lundy** • *Department of Pathology and Laboratory Medicine, Brown University, Providence, Rhode Island*

**Carbone, David** • *NCl-Navy Medical Oncology Branch, National Cancer Institute, Bethesda, Maryland*

**Chopra, Dharam P.** • *Institute of Chemical Toxicology, Wayne State University, Detroit, Michigan*

**Chung, S. I.** • *National Institute of Dental Research, National Institutes of Health, Bethesda, Maryland*

**Colburn, Nancy H.** • *Cell Biology Section, LVC, NCI-FCRDC, Frederick, Maryland*

**Dritschilo, Anatoly** • *Department of Radiation Medicine, Georgetown University Medical Center, Vincent T. Lombardi Cancer Research Center, Washington, DC*

**Fahl, William** • *McArdle Laboratory, University of Wisconsin, Madison, Wisconsin*

**Fusenig, N.** • *Institute of Biochemistry, German Cancer Research Center, D-6900 Heidelberg, Germany*

**Greenberger, Joel S.** • *Department of Radiation Oncology, University of Massachusetts Medical Center, North Worcester, Massachusetts*

**Harris, Curtis C.** • *Laboratory of Human Carcinogenesis, National Cancer Institute, Bethesda, Maryland*

**Haugen, Aage** • *Department of Toxicology, National Institute of Occupational Health, Oslo 1, Norway*

**Jay, Gilbert** • *Laboratory of Virology, American Red Cross, Rockville, Maryland*

**Kaufmann, David G.** • *Department of Pathology, University of North Carolina School of Medicine, Chapel Hill, North Carolina*

**Kieff, Elliott D.** • *Department of Microbiology and Molecular Genetics, Harvard Medical School, Boston, Massachusetts*

**Kumar, C. C.** • *Department of Tumor Biology, Schering Research, Bloomfield, New Jersey*

**Lechner, John** • *Cellular and Molecular Toxicology, Inhalation Toxicology Research Institute, Albuquerque, New Mexico*

**Little, John** • *Harvard School of Public Health, Boston, Massachusetts*

**McCormick, J. Justin** • *Carcinogenesis Laboratory, Fee Hall, College of Osteopathic Medicine, Michigan State University, E. Lansing, Michigan*

**Milo, George E., Jr.** • *Department of Physiological Chemistry, Ohio State University, Columbus, Ohio*

**Minna, John** • *NCI-Navy Medical Oncology Branch, National Cancer Institute, Bethesda, Maryland*

**Namba, Masayoshi** • *Department of Pathology, Institute for Cancer Research, Okayama University School of Medicine, Okayama 700, Japan*

**Paraskeva, Chris** • *Department of Pathology & Microbiology, School of Medical Sciences, University of Bristol, UK*

**Reznikoff, Catherine A.** • *University of Wisconsin, Clinical Cancer Center— K-4/536, University of Wisconsin, Madison, Wisconsin*

**Rheinwald, James G.** • *Dana-Farber Cancer Institute, Boston, Massachusetts*

**Rhim, Johng S.** • *Laboratory of Cellular and Molecular Biology, NCI/NIH, Bethesda, Maryland*

**Rutkowski, J. Lynn** • *Pediatric Neurology, University of Michigan, Ann Arbor, Michigan*

**Sager, Ruth** • *Dana-Farber Cancer Institute, Boston, Massachusettes*

**Sanford, Katherine K.** • *National Cancer Institute, Bethesda, Maryland*

**Schlegel, Robert** • *Department of Pathology, Georgetown University Medical Center, Washington, DC*

**Srivastava, Shiv** • *Department of Pathology Uniformed Services University of the Health Sciences, Bethesda, Maryland*

**Stampfer, Martha R.** • *Lawrence Berkeley Laboratory, Berkeley, CA*

**Stoner, Gary D.** • *Department of Pathology, Medical College of Ohio, Toledo, Ohio*

**Sukumar, Sara** • *The Salk Institute, San Diego, California*

**Thraves, Peter J.** • *Department of Radiation Medicine, Georgetown University Medical Center, Vincent T. Lombardi Cancer Research Center, Washington, DC*

**Weichselbaum, Ralph R.** • *Department of Radiation and Cellular Oncology, Michael Reese Hospital, University of Chicago, Chicago, Illinois*

**Willey, James C.** • *University of Rochester School of Medicine, Rochester, New York*

**Woodworth, Craig D.** • *Laboratory of Biology, Division of Cancer Etiology, National Cancer Institute, Bethesda, Maryland*

**Yang, Tracy C.** • *NASA Johnson Space Center, Houston, Texas*

# Registrants

J. Ainsworth
R. Albert
A. P. Albino
A. Albor
I. Al-Nabulsi
B. L. Allen-Hoffman*
L. Amundadottir
F. Angelosanto
P. Anklesaria
M. Babich
V. Band*
J. C. Barrett*
L. Bergstraesser
W. F. Blakely
C. Branting
A. Braun
L. Braun
P. Briscoe
A. Brown
V. A. Brown
D. Carbone*
R. L. Chang
L. L. Chen
D. P. Chopra*
S. Choudhury
S. Chrysogelos
S. I. Chung
S. L.-N. Chung
N. H. Colburn*
M. Conrad
J. Cortesi
R. E. Cuca

R. Dickson
L Dirscherl
J. Doniger
A. Dritschilo*
D. Duhamel
V. C. Dunkel
K. Dutt
D. El-Ashry
P. Ehrenberg
W. Fahl*
P. Fang
R. Faris
T. J. Fitzgerald
D. Flessate
N. E. Fusenig*
K. Gaido
P. Garcia-Morales
H. Gerstenberg
D. Goldstein
M. Gottardis
R. C. Grafstrom
J. S. Greenberger
R. Gudi
M. Gurley
C. C. Harris*
A. Haugen
F. Hendler
A. Hruszkewycz
M. T. Huang
R. Husain
A. Inamdar
R. Isfort

G. Jay*
M. D. Johnson
T. J. Jorgensen
M. Jung
C. R. Kahn
U. N. Kasid
D. G. Kaufman*
E. Kearsley
F. Kern
D. Kiang
E. Kieff*
W. K Kim
A. R. Kinsella
D. Koval
R. Kremer
M. Kuettel
C. C. Kumar*
J. Kurebayashi
J. Laborda
I. Lacaci
J. N. LaPeyre
A. Lauber
S. Lavu
J. F. Lechner*
I. H. Lee
J. D. Lee
M. S. Lee
K. C. Lee
J. Leighton
C. C. Lin
M. E. Lippman
M. M. Lipsky

J. B. Little*
C. Louden
D. Lu
Y. P. Lu
B. D. Lyn-Cook
M. B. Martin
J. J. McCormick*
R. Miller
G. Milo*
M. Namba*
D. M. Nanus
R. Narayanan
S. Niemi
V. Notario
C.-H. Pan
C. Paraskeva*
B. Patel
G. Pearson
D. Pelroy
J. Plante
P. Posch
S. C. Prasad
A. Rahman
N. Ramakrishnan
P. Ramsamooj
D. S. Reinhold
M. J. Renan
C. A. Reznikoff*
J. Rheinwald*
J. S. Rhim*
J. A. Rhim
L. Rosenthal
J. L. Rutkowski
P. A. Ryan
M. Saceda
Peter G. Sacks
Z. Salehi
K. K Sanford*
A. Saran

N. Sato
R. E. Savage, Jr.
M. J. Sawey
J. M. Scheid
J. H. Schiller
R. Schlegel*
E. Shi
S. ShiShang
J. Siddiqui
M. Smulson
S. Southard
J. W. Spalding
J. Sparkowski
T. Sreenath
A. Srinivasan
S. Srivastava*
M. R. Stampfer*
C. Stevens
G. D. Stoner*
P. Strudler
L. N. Su
S. Sukumar*
Y. Sun
S. Taduru
M. Takeshita
R. W. Tennant
A. R. Thierry
J. Thompson
P. J. Thraves*
J. Torri
J. Torrisi
T. Tsutsui
J. Tuturea
M. M. Webber
R. R. Weichselbaum*
R. W. West
H. Wey
P. Whittaker
J. C. Willey

T. Winters
J. Wise
C. D. Woodworth*
P. K. Working
J. Wray
D. Yang
J. H. Yang
T. C. Yang*

*Speaker

# Index